Natural remedies, clean beauty and green cleaning with eight miracle ingredients

CUPBOARD HEROES

PENNY STANWAY

WATKINS
Sharing Wisdom
Since 1893

CUPBOARD HEROES
By PENNY STANWAY

First published in the UK and USA in 2026
by Watkins, an imprint of Watkins Media
Limited, Unit 11, Shepperton House,
83–89 Shepperton Road, London N1 3DF

enquiries@watkinspublishing.com

Editorial Director: Ella Chappell
Commissioning Editor: Sophie Blackman
Managing Editor: Daniel Culver
Head of Design: Karen Smith
Typesetting/Proofreading: JCS Publishing
Partnership
Design Concept: Francesca Corsini
Production: Uzma Taj

Typeset in Gravita HUM
Printed and bound in China

The manufacturer's authorised
representative in the EU for product
safety is: eucomply OÜ – Pärnu mnt 139b-14,
11317 Tallinn, Estonia,
hello@eucompliancepartner.com,
www.eucompliancepartner.com

A CIP record for this book is available from
the British Library

ISBN: 978 1 78678 985 3 (paperback)
ISBN: 978 1 78678 986 0 (e-book)

10 9 8 7 6 5 4 3 2 1

www.watkinspublishing.com

FSC
www.fsc.org
MIX
Paper | Supporting
responsible forestry
FSC® C104723

CONTENTS

INTRODUCTION

Many of us keep apple cider vinegar, lemons, bicarbonate of soda, olive oil, honey, garlic, spices and teas in our cupboards at home. Indeed, these are some of the ingredients most used by both home and professional chefs. But they also have a huge range of uses and benefits beyond the stove. Read on to hear how these eight ingredients deserve the title "cupboard heroes" on many levels. We are all familiar with the ways in which some of our "heroes", such as lemons, olive oil and garlic, can transform drab dishes into something special. But what many don't know is that each of the eight heroes can also benefit your skin, your hair, your home and – most importantly – your health. Time was when many of them were considered only as folk remedies, but continuing medical research is uncovering a wealth of evidence showing they can help prevent or treat a wide variety of illnesses. These include the many diseases associated with chronic inflammation – including Alzheimer's disease, cancer, type 2 diabetes, heart disease and Parkinson's disease – that can ruin a person's chance of having a good "health-span", meaning the number of years spent in good health.

Not only do the cupboard heroes provide natural ways of helping prevent or treat health problems, but they also offer choice: something paramount to many of us these days. From Generation-Zs (born 1997–2012), right through to Baby boomers (1946–64), people more than ever want to know what they themselves can do that will not only be safe and sensible but, most important, will have a good chance of helping with their ailments. They also want to understand why this might be. Many of us prefer to consult a doctor only when necessary – and knowing which simple things might help, and how, can give us the agency and confidence to look after ourselves better.

It goes without saying that conventional medical treatments such as medications and surgery can be very useful – indeed, they can save lives. But they can be costly and have unwanted side effects. The good thing is that we don't have to choose either medical care or "natural" healthcare options ... we can use and benefit from both.

Between 2010 and 2013, I wrote a series of eight books, entitled "The Miracle of ..." either Apple Cider Vinegar, Lemons, Bicarbonate of Soda (Baking Soda), Olive Oil, Honey, Garlic, Spices or Teas. It's with great interest and pleasure that I've updated the health-promoting, curative, beauty-care and home-care properties of each of these enduringly popular items for this new book, *Cupboard Heroes*, that combines all eight "heroes" in one handy volume.

I hope you enjoy using them for beauty, cleaning and health!

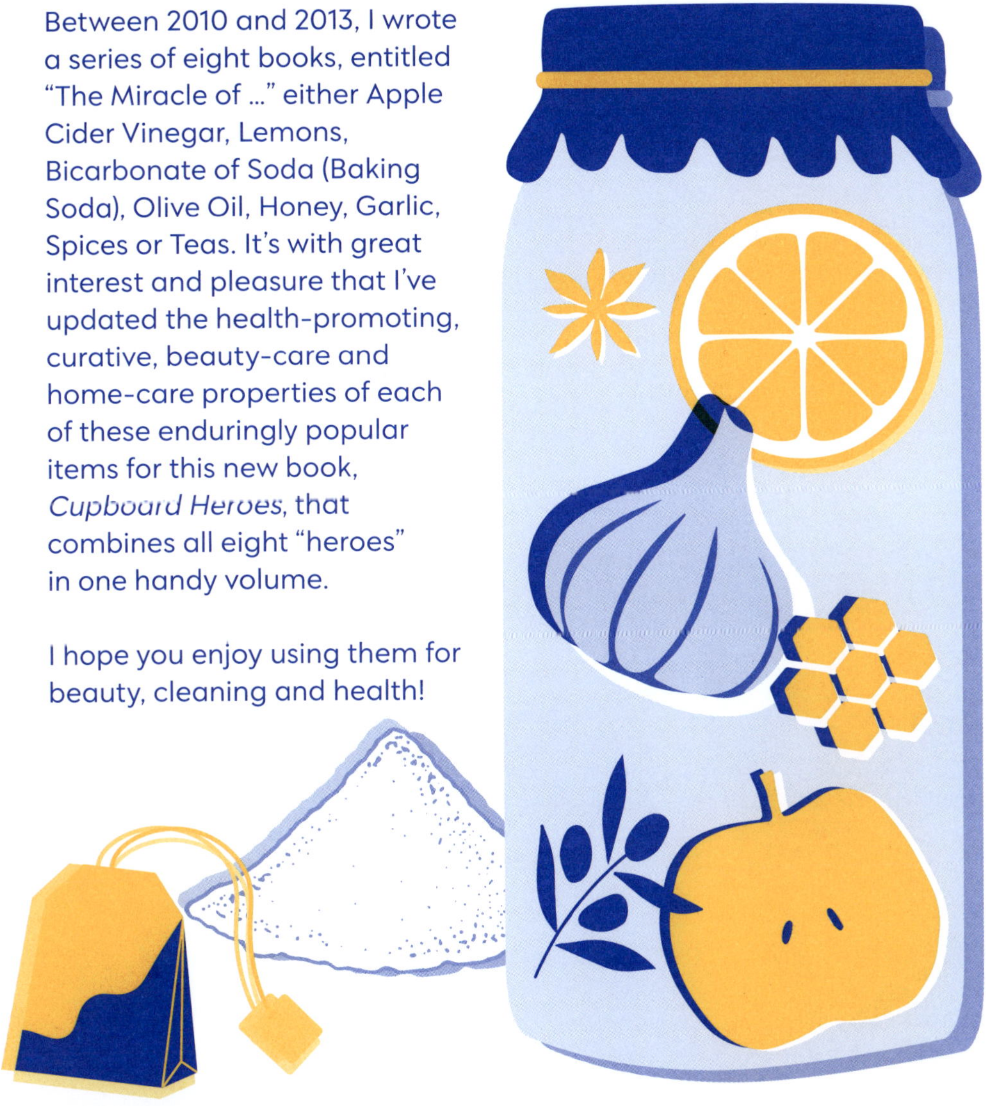

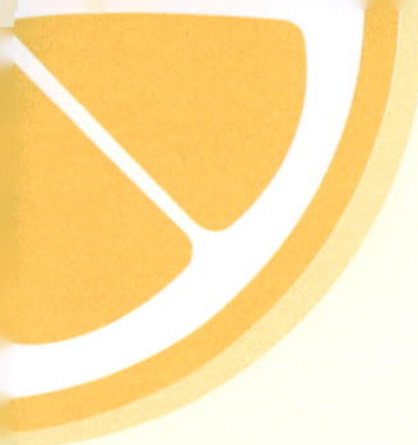
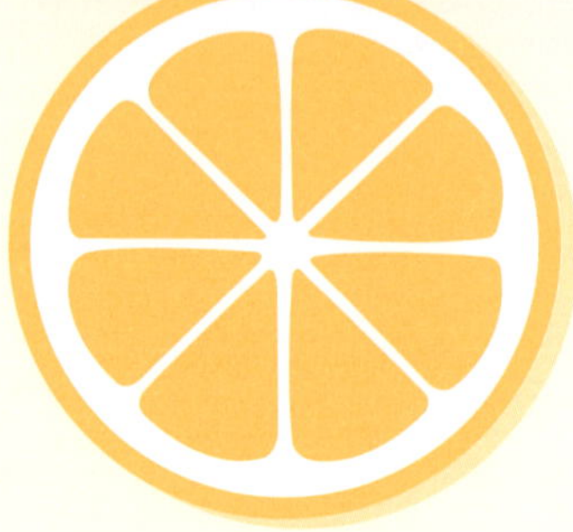

CHAPTER 1
EIGHT MIRACLE INGREDIENTS

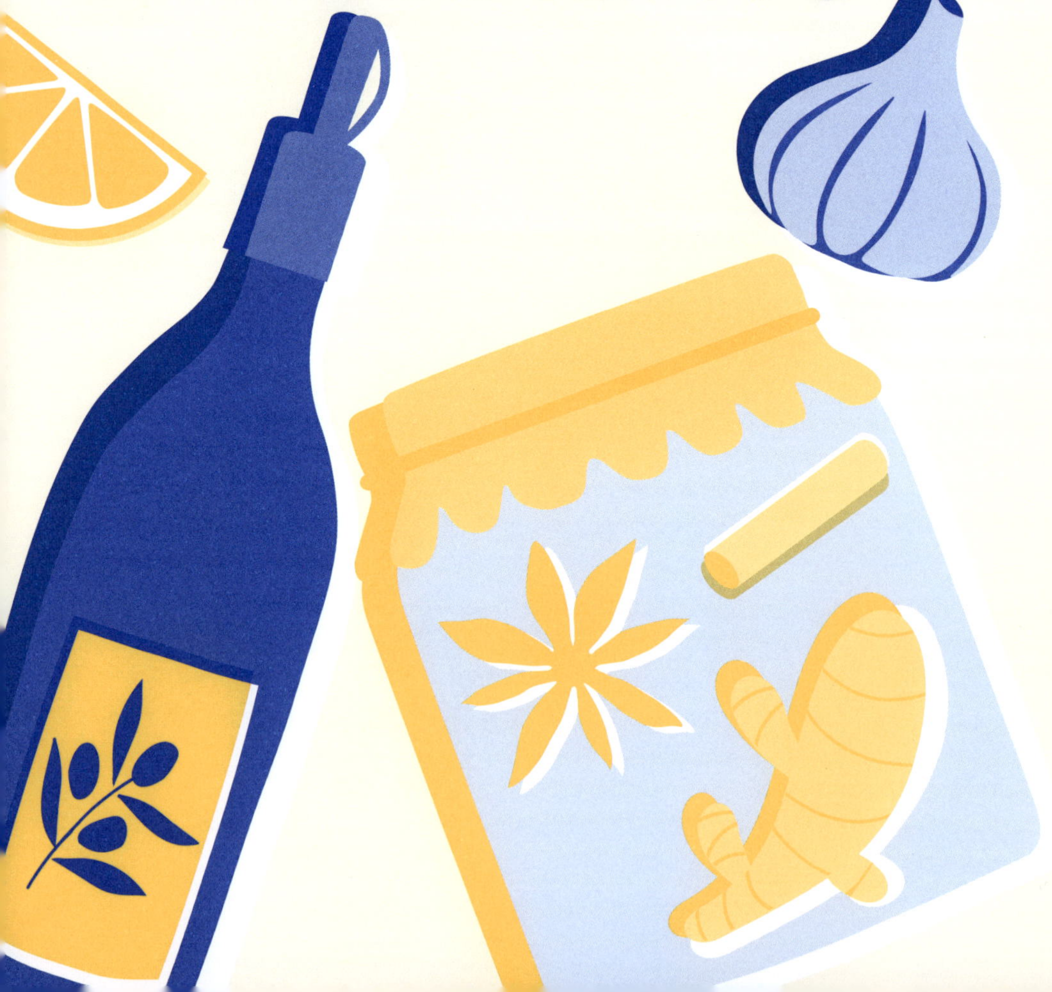

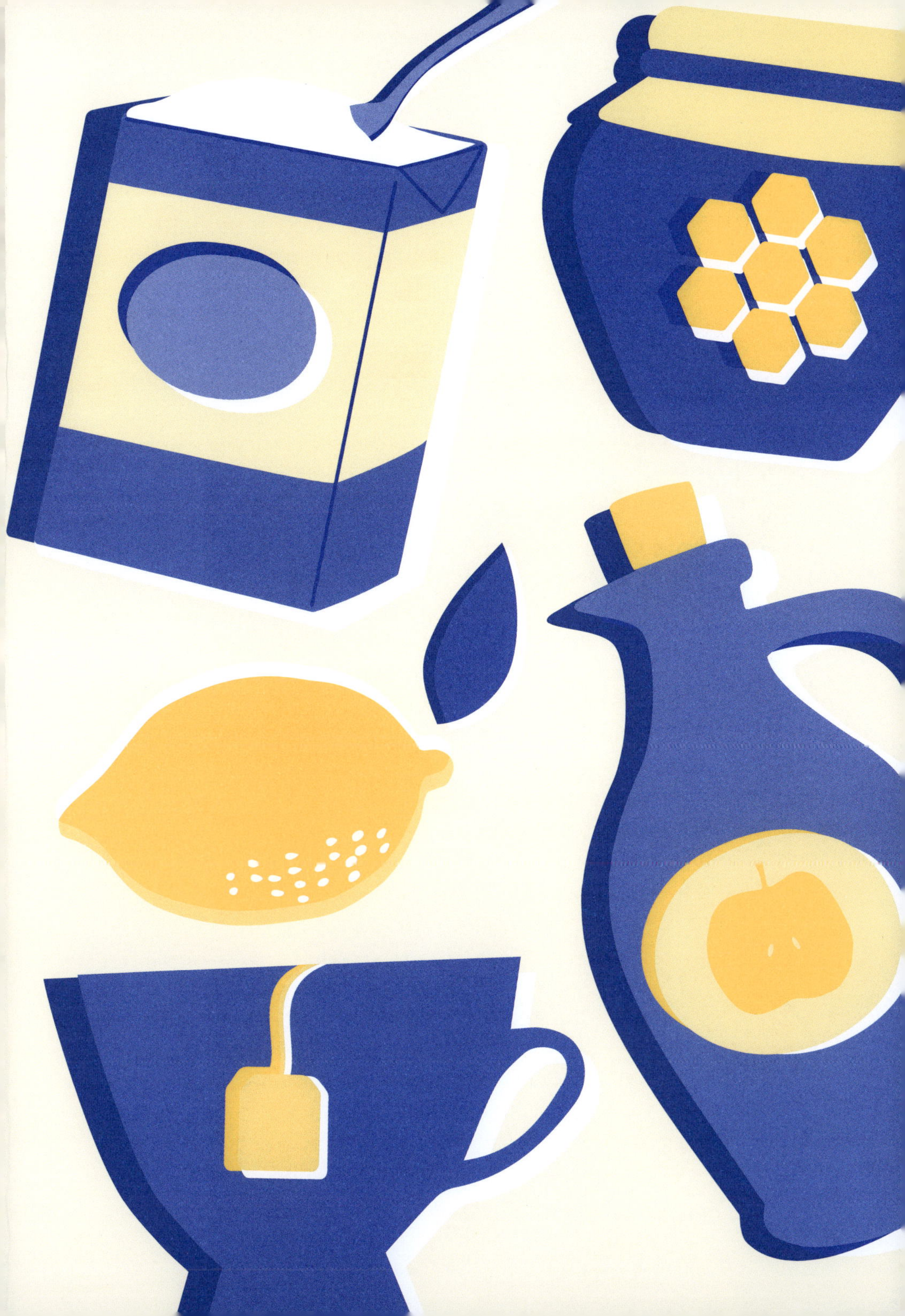

APPLE CIDER VINEGAR

Archaeologists believe that apple trees originated around the Caspian and Black seas, and that people ate apples as long ago as 6500 BC. Apple cultivation spread to Europe and in the 16th century King Henry VIII instructed his fruiterer to search the world for the best varieties, so he could set up his own orchards. Apple cultivation spread to the US, Australia, New Zealand, South Africa and South America. Historians are unsure when people first enjoyed cider but know it was a popular drink in Britain in the 1st century BC. But archaeologists say apple cider vinegar has been used for much longer, since traces of it exist in Egyptian urns dating from 3000 BC.

Making apple cider vinegar

To make apple cider vinegar, apple juice is fermented so its sugars become alcohol, turning it into cider. Then a second fermentation turns this alcohol into the acetic acid that characterizes cider vinegar.

Non-organic apple cider vinegar has been pasteurized – heated to at least 140°F (60°C) so the vinegar is no longer "raw". It has also been filtered and, perhaps, treated with chemicals, to extend its shelf life. Pasteurization destroys micro-organisms such as bacteria, as well as enzymes. Added chemicals may include pesticides sprayed on to the trees from which the apples came, as well as preservatives (such as potassium metabisulphite or potassium sorbate) that suppress the future growth of yeasts and moulds. Cider vinegars made this way are clear, rather than cloudy.

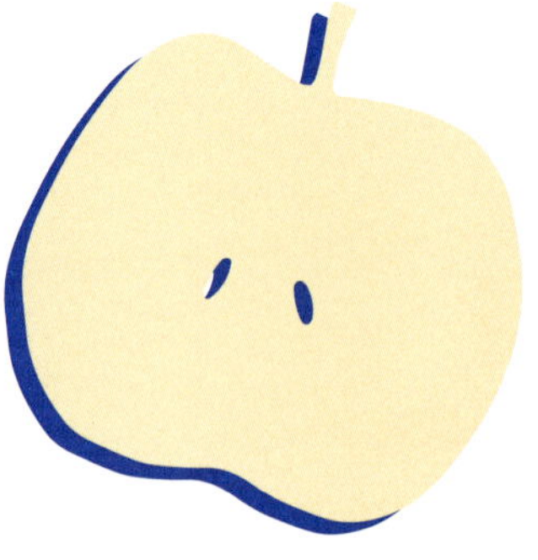

Organic – also called "raw" – apple cider vinegar has not been pasteurized, filtered or treated with chemicals, so may contain beneficial bacteria and yeasts, as well as enzymes and more nutrients than in the pasteurized version. Its cloudy appearance results from the presence of live bacteria and yeasts, together known as the "mother". Because of all this, many consider organic cider vinegar more beneficial to health than other cider vinegars. Despite the lack of interventions, organic apple cider vinegar is usually more expensive.

CAUTION: It's possible, though unproven, that certain bacteria in organic apple cider vinegar might harm pregnant women or other people with lowered immunity.

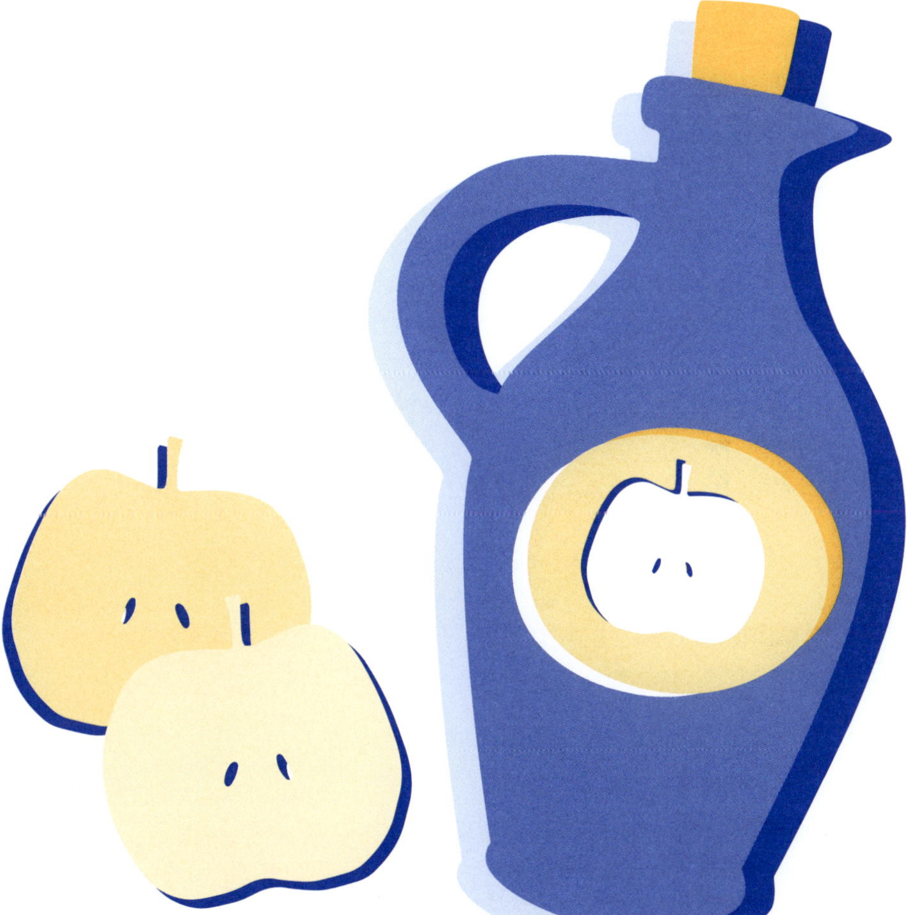

LEMONS

Because of their vibrant yellow colour, shiny, grained peel and distinctive ovoid shape, many artists throughout history have been inspired to portray lemons in paintings, ceramics, mosaics, reliefs, sculptures and fabrics. Artists often used lemons as symbols of friendship, longevity, love and, since they were once very expensive, status.

Conversely, to some viewers the image of a cut lemon might insinuate that something is sour, faulty or otherwise amiss. And in popular parlance, calling someone or something "a lemon" suggests all is not as it should be. Lemons are nearly always extremely sour because they contain a lot of acid. However, this very acidity not only aids good health but also helps account for the usefulness of lemons in beauty and home-cleaning products.

Anatomy of a lemon

A lemon has three layers: the peel, the pith and the pulp. It also houses pips within the pulp.

- **The peel** is the tough, shiny, textured, vibrant yellow (or green) outer layer. The peel's thickness varies according to a lemon tree's variety and growing conditions. Cellulose fibre makes up 30 per cent of the peel. It also houses lemon-oil glands, which open via pores on to its surface. A lemon's natural growth, together with abrasion of its peel, can expose the most superficial oil glands, giving a grainy effect to the lemon's surface.
- **The pith** is the peel's soft, spongy white lining. It's mainly composed of fibre but also contains small amounts of antioxidants (such as polyphenols and limonin). The antioxidants we get from lemons (and other fruits and vegetables) help protect our body's cells from inflammation and diseases such as cancer.
- **The pulp** fills the lemon and is separated by membranes into between eight and ten segments, each containing tiny ovoid sacs filled with yellowish juice. The juice forms 20–25 per cent of a ripe

lemon's weight and contains 90 per cent of its vitamin C, small amounts of other antioxidants, and various vitamins, minerals and organic acids.
- **The pips** are the bitter, whitish seeds in the pulp of most lemons. Their contents include salicylic-acid salts (as in aspirin), limonin and a little lemon oil.

Nutrients and antioxidants

Lemons contain a wealth of health-promoting nutrients, and their antioxidants and acids help explain why they are so beneficial. Lemons are one of our best food sources of vitamin C. Even a small (100g/3½oz) lemon contains 60–100mg of vitamin C, so a lemon a day can provide most, if not all, of an adult's daily requirement. If you need more antioxidants than usual – for example, in later life, or if you have an infection, feel stressed or smoke (one cigarette destroys 25mg of the average adult body's vitamin C) – the solution is to eat more antioxidant-rich foods. Including lemons in your diet is a good start!

FLAVONOIDS

Lemons are rich in polyphenols (beneficial plant compounds) such as flavonoids. Some lemon flavonoids are dubbed "super-flavonoids" as they are particularly powerful antioxidants. The most common super-flavonoids in lemons are luteolin, nobiletin, quercetin and tangeretin; others include apigenin, eriocitrin, hesperidin and naringenin. Lemon peel is 20 times richer in super-flavonoids than is its juice, and is also richer in other flavonoids, so it's well worth finding ways of including small amounts of it in your diet.

Flavonoids deliver a host of benefits:

- They help counter inflammation and infection.
- They improve the absorption of vitamin C and protect it from oxidation.

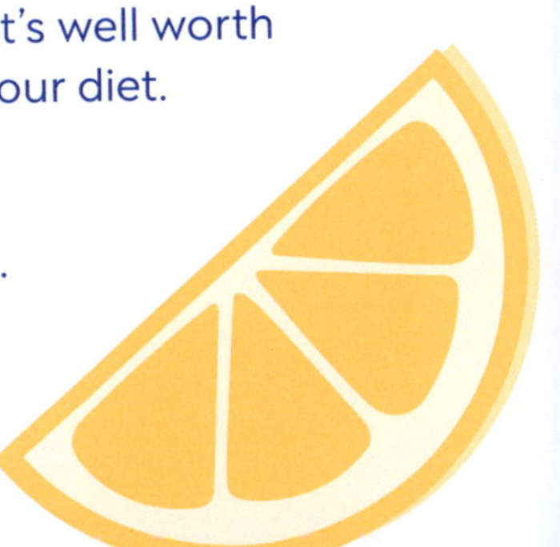

- They strengthen the walls of capillaries (our tiniest blood vessels), so maximizing their potential volume and encouraging good blood flow.
- They discourage cancer: naringenin, for example, helps prevent damage to our cells' DNA (genetic material), enhances its repair and has oestrogen-balancing effects.
- They lower LDL cholesterol (the potentially damaging type) by up to 40 per cent, possibly by reducing its production in the liver. This helps keep arteries healthy and blood flowing freely.
- In high enough amounts, they can discourage heart disease.
- They help counter the production of fat cells.

PIGMENTS AND LIMONOIDS

As a lemon ripens, its colour changes from green to yellow, thanks to the hormone-controlled replacement of chlorophylls by carotenoids (such as beta-carotene). Carotenoids are hugely valuable as they are converted in the body into vitamin A, which promotes eye health and discourages infection.

Lemon peel contains little bubbles of lemon oil, half to three-quarters of which is a terpene called limonene. This yellow oil tastes bitter and citrusy. It also has anti-inflammatory, antioxidant, antibacterial, antiviral, antifungal and, perhaps, anti-cancer properties. Lemon peel, pulp and seeds contain limonoids, which are bitter triterpenes with benefits similar to those of limonene. Other health-giving constituents include vitamins B and E, certain minerals (particularly potassium but also calcium, copper, iron, magnesium, manganese, phosphorus, selenium and zinc), organic acids (mainly citric and malic) and small amount of simple sugars (glucose, fructose and sucrose).

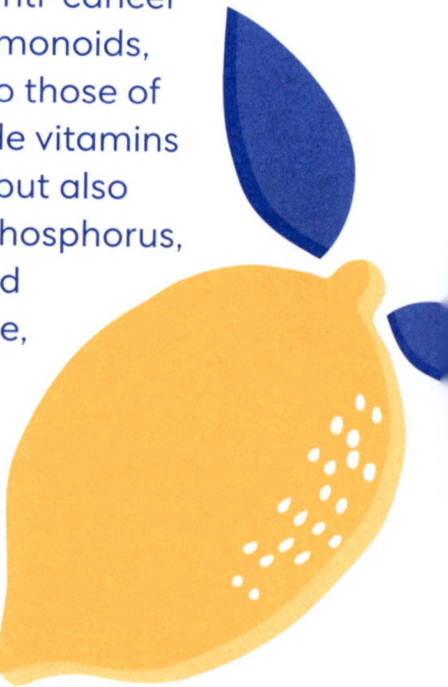

VALUABLE FIBRE

A lemon's peel, pith, pips and pulp membranes are rich in valuable fibre. Many people don't eat enough fibre – in the US, for example, the average adult intake of fibre is only half the recommended amount of 25g (0.88oz) for a woman, or 38g (1.3oz) for a man. Lemons' two types of fibre are cellulose, which strengthens cell walls, and pectin, which binds cells together. Pectin is an antioxidant that dissolves in water in the digestive tract to form a gel. About 90 per cent of this is then fermented by "good" bacteria, releasing butyric acid and other short-chain fatty acids. These acids are valuable to our health because they:

- Aid absorption of calcium and other minerals from the bowel
- Suppress the liver's cholesterol production
- Reduce absorption of cholesterol from the bowel into the blood
- Boost the proportion of HDL cholesterol (the "good" type) in blood
- Encourage apoptosis ("suicide") of bowel-cancer cells

CHOOSING LEMONS FOR CONSUMPTION AND SKINCARE

Choose fresh, healthy lemons. These look, smell and taste good and have plenty of juice, nutrients and other health-promoting substances. When selecting a lemon, check that it:

- Feels firm, full and heavy but has some "give" when pressed – avoid a hard or shrivelled lemon (as it may be old and desiccated) or a soft and squidgy one (as it may be decaying)
- Is well-shaped and free from scabs, streaks, spots or other discolouration, as this could be associated with viral, bacterial or fungal infection, or damage during harvesting, washing or storage
- Is free from scars, which could result from wind, pesticide sprays or fumigation
- Has rind that is free from pitted or sunken areas, which could result from excessive oil-spraying before harvest, or excessive chilling, mechanical brushing or humidity afterwards
- Has bright, shiny yellow peel, showing it is well ripened; a greenish or pale yellow lemon will be more acidic
- Has a uniform colour, indicating that the peel is not infected and the lemon has been well handled
- Has unbroken peel, since a break could have enabled intrusion by infecting micro-organisms

- Ideally has a coarsely "pebbled" rind, indicating it is likely to store well
- Has rough, thick peel if you particularly want its zest, as the yield will be greater
- Has thin, smooth peel if you particularly want its juice, as the yield will be greater
- Is unwaxed if you particularly want its peel, as this will be free from the wax, fungicide and other substances commonly sprayed on lemons during commercial storage

When you cut into a lemon, check that it is juicy. Dryness indicates it has been kept for too long or is unhealthy. Check too that its pith and membranes are whitish and its pulp pale yellow, as discolouration can signify a fungal infection. Discolouration can also result from excessive chilling after a lemon has been harvested.

Storing lemons

You can store a lemon for three weeks – perhaps longer – in a sealed plastic bag or tightly lidded jar in the refrigerator, or for one to two weeks at room temperature and out of direct sunlight. You can keep lemon juice in an airtight container in the refrigerator for up to five days. Or you can put the juice into ice-cube trays and freeze them for use at a later date. Lemon zest can be stored in an airtight container in a cool, dry place, or put in an airtight freezer bag and frozen. Lemon slices or wedges can be pre-prepared and kept in a plastic bag in the refrigerator for three or four days.

Washing lemons

Before grating or cutting the rind of a waxed lemon for use in drinks or food, or before liquidizing it whole, brush or rub it with hot water and washing-up liquid for a minute, then rinse really well with water. This is sensible because most lemons are sprayed after harvest with an aqueous emulsion of wax (such as carnauba wax)

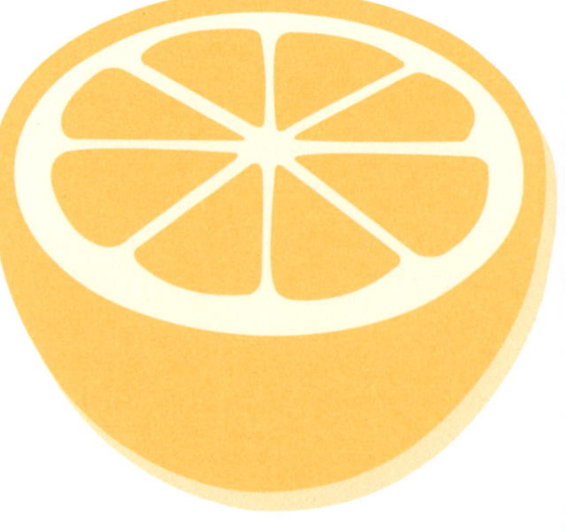

plus a pesticide, to prevent them drying out and to help avoid infection. Alternatively, dip the lemon in just-boiled water for half a minute to dissolve the wax, then remove the lemon and brush it under running water.

Lemon juice

When using lemon juice for skin and haircare, domestic cleaning and, indeed, preparing foods and drinks, here's how to extract the most juice from the fruit. A lemon needs to be at room temperature if you are to get the maximum volume of juice from it. If it has been kept in a fridge, remove it a couple of hours before juicing it, or put it in a bowl and cover it with just-boiled water for half a minute. Next, roll the lemon with your hand on a flat surface to break down the lemon's internal membranes and so help release the juice. Finally, squeeze out the juice using one of the following:

- Your hands
- A citrus reamer (a plastic, wooden, metal or ceramic ribbed rounded-cone-shaped device that you twist into the cut surface of ½ a lemon)
- A citrus trumpet (a metal gadget that you screw into a whole lemon then squeeze the lemon juice into it by hand)
- A lemon squeezer (a glass, ceramic or metal ribbed device with a pip catcher and a juice-collecting area)
- An electric lemon squeezer

You can add the leftover lemon pulp to the juice if you like. Note that bottled lemon juice available in stores can be handy but does not taste nearly as good as fresh juice. One reason is that its contents are slightly different from those of fresh juice. For example, bottled juice has less vitamin C. It's also likely to contain preservatives such as sodium benzoate or sodium metabisulphite (which can trigger an allergic reaction in certain people). On the plus side, bottled juice is usually cheaper than fresh juice. It also lasts longer, so you may like to use it in home-made cleaning products (pp.314–17).

SODIUM BICARBONATE (BICARBONATE OF SODA, BAKING SODA)

This fine, white crystalline mineral powder has many uses: domestic, commercial and health-promoting. "Sodium bicarbonate" is its generic (scientific) name but it is also known as "bicarbonate of soda", "sodium hydrogen carbonate" and, traditionally, as "baking soda", "bread soda" or, simply, "bicarb".

In this book I refer to it as "sodium bicarbonate" when talking about health matters (because this is what doctors call it) and as "bicarbonate of soda" when dealing with beauty and homecare hints (because this is what it is most often known as domestically in the UK).

When purchasing the ingredient from supermarkets and grocery stores, look for "bicarbonate of soda" In Australia, New Zealand and the UK, and for "baking soda" in the US. It is also available as "sodium bicarbonate" from pharmacies or in bulk online.

CAUTION: Don't confuse sodium bicarbonate with baking powder, a culinary product that also contains cream of tartar (also known as potassium hydrogen tartrate) or a "filler" such as cornflour or rice flour, which is used to thicken soups and sauces. Certain other chemicals may sound confusingly similar; they include:

- Caustic soda (sodium hydroxide)
- Sodium chloride (salt)
- Washing soda (sodium carbonate or soda ash)

It is vital never to confuse any of these with sodium bicarbonate, so make sure that you clearly label any container of white powder you are storing in your larder.

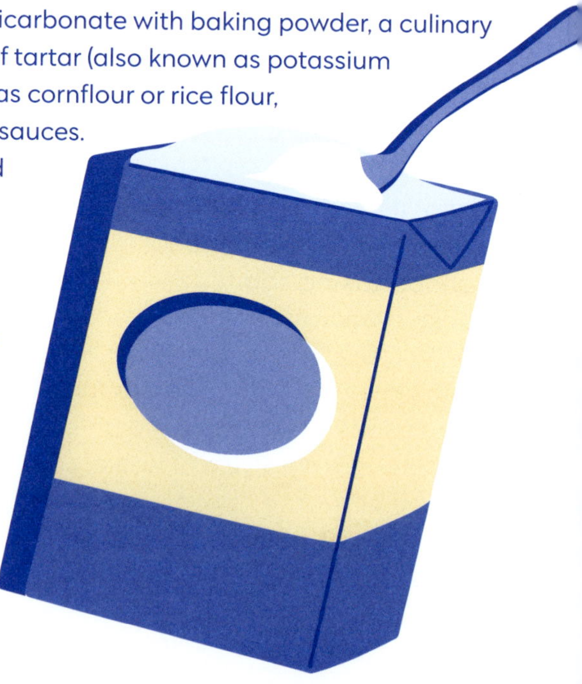

Sodium bicarbonate is present (with sodium carbonate) in natron, a mineral deposited from salt lakes. Ancient Egyptians used this to clean their homes, their teeth and, when mixed with oil, their skin. They also used it to mummify dead bodies. Sodium bicarbonate can also be mined from certain rock as deposits of nahcolite, and is also present in the water of many hot springs. Today, though, it is mostly produced in factories, mainly by mixing salt, ammonia, calcium carbonate and carbon dioxide in water. 100,000 tonnes (110,231 tons) are produced this way each year in countries including the USA, Italy, Egypt and China.

Sodium bicarbonate is mildly alkaline in water but is also amphoteric, meaning it reacts with both acids and alkalis. It is useful in many commercial and domestic situations. It is present, for example, in baking powder and self-raising (self-rising) flour as a cake- and bread-raising agent. It is also used to make soaps, domestic cleaning and deodorizing products, medications, water-softeners, "dry" fire extinguishers and pesticides. It can also be used to make toothpastes and "bath bombs" and to coat dental floss.

Our body's own, internally-produced sodium bicarbonate is a vital part of its acid–alkali balancing systems that keep us healthy. And by eating a healthy diet (which some people call an "alkaline diet") and, perhaps, taking sodium bicarbonate or applying it to our skin, we can help to treat certain common ailments.

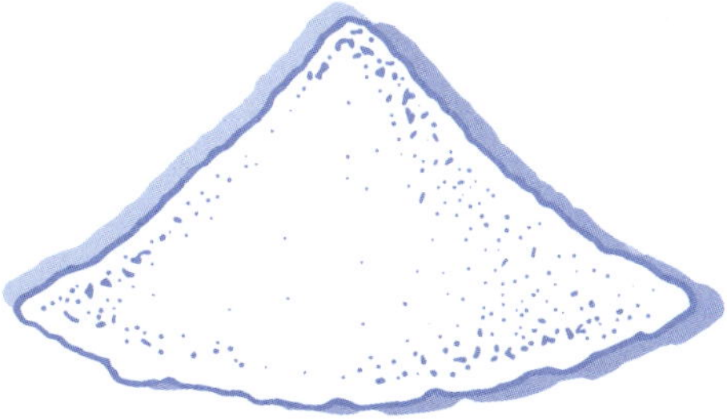

OLIVE OIL

Is olive oil truly a miracle? Arguably it is – if we define a miracle as an amazing or wonderful occurrence. For example, its colour is attractive, its smell delightful, its flavour luscious, its feel in the mouth and on the skin sensual. In addition, olive oil as part of a healthy diet can help to prevent and treat many ailments, thanks to constituents such as its monounsaturated fats and antioxidant polyphenols.

So valuable a commodity has olive oil been over the centuries, it is easy to understand why Homer called it "liquid gold" in *The Odyssey*, and why Hippocrates – the "father" of medicine – referred to it as the "great healer".

All in all, olive oil is highly prized as a food, a medicine and a beauty aid. An unofficial industry benchmark for high-quality olive oil (one made with good olives and a good production process) is a free fatty acid level of 0.3 per cent or less.

Types of olive oil

The *Codex Alimentarius* is a collection of international food standards, guidelines and codes of practice set up to protect consumers' health and ensure fair practice in the food trade. It defines four grades of edible olive oil. These are:

1. Virgin and extra-virgin olive oil
2. Olive oil
3. Refined olive oil
4. Olive pomace oil

Most regulatory authorities worldwide base their grading on these four grades, perhaps with some variation.

EXTRA-VIRGIN AND VIRGIN OLIVE OILS

These are created by pressing or other physical means, under conditions that don't alter the oil, from olives that have had no treatment other than washing, decanting, centrifuging (spinning) and filtering. The less acidic the oil and more concentrated its polyphenols, the better its quality.

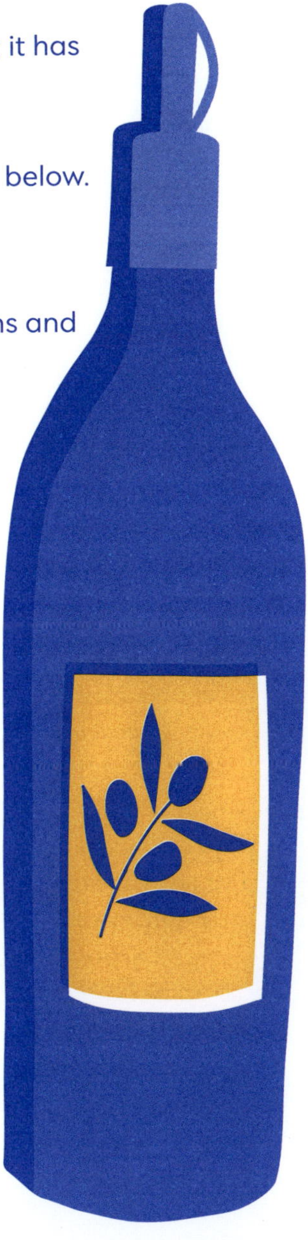

"OLIVE OIL"
This is a blend of refined olive oil and virgin olive oil; it has little or no odour or flavour.

REFINED OLIVE OIL
This is obtained by refining lampante olive oil – see below. This oil has no odour or flavour.

OLIVE POMACE OIL

- **Olive pomace** is the solid mass of olive pulp, skins and stones remaining when most of the oil has been pressed from olives. Olive pomace oil is usually obtained by treating olive pomace with a solvent such as trichloroethylene.
- **Crude olive pomace oil** is edible only if refined by removing its free fatty acids (and therefore its acidity) without altering its fats. One method is to centrifuge it, then heat it in a vacuum to evaporate its fatty acids.
- **Blended olive pomace oil** is a mixture of refined olive pomace oil and virgin olive oil.

LAMPANTE OIL
In its raw state, this is considered unfit for human consumption because of its poor quality and unpleasant taste. It is used in industry. The word "lampante" comes from the Italian for "lamp", as this l oil can be burnt in oil lamps to produce light.

The following chart shows the maximum free acidity and the polyphenol content of several of the types of olive oil available. A polyphenol content of 220mg/kg or more is considered "high".[1]

TYPE OF OLIVE OIL	MAXIMUM FREE ACIDITY (G/100G)	POLYPHENOL CONTENT (MG/KG)
Extra-virgin olive oil	0.8	350 or more
Virgin olive oil	2	120–220
Olive oil	1	60–70
Refined olive oil	0.3	About 60

Benefits of olive oil

1. Olive oil is high in monounsaturated fatty acids and low in polyunsaturated and saturated fatty acids.

This tends to lower LDL ("bad") cholesterol and increase HDL ("good") cholesterol. Olive oil has the highest percentage of monounsaturated fat of all the edible plant oils, and is the best culinary oil or fat for encouraging a healthy cholesterol ratio. Monounsaturated fats decrease the body's production of inflammatory compounds; while polyunsaturated fats, saturated fats and trans fats do the opposite.

2. It has a better balance of omega-6 and omega-3 fatty acids than do most other common culinary oils.

The amounts of these in olive oil (as in most other common culinary oils) are relatively small, and the ratio of omega-6s to omega-3s is overbalanced toward omega-6. Nonetheless its omega-3s are useful, and the omega-6 to omega-3 ratio is more favourable than that of many common oils, including corn and sunflower.

3. It contains antioxidants such as vitamin C, many polyphenols (including flavonoids and flavonols) and compounds called terpenes and terpenoids which have various helpful functions in the body.

These components discourage oxidation of LDL cholesterol. This is good because oxidized LDL cholesterol inflames artery walls, encouraging cardiovascular disease – for example, heart attacks and strokes. The components include polyphenols (such as quercetin, which is a flavonoid, and chlorophyll, which is a plant pigment), as well as squalene and vitamin E. Squalene, a terpenoid our body uses to make cholesterol, is present in higher concentrations than in other vegetable oils. It may also promote liver function and bile secretion; enhance immunity; have anti-ageing, anti-fatigue, antibacterial and anti-inflammatory actions; improve vision; and promote wound healing. The amounts of polyphenols are small, with extra-virgin olive oil having the most. Nevertheless, they are worth having because:

- They discourage cancer, heart attacks, strokes and inflammatory diseases.
- They protect vitamin C by improving its absorption and helping prevent its oxidation.
- They strengthen the walls of capillaries (tiny blood vessels), so maximizing the capillaries' potential volume and thereby promoting good blood flow.

4. It contains the fat-soluble vitamins E and K.
One tablespoon of extra-virgin olive oil has 1.9mg of vitamin E, which is 13 per cent of the recommended daily intake for adults and more than in other grades of olive oil. All grades of olive oil contain vitamin K, the only richer sources being green, leafy vegetables. Vitamin E helps protect cells from damage and aids our immunity, while vitamin K enables healthy blood clotting and aids our body's use of calcium, so encouraging strong bones.

5. It contains organic acids and alcohols.
Olive oil's caffeic and gallic acids stimulate the release of bile from the gallbladder into the intestine. This is beneficial to us, as bile helps overcome the acidity of the food residues that have just left the stomach, enabling the further digestion that requires an alkaline environment. Olive oil's phenylethanol is an alcohol that stimulates production of fat-digesting enzymes in the pancreas.

6. It contains sterols.
Olive oil's very small amounts of sterols include cholesterol, campesterol and beta-sitosterol. Some are useful to us – for example, not only is beta-sitosterol an antioxidant, it also reduces the reabsorption of cholesterol excreted by the liver into the intestine, so lowering the amount of cholesterol in the blood and liver.

HONEY

This fragrant food is made by honeybees. In ancient times it was considered to be a food of the gods, a symbol of wealth, health and happiness and even an elixir of immortality. The Bible's Old Testament promised Israelites "a land flowing with milk and honey". Mohammed claimed honey was a remedy for every illness. Egyptian doctors used honey-containing remedies 5,000 years ago. And Hindus still use it today as one of five foods traditionally offered in worship or welcome.

The word "honey" comes from "oneg", Hebrew for "delight". Honey is also known as the "food of love". Indeed, the word "honeymoon" references the ancient Viking custom in which bride and groom consumed honey cakes and mead (a drink made by fermenting honey) for a month after betrothal.

History of honey

A 100-million-year-old bee was recently found preserved in amber. We know people have eaten honey for thousands of years, but they have probably done so for much longer. They began by collecting honey from wild bees' nests, then progressed to keeping bees. Early in its history, beekeeping was especially popular in Europe and so common in ancient Britain that the country was known as the "land of honey".

At first, honey was the only available sweetener other than date, fig or maple syrup. Alexander the Great brought sugar cane from India to Greece in the 4th century BC, but only the rich could afford sugar from this "honey reed". When the mass cultivation of sugar cane and sugar beet began in the 18th century, sugar became more affordable and honey less important.

Honey production and consumption

The worldwide production of honey in 2022 was 1.83 million tonnes (2 million tons). China was the main producer, with 25 per cent of global production, followed by the European Union with 16 per cent. Other honey producers include Turkey (6 per cent); Argentina, India, Iran and Russia (4 per cent each); Brazil, Mexico, Ukraine and the US (3 per cent each); and Canada, Korea, Spain and Tanzania (2 per cent each).

Honey consumption in 2022 was greatest in the Central African Republic, at 3.1kg (6lb 9oz) per person per year, while people in Saint Lucia ate virtually no honey. In Canada, honey consumption per person per year was 0.86kg (1lb 14oz), while in the UK it was 0.87kg (1lb 15oz); in the US 0.58kg (1lb 4oz); in Australia 0.52kg (1lb 2oz); and in China 0.2kg (7oz).

About 85 per cent of globally produced honey is used as "table honey" – a spread, drizzle or sweetener for use by consumers; the rest is used by the food industry for bakery, confectionery and breakfast cereals, for example. There is also a small market for honey in the pharmaceutical and tobacco industries.

CAUTIONARY NOTE: Many honeybees are dying today because of the continued use of certain pesticides that can kill pollinating insects, leading to the loss of wild flowers and resulting malnutrition of bees. Hopefully, further research and legislation will guarantee the survival of the honeybee so our supplies of honey – and, most important, the pollination of our food crops and other crops by honeybees – will continue.

Types of honey

Honeys vary in colour, thickness, clarity, scent and flavour depending on their nectar and honeydew sources, and the types of processing and storage. Bees use both nectar and honeydew to make honey. Honeydew is a sweet, dark or greenish liquid or crystalline substance excreted by aphids (greenflies), leafhoppers and scale insects that eat sap. Droplets of honeydew glisten like dew on leaves, stems and branches, hence its name.

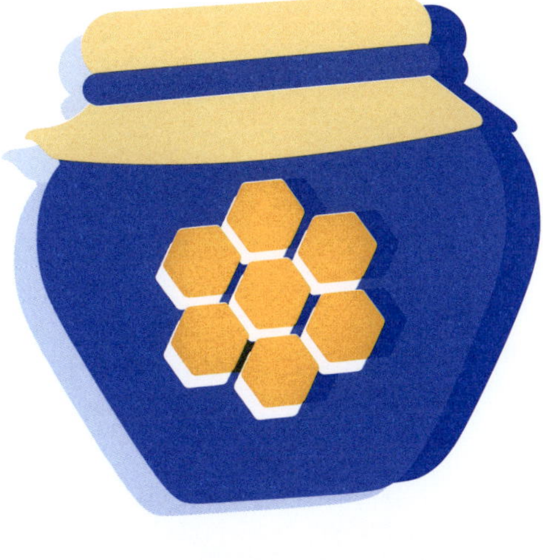

Multifloral and blended honeys are the most commonly available sorts, although people increasingly pay a premium for monofloral, raw or organic honey, and there is growing interest in darker, stronger-tasting honeys. Just as wine or olive oil aficionados delight in the differences between wines or oils from different seasons, producers and varieties of grape or olive, so too do honey lovers enjoy different honeys.

- **Colour:** The US Department of Agriculture identifies seven colours of honey: water-white, extra-white, white, extra-light amber, light-amber, amber and dark-amber. Certain honeys even have yellow, pink, red, green, blue or even black tones.
- **Consistency:** Honey is runny (uncrystallized) or thick (crystallized) depending on its source plants, processing and age. Most honeys start off runny, but almost all thicken in time, some much faster than others. Worldwide, most consumers prefer thick honey, apart from Americans, who tend to prefer runny honey.
- **Clarity:** Cloudiness in a runny honey generally results from pollens. Frosting around its edge is caused by small air-filled spaces developing during crystallization. Cloudiness can also come from suspended particles of wax, propolis, bee parts and dust. Thick honey is opaque.

RAW HONEY

Raw honey has higher levels of enzymes, scent and flavour compounds than does heated honey. And there is no risk of any other constituents having been altered by heat. Raw honey is available from beekeepers, farmers' markets and gourmet or organic food stores.

To extract raw honey, it is gently poured or mechanically removed from the comb, then left for about a week so risen debris and bubbles can be skimmed off, or strained through a wide stainless-steel mesh. Honey labelled "raw" should not have been heated. Even using an electric knife to cut wax cappings from honeycomb could adversely affect the honey. Any honey that is very clear has almost certainly been heated to enable filtering, so isn't truly raw. Raw honey must also not have been filtered, creamed or irradiated.

CAUTION: Don't give raw honey to babies under the age of one (or rub it on their gums during teething) as there is a chance that it might contain spores of *Clostridium botulinum* bacteria, which could cause botulism poisoning. Buy raw honey from trustworthy suppliers, for example, beekeepers at farmers' markets or reputable stores.

ORGANIC HONEY

Certified organic honey is free from pesticides and antibiotics. Regulations vary from country to country, but European Union certification, for example, requires that:

- The land within 3km (1.9 miles) of the hive must be uncultivated or organically cultivated.
- The land on which the hives are kept must be unaffected by significant pollution.
- The hive must be kept on land certified as organic.
- The hive must be made from natural, untreated timber.
- The hive must have been managed organically for 12 months or more.
- The wax used must be organic.
- The bees must be fed with organic honey or sugar.
- The bees must be fed only between the last honey harvest and the 15 days before the first nectar flow.
- The priority for disease control is to build health and vitality through positive management. Unrestricted use of herbal treatments and natural acids (lactic, formic, oxalic) is allowed. After using a prescribed medication such as an antibiotic, the wax must be replaced, and organic status is withdrawn for a year.
- While labelling regulations vary, ideally a label should record a honey's weight, whether it has been heated, whether it is monofloral or blended, its country of origin, and where it was packed. A best-before date and the producer's name and address may be given. Any added ingredients (such as flavourings) should be listed, along with their percentages.

Monofloral, blended and honeydew honeys

Blended honeys are the main type you will see in stores. Mixed floral (multifloral or polyfloral) honeys are also widely available.

MONOFLORAL HONEY

This is honey made mostly from one particular species of plant. This plant may grow in profusion (for example, rapeseed and ling heather), or it may be a prolific nectar-producer with easily accessible nectar (for example clover and milkweed). To ascertain whether a monofloral label is warranted, beekeepers aim to note the flowers their bees visit. If most are of one species, the honey harvested within a day or two of the flowers' nectar flow ceasing can be called a monofloral honey.

MIXED FLORAL HONEY

Most honeys are made from the nectars and honeydews of many plant species. Examples include summer, autumn, jungle and rainforest honeys, and wildflower honeys. Clover honey's flavour lends such a characteristic stamp to a multifloral honey that this is sometimes sold as "clover honey".

BLENDED HONEY

Blending honeys, sometimes from different countries, can alter the resulting honey's colour, flavour and texture. For example, it can lighten the colour, reduce bitterness (for example, from almond honey) and, if one constituent honey is prone to early crystallization, keep it runny.

HONEYDEW HONEY

Any honey can contain some honeydew, but "honeydew honey", unsurprisingly, contains more. It's sometimes sold as "forest" or "tree" honey. Summer and autumn honeys are the most likely to contain honeydew. Honeydew honey tends to be dark, with strong fig, aniseed or woody flavour notes, depending on its sources.

Tree sources of honeydew include beech, cedar, chestnut, citrus, fir, hickory, juniper, larch, lime, maple, oak, pine, poplar, spruce and willow. Honeydew honey from fir, larch, linden, oak and spruce trees is rich in a sugar called melezitose, which makes it harden fast. Plant sources of honeydew include alfalfa, beans, clover and wheat.

Storing and using honey

- Keep honey in a dark place, or in an opaque or dark glass jar, to preserve its antimicrobial power.
- Store honey at a cool room temperature.
- Honey stored in the refrigerator thickens. If borage honey is refrigerated, it develops a chewy texture like that of toffee. Most runny honeys crystallize fastest at 14°C (57°F). Freezing honey prevents changes in its composition, and the process of freezing runny honey prevents natural crystallization.
- In general, properly stored honey keeps well. But storing honey for six months diminishes its antioxidant power by 30 per cent. And storing it for two years begins to reduce its antibacterial power.
- Liquefying thick honey makes it easier to pour and mix. To do this, stand a glass or a ceramic container of honey in hot but not boiling water for 15 minutes and stir occasionally. Or microwave an open glass jar of honey on low for 30 seconds, stir and repeat if necessary.
- When measuring honey, coat the spoon or the inside of the measuring bowl or cup with vegetable oil so the honey can slip out easily.

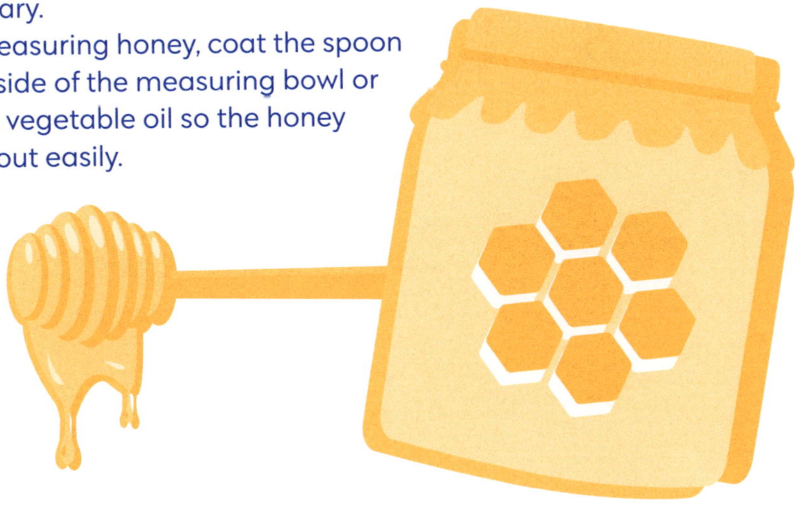

GARLIC

All over the world, garlic is valued as a flavouring ingredient, a food and a medicine. It belongs to the *Alliaceae* family, whose 750 species include onions, shallots, chives, leeks and ornamental alliums. The word "garlic" originates from the Old English for "spear" (gar) and "leek" (leac). Its Latin botanical name, *Allium sativum*, comes from the Greek for "avoid" (presumably because of its smell!) and "cultivated". In English alone its many other names include "prince of herbs", "food of love", "nectar of the gods", "devil's posy", "camphor of the poor", "poor man's treacle" ("treacle" from the Latin *theriaca*, meaning "antidote to poison" or "heal all"), "onion stinker" and "stinking Jenny/stinking lily/stinking rose".

Today's garlic originated as a wild form in Central Asia more than 10,000 years ago. Over the centuries, it was cultivated then traded along the spice and silk routes between China, the Middle East and the Mediterranean. Eventually it reached Africa, Europe, Australia and the Americas. Today, China produces more than 21 million tonnes (23 million tons) a year, which is nearly three-quarters of the global crop. Other top producers, in order of harvest-size, include India, South Korea, Egypt, Russia, the US (especially California), Spain, Argentina and Burma.

Garlic's flavour is hard to classify – it's variously described as pungent, tangy, full, nutty, sweet and musky. Not everyone likes it – some people dislike its flavour as well as the scent that emanates from the mouths (and bodies) of garlic eaters.

The power of garlic through history

From the time of Ancient Egypt, around 4000 BC, to the end of the 19th century, garlic was the most widely used medicinal plant in the world. It remains a popular traditional remedy for many ailments today. Garlic supplements are among the top-selling herbal supplements in the Western world, and thousands of scientific studies have investigated how garlic can promote good health.

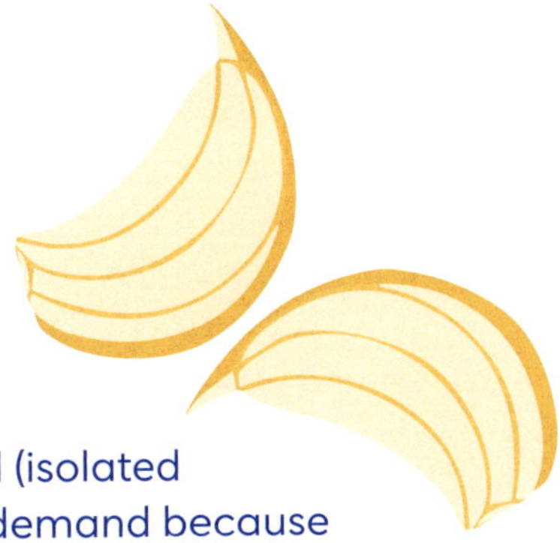

Historically, garlic was also used in the art world: during the 13th–17th centuries, gilders used its sticky juice to attach gilding to picture frames and furniture. Nowadays, it is used in industry, too. Garlic oil (isolated by distilling garlic cloves with water) is in big demand because it contains compounds needed for the production of industrial chemicals called alkenes. Alkenes are used for making high-end lubricants, sealants for the glass industry, and binders used in solid propellants for rockets, as well as in the vulcanization of rubber.

Over the millennia, magical powers have been attributed to garlic, and it has been said to protect against vampires, werewolves, witches, sorcerers, demons and evil spirits! Even today some Greek midwives have garlic in the delivery room to divert the "evil eye" away from the newborn baby, and in some countries people hang garlic outside their homes to protect their families.

NOTE: There are two special things about garlic. First, more than 160 of a garlic bulb's thousands of constituents are bioactive, meaning they can affect the working of the body. The amounts are tiny but can nevertheless contribute to health, especially if consumed regularly. Second, garlic's odour, flavour and tingle on the tongue are unique.

WHAT HAPPENS TO GARLIC IN THE BODY?

When you consume garlic, its water-soluble and oil-soluble compounds affect the body in different ways:

- Garlic's water-soluble compounds have small molecules that easily diffuse from the intestine into the capillaries (tiny blood vessels) in the intestinal wall; these capillaries empty into the hepatic portal vein which takes blood to the liver. One such compound, gamma-glutamyl cysteine, is converted into S-allyl cysteine, which can be measured in the blood, liver and urine and contributes heavily to the health benefits of garlic.

- Garlic's oil-soluble compounds (allicin and allicin derivatives) have large molecules, so only very small amounts can diffuse from the intestine into the capillaries. Any allicin that enters the blood either quickly breaks down into sulphur-containing compounds responsible for most of garlic's health benefits in the body, or enters cells.

WHAT HAPPENS TO GARLIC ON THE SKIN?

When you apply garlic to the skin, some of its sulphur compounds penetrate it and enter the blood. So if garlic is rubbed on to the soles of the feet, for example, the person's breath will be scented with garlic within 10 minutes or so.

Health-promoting effects of garlic's sulphur compounds

The sulphur compounds in garlic are hugely important to health, and garlic is four times richer than onions in these vital ingredients. Scientists believe that sulphur compounds such as alliin, gamma-glutamyl cysteine, S-allyl cysteine and allicin derivates (such as allyl sulphides, ajoene and vinyl dithiins) account for most of garlic's health-promoting effects, promoting benefits such as:

- Anti-cancer
- Anti-clotting
- Anti-diabetic
- Antimicrobial
- Anti-obesity
- Antioxidant and anti-inflammatory
- Cholesterol-lowering
- Detoxifying
- Digestive-juice-stimulating
- Immunity-enhancing
- Smooth muscle-relaxing

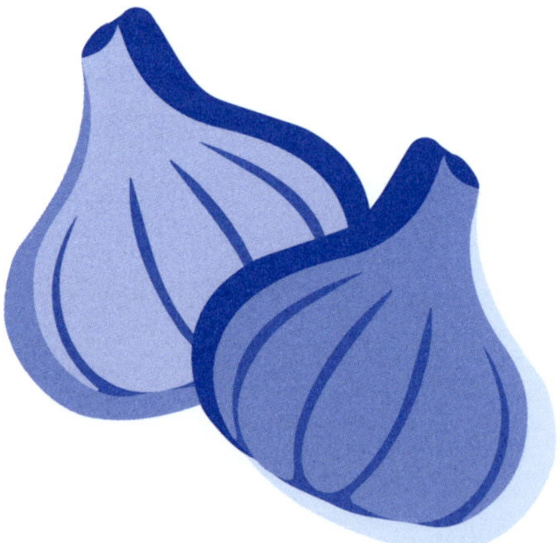

Other constituents of garlic

Besides sulphur compounds, garlic cloves contain water (which accounts for over half their weight), proteins, free amino acids, oils, fats, carbohydrates, vitamins, other minerals and certain other constituents.

PROTEINS AND AMINO ACIDS

The 17 "free" amino acids in garlic (meaning those amino acids not chemically combined with other amino acids to form proteins or peptide chains) include arginine (an antioxidant that helps to maintain healthy blood pressure and is being studied for its anti-cancer potential) and four sulphur-containing amino acids: cysteine, cystine, methionine and taurine (essential for our body's structural proteins, including keratin in nails and hair, and collagen in joints).

VITAMINS

Garlic's main vitamins are B6 and C; others include A, B1, B2, B3, biotin (B7) and E. The S-allyl group common to many of garlic's sulphur compounds aids absorption of vitamin B1.

MINERALS

Garlic is rich in phosphorus, potassium, selenium, sulphur and the trace elements germanium and manganese.

Garlic is the richest in selenium of all vegetables. Interestingly, its roots can extract selenium even when the concentration of this mineral in soil is poor. While a large clove contains only 1.6 per cent of the US Recommended Dietary Allowance (RDA) for selenium, a large clove grown in selenium-enriched soil can contain four times this RDA. Garlic's sulphur content enhances the antioxidant power of its selenium.

Garlic is also the richest in sulphur of all vegetables, containing at least four times as much as do onions and cabbage, for example. Our body's sulphur is distributed among certain enzymes and bile acids, as well as insulin, biotin, collagen, elastin, proteoglycans ("mucopolysaccharides", in connective tissues and joint fluid), coenzyme A, lipoic acid and the antioxidant enzyme glutathione.

LESSER-KNOWN COMPONENTS OF GARLIC

Garlic also includes:

- **Flavonoids** – including myricetin and apigenin (currently being investigated for its anti-cancer effects). Many, notably quercetin, allicin and anthocyanins, are powerful antioxidants. Quercetin also has antihistamine and antiviral properties, can lower blood sugar by stimulating insulin production, and can strengthen capillaries. Allicin helps to prevent the formation of those prostaglandins that encourage inflammation, blood clotting and cancer growth; it also has antimicrobial effects and enhances nerve growth

- **Anthocyanins** – flavonoid derivatives, and polyphenols (types of phenolic compounds) that include caffeic acid, ferulic acid and tannins (which have antioxidant properties)
- **Plant hormones** – for example, glucokinin ("plant insulin"), which is thought to lower blood sugar and so protect the pancreas from exhausting itself by having to produce a large amount of insulin
- **Saponins** – steroid-like substances thought to have cholesterol- and blood pressure-lowering actions and to encourage healthy proportions of micro-organisms in the bowel. They are also thought to help protect against bowel cancer by breaking down the cholesterol-rich membranes of its cells. Certain saponins have anti-inflammatory, antimicrobial and anti-parasitic activities
- **Terpenes** – odoriferous compounds in garlic's oil, including citral (lemon-scented), geraniol (rose-scented), linalool (with a sweet, woody, lavender scent) and phellandrenes (with a peppery, minty or citrus scent)

Using garlic

Separate only the cloves you need.

PEELING

Fresh cloves are harder to peel. Make peeling easier by soaking cloves in water for an hour, or boiling them in water for 20 seconds. Cut each clove above its base then peel off its papery skin ("wrapper") with your fingertips or a knife. Alternatively, put a clove on a chopping board and press it with the flat surface of a broad sturdy knife blade to break its wrapper and make it easier to peel. Or use a polyurethane garlic peeler (which looks like a piece of giant macaroni). Put it on a worktop and insert some cloves, then roll it backward and forward several times. Discard any cloves that look greyish or yellowish, or are dry and stringy inside.

CRUSHING OR CHOPPING

The smaller the pieces of garlic, the greater the damage, the larger the potential yield of allicin and the stronger its scent and flavour. The longer you leave crushed or chopped garlic to stand, up to 90 minutes, the more allicin it yields (p.79). To crush a clove, choose one of the following options: chop it then squash the pieces with the flat surface of a broad sturdy knife blade; just squash it; use a garlic crusher; or use a pestle and mortar. You don't have to peel a clove before crushing it, though many people find it easier to do so.

SOAKING

Some people soak crushed or chopped garlic in milk, vinegar or alcohol, or boil cloves in water or milk, before use. This makes the flavour milder because sulphur compounds diffuse into the liquid. But you then lose some of the health benefits unless you consume the liquid too.

JUICING

To extract garlic juice, whizz peeled cloves in a blender until smooth. Spoon the purée into a fine sieve over a bowl and use a wooden spoon to force the juice through. By adding water to the juice you can make "garlic water" for bathing skin infections or wounds (p.81). One garlic bulb produces up to 4 tablespoons of juice.

Storing garlic

What is the best way to store garlic and extend its lifespan once you bring it home? Cool, moist conditions encourage sprouting, while hot, dry conditions make garlic bulbs dry out faster.

Many people store garlic in the refrigerator, but this is too cold. The optimal conditions for storing garlic are to keep it uncovered or loosely covered in a dark, dry place at 10–20°C (50–68°F) and ideally at 13–14°C (56–58°F). Why does garlic need these conditions?

- This temperature discourages sprouting, rotting and drying out.
- Good ventilation provides garlic with the oxygen its cells need to breathe, helping to keep them healthy and rot-resistant. Try storing your garlic in a purpose-made terracotta "garlic-keeper" pot, or a net bag. Never store fresh garlic in plastic bags as this would make it more likely to rot.
- Darkness helps to prevent drying or greening.
- Air humidity should be 40–60 per cent (ideally 45–50 per cent); any higher encourages rotting and root growth: any lower dries garlic faster.

Inspect stored garlic frequently and remove any soft or mouldy bulbs or cloves. Separated cloves dry and rot faster, so break off only those you intend using immediately. Crystals forming on stored garlic consist of its sulphur compound allicin.

Preserving garlic

Although nothing can replace fresh garlic for the best flavour and health benefits, preserved garlic is a useful standby and contains many health-promoting constituents. You can preserve garlic by drying, freezing, or steeping in oil, vinegar or wine.

DRYING GARLIC

As garlic dries, its flavour intensifies. Garlic bulbs dry out in 4–10 months at room temperature. There are three methods of drying garlic faster:

- Dry 5mm- (¼in-)thick slices at warm room temperature in a dry, well-ventilated, non-sunny space. They should dry out in 1–2 weeks
- Use a food dehydrator, following its instructions
- Dry cloves in the oven at no more than 50°C (122°F) for several hours until dry and crisp. (Higher temperatures destroy alliinase – the enzyme that releases allicin, which helps give garlic its odour, flavour and health-promoting properties)

Keep dried garlic in an airtight container.

FREEZING GARLIC

You can freeze garlic for several months using the following methods:

- Freeze peeled cloves in a plastic freezer bag. This changes the cloves' texture slightly
- Freeze garlic juice in an ice-cube tray, then transfer the cubes into a plastic freezer bag
- Freeze chopped garlic in a plastic freezer bag. When you want to use it, grate or break off what you need
- Freeze peeled cloves covered with oil in a covered freezer container
- Freeze crushed garlic mixed with extra-virgin olive oil (about 6 tbsp oil for the cloves from one medium bulb). Freeze this purée in a plastic freezer bag. When you want to use it, scrape off what you need

Remember to label and date each batch.

GARLIC BREATH

One potential disadvantage of consuming garlic for health or pleasure is the "garlic breath" effect, as this can be quite noticeable to others. To reduce the pungency of garlic breath, try the following:

- Add milk to garlic before cooking it (recent research found this halved the expected intensity of garlic breath)
- Drink 200ml (7fl oz/generous ¾ cup) of milk before consuming garlic
- Chew raw fruits or vegetables; herbs such as mint or basil; or caraway, fennel or cardamom seeds
- Eat cooked rice or eggs
- Clean teeth to remove garlic debris
- Rinse your mouth with ½ a glass of water containing a teaspoon of bicarbonate of soda
- Use a commercial mouthwash

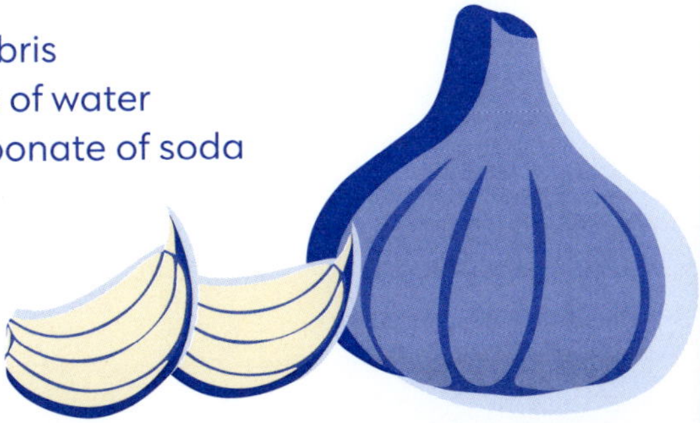

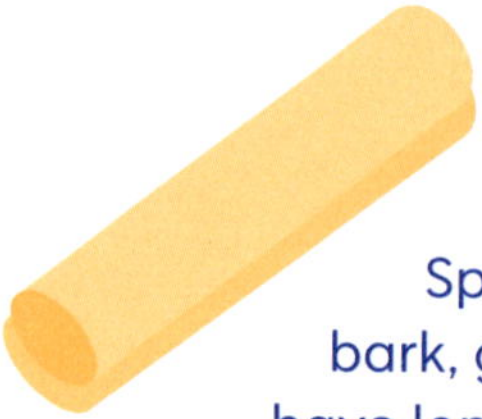

SPICES

Spices come from the aromatic seeds, fruits, flowers, bark, gums, roots or rhizomes of particular plants. They have long been valued as perfumes, in foods and as medications. The earliest written records of spices are in recipes containing garlic, cumin and coriander written on clay tablets found 3,774 years ago in Mesopotamia – the land between the Tigris and Euphrates rivers, today comprising Iraq and parts of Iran, Kuwait, Syria and Turkey. Pepper was recorded in Sanskrit and Chinese texts 12,000 years ago.

Trading and usage

Trading in coveted spices led over centuries not only to vast riches for individual traders, cities and even countries, but also to wars over trade routes and to the "discovery" by Europeans of the Americas. People in cooler climes were familiar with home-grown spices such as caraway, celery, coriander, cumin, dill, fennel, juniper, horseradish, lovage and mustard, but they coveted exotic spices such as cinnamon, ginger and pepper.

The world's 70–80 commercially produced spices are widely available today. Chilli, cloves and pepper are the most traded. Saffron is by far the most expensive because the orange-yellow strands – the pistils from autumn-crocus flowes – are hand-picked. Vanilla and cardamom come second and third.

Spices can not only make food taste wonderful but they can also benefit our health (see Chapter 2) and skin (see Chapter 3) and make our homes and domestic cleaning products smell fragrant (see Chapter 4).

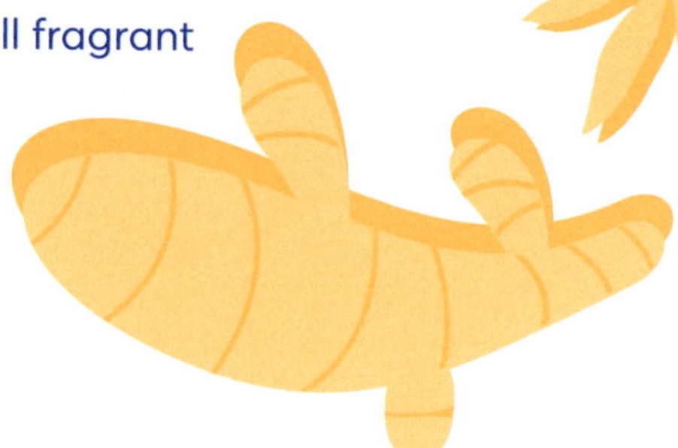

TEA

A cup of tea is a daily delight to billions, and the habit of tea-drinking is deeply embedded in many cultures, whether as a quick and restorative pick-me-up, for leisurely enjoyment, or during a calming, contemplative Japanese tea ceremony. A staggering five billion cups of tea are drunk each day around the world, but the amounts vary hugely country by country. The brew commonly called "tea" originates from the downy leaf buds and thin leathery leaves of *Camellia sinensis*. Tea bushes and trees are cultivated mainly in tea plantations – known as "tea gardens" – in China, India, Sri Lanka and Kenya. Certain other countries, including Japan, Malawi, Nepal and Vietnam, also produce tea.

Processing darkens the green leaves, hence the term "black tea"; adding milk to a brew of black tea turns it light brown. For this reason and also to distinguish black tea from the many "herb teas", I will call it "*Camellia-sinensis* tea", or simply "tea". Interestingly, the "green tea" beloved for its health benefits is created by more minimal processing of the same *Camellia sinensis* leaves; this changes their green colour very little. So familiar is the name "green tea" that I will call it that, rather than "*Camellia-sinensis* green tea".

The various teas made from *Camellia sinensis* have countless benefits. For instance, they can alleviate the symptoms of many diseases and help prevent obesity, circulatory diseases, type 2 diabetes and certain cancers (bladder, breast, endometrium, large intestine, lung, oral cavity, ovary, prostate, skin).

History of tea

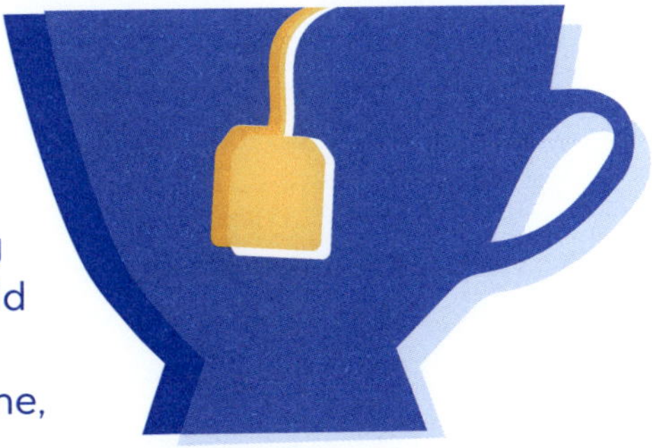

Camellia-sinensis tea bushes and trees originated in China 60–70 million years ago. At some point in time, people discovered that chewing and swallowing the fresh leaves of wild tea tasted good and boosted their energy. Somewhere in the mists of time, someone thought to pour hot water over these leaves and drink the resulting brew. Tea-drinking was first documented some 2,500 years ago, and by about 2,000 years ago, tea was held in such high esteem that it was reserved only for emperors and other VIPs.

Around 1,500 or so years ago, green tea was being drunk by ordinary people and had become a locally traded commodity. The practice of oxidizing green tea to make black tea, or fermenting it to make *puerh* (pronounced "poo-er") tea (p.42), began during the Ming Dynasty (1368–1644). This allowed tea to stay wholesome when transported over long distances – for example, the 930 miles (1,500km) to Tibet along what became known as the "Tea Road".

Portuguese traders took green tea to Europe in the 1580s; the Dutch took tea to New Amsterdam (later known as New York) around 1650, and to England in 1669. In the 1860s, an undercover agent of England's East India Company travelled to China, then leaked to India the secret of how black tea was made. Black tea soon became the favourite in Europe and India, but green tea has remained the first choice in eastern Asia. This explains why it's the second-most popular drink – after water – in the world.

Other names

Camellia sinensis, also called *Thea sinensis*, belongs to the botanical family *Theaceae*. It's sometimes described as "true tea", to distinguish it from the many other herb teas. It has more than 3,000 subvarieties and cultivars, but two main varieties:

- *Camellia sinensis* var. *sinensis*, the small-leafed "China bush" that is resistant to cold temperatures
- *Camellia sinensis* var. *assamica*, the large-leafed "Assam bush" that may become a tree and needs plenty of warmth

The word tea comes from *tay* in the Min Nan language of parts of China. Variations include *thé* in French and *té* in Spanish. *Cha* is Mandarin for tea in China and a nickname for tea in English-speaking countries. Japan and Portugal also use the word *cha*, while versions of it include *chai* in India and Russia.

Tea and *cha* derive from *tu* and *jia* in different languages of ancient China, both of which come from the even older *d'a*.

Types of *Camellia-sinensis* tea

Freshly-picked leaves and buds are processed in several ways to produce the six types of *Camellia-sinensis* tea – black, green, purple, oolong, white and *puerh*. Each of these could be made from any tea bush or tree, but Assam is favoured for black tea and China for green and white teas.

Of all the tea produced around the world, 78 per cent is black, 20 per cent green and most of the remainder oolong. Only China produces all six types, although three-quarters of its total production is green. Almost all India's teas are black, and almost all Japanese ones green.

Processing

Each type of tea is produced in a particular way. The main processes are:

Withering – softens leaves to help them stay whole, retain their aromatic constituents and, when rolled, hold their shape. It also boosts sweetness by converting some of their complex sugars into simple ones. And it increases their range of aromatic compounds.
Rolling, tossing or tumbling – bruises leaves and twists or curls them, so releasing and activating oxidation enzymes. A well-rolled leaf is long, thin and "wiry".
Sifting – separates whole leaves from broken ones and sifts leaves into different sizes.
Machine-cutting – chops broken or lower-quality leaves into even-sized fragments. This allows their constituents to infuse into water at the same rates, enabling predictable steeping times and flavours for their brews.
Oxidation – this enzyme-enabled chemical process is the main factor that differentiates teas. Oxidation of chlorophyll removes the leaves' green colour. Oxidation of polyphenols called catechins into other polyphenols called theaflavins and thearubigins, colours the

leaves red and brown and makes them less astringent. Theaflavins are more astringent than thearubigins.

- Green tea is minimally oxidized, so the leaves keep their green colour and their catechins (types of flavonoid) are largely undiminished. This tea is by far the richest tea in catechins and the poorest in the polyphenol pigments theaflavins and thearubigins.
- Oolong and white teas are partially oxidized, so have middling amounts of catechins and thearubigins. White teas have middling amounts of theaflavins; oolongs none, though they do contain thearubigins from other sources.
- Black teas are fully oxidized, so are the richest in theaflavins and thearubigins. These pigments account for the amber, reddish and brown colours of these teas.

Firing or steaming – the heat of these halts oxidation at the time required for the type of tea being produced. It also prevents fermentation by killing bacteria and fungi. The higher temperatures used for certain teas affect their flavour by creating new aromatic compounds, increasing carboxylic acids, caramelizing sugars and producing complex and nutty or otherwise attractively flavoured constituents.
Ageing – to further develop their flavour.

Black *Camellia-sinensis* teas

Mainly produced in India, Sri Lanka and Kenya, these constitute about 90 per cent of the *Camellia-sinensis* tea drunk in Europe and the US, and are the teas most commonly consumed in India and the Middle East. They are black because they are fully oxidized. Their astringency, body and flavour are stronger than that of other *Camellia-sinensis* teas. Their flavour is commonly described as earthy and smoky, while some are fruity or citrusy. They have a hint of bitterness and may have a slight sweetness.

Green *Camellia-sinensis* teas

These are mostly produced in China and Japan and account for most of the tea drunk there, but only 20 per cent or so of that in Europe and the US. They are also popular in North Africa and South America. These teas' whole leaves are sometimes powdered.

Green tea may contain rolled bud sets, called "swords" or "needles"; these may float upright in a cup of tea. Its rolled leaves are described as "blades", "strips" or "twists". Tumbling of the leaves during processing forms them into balls called "pearls", "pellets" or "semi-balls", depending on their tightness and shape. The smallest and tightest are best as their shape helps prevent their essential oil, and therefore their flavour, from evaporating. Some green teas are tied into balls.

Matcha is a bright-green tea produced by growing *Camellia sinensis* bushes in shade (to increase their green chlorophyll) then powdering their dried leaves. It is particularly antioxidant-rich, has a fresh, grassy aroma, and umami is one of its flavour notes.

"Purple" *Camellia-sinensis* teas

This is made from tea plants which have a genetic mutation that produces more of the purple pigment anthocyanin in their leaves. A brew made from this tea has a light pink tint that intensifies if you add a little lemon juice. The purple leaves contain more antioxidants than any other tea leaves! Their anthocyanin gives them their colour and is a powerful antioxidant (and, interestingly, is also found in blueberries).

This tea has antiviral, anti-inflammatory and anti-cancer properties; it reduces cholesterol, boosts cognitive function and helps prevent colds and flu. It has half the caffeine of green tea and even less than that in black tea.

Oolong *Camellia-sinensis* teas

Most of these whole-leaf teas come from the south-east coasts of China and are the main teas drunk there. They are made from shoots of up to three leaves, perhaps with buds. Their processing includes withering, bruising, exposing them to air so they oxidize, firing (also called "fixing" or "kill green") to stop oxidation, rolling (to produce the twisted leaves that characterize oolong teas), drying and roasting. The degree of oxidation determines their flavour and aroma: the more heavily oxidized a tea, the more robust and earthy its flavour and the "fuller" its mouth-feel or "body" (meaning the greater its viscosity and its weight on the tongue).

Oolong tea is more strongly flavoured than green teas but less so than black teas. Some leaves are rolled into long curves, others pressed into ball shapes. Heavily oxidized oolongs are called black-dragon (wulong) teas.

White *Camellia-sinensis* teas

So called because of the silvery-white down on their buds that persists after processing, these Chinese teas are made from early-spring buds. The best white teas contain only buds.

Their processing usually simply involves withering the buds. This produces partial oxidation of only 5–12 per cent, so white teas are nearly as rich in antioxidants as are green and *sheng puerh* teas. Some lower-quality white teas are fired as well.

White teas have a mild, delicate, refreshing flavour with some similarities to that of black tea but little or no astringency.

Puerh teas

The processing of these teas gives them a sweet, mellow, earthy flavour.

- *Sheng* ("raw") *puerh* tea is made by withering, roasting, rolling and sun-drying the leaves. It has a grassy, sometimes bitter, flavour.
- *Shou* ("cooked" or "ripe") *puerh* tea is made by withering, roasting, rolling, sun-drying, wetting, covering, then leaving the leaves to ferment for up to 40 days. It has an earthy flavour.

Colours of *Camellia-sinensis* tea

Dried teas and their brews come in a variety of colours: Black tea leaves are dark brown; green tea leaves are olive green; white tea leaves are greenish or silvery; oolong tea leaves may be green, brown, greyish-black or mottled; purple tea leaves are charcoal grey, or purple, and *puerh* tea leaves are dark or greenish-brown.

WHAT COLOUR WILL YOUR BREW BE?

The colour you end up with when your choice of tea is brewed with hot water can be surprising, as we can see from these examples:

- Most black teas – light golden to very dark brown
- Certain black teas – deep or cherry red
- Oolongs and certain black and white teas – green to copper
- Certain white teas – pale honey to pale orange
- Certain white teas – light green
- Green teas – light to dark olive green
- Purple tea – light pink
- Japanese green tea – bright olive green
- Japanese powdered green teas – vivid green
- *Sheng puerh* – gold
- *Shou puerh* – dark red to black

Flavoured *Camellia-sinensis* teas

Certain teas are sprayed in tea factories with mango, apricot or orange flavours, or stored with jasmine, osmanthus or other flowers. These give rise to some well-loved variations of black tea, for example:

Earl Grey tea is made by adding a little bergamot orange essential oil to black tea.

Jasmine tea is produced by layering and lightly heating fresh jasmine flowers with green tea leaves (10 times as much jasmine as the weight of tea!). This allows some oxidation and continues for 12 hours. The process is repeated up to eight times using fresh flowers. Jasmine tea has some of the colour of black tea, but the flavours of green tea, plus extra aromatics. Jasmine or other green tea is commonly offered in Chinese restaurants in the West to accompany food, but the Chinese themselves drink it only between meals.

"Herb teas"

This is the term commonly used to describe teas made by infusing the leaves or other parts of plants other than *Camellia sinensis*.

Some of the 27 teas below make enjoyable everyday drinks. Some are good for personal care or home care. All are valued medicines. Most are straw, golden, light olive or light brown in colour, while hibiscus tea is pinkish-red and peppermint tea greenish-brown.

Unlike *Camellia-sinensis* tea, which contains caffeine, teas made from the herbs below are caffeine-free.

WHAT PART OF THE PLANT DOES YOUR TEA COME FROM?

Different "herb teas" are made from different parts of various plants, for example:

All aerial parts (the parts above ground) – lemon balm, passionflower, rosemary and verbena teas.

Flowers – calendula, chamomile, elderflower, hibiscus, lavender, linden, red clover and rosehip teas.

Fruits – rosehips and *Vitex agnus castus* teas.

Leaves – chickweed, dandelion, nettle, peppermint, rooibos, rosemary and thyme teas.

Roots and/or rhizomes (underground stems) – black cohosh, dandelion, dong quai, echinacea, ginseng and valerian teas.

Seeds – barley and corn teas.

NOTE: The "Notable contents" section in each of the following list of teas highlights the main bioactive constituents of each tea; for more information, see Chapter 2.

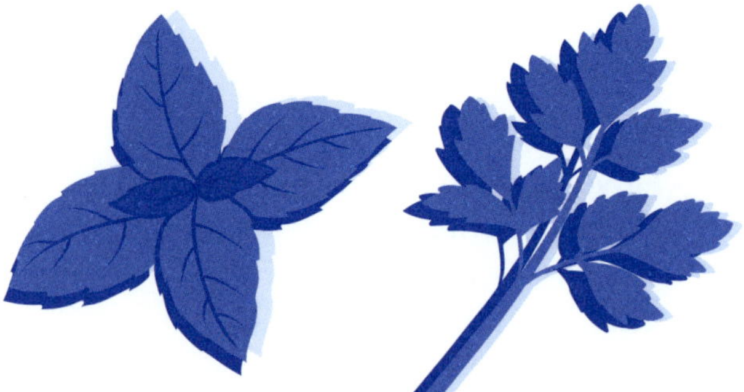

BARLEY AND ROASTED-BARLEY TEAS

Made from the hulled (pearl barley) or unhulled (pot barley or barley groats) grains of *Hordeum distchon*, a plant in the grass family.

- **Other names** – Barley tea is called barley water in the UK; roasted-barley tea is popular in Korea (as *boricha*) and Japan (as *mugicha*)
- **Flavour** – Barley tea: sweetish and slightly bitter; roasted-barley tea: "toasty" and a little like coffee but not as bitter
- **Notable contents** – Barley tea: alkaloids; betaine; the mineral selenium; the phyto-oestrogen trigonelline. Roasted-barley tea: as above, plus complex flavour constituents ("Maillard-reaction compounds") created by roasting; (the Maillard reaction is a chemical reaction that gives browned food its distinctive flavour)
- **Used for** – Barley tea: everyday drink; medicine; roasted-barley tea: everyday drink

BLACK COHOSH TEA

Made from the rhizomes and rootlets of *Cimicifuga racemosa*, a perennial plant in the buttercup family.

- **Other names** – black snakeroot; bugbean; rattleroot; squaw root (a name also given to blue cohosh, which is different)
- **Flavour** – acrid and bitter
- **Notable contents** – acids; flavonoids; glycosides; phyto-oestrogens; resin; salicylates
- **Used for** – medicine

BUTTERFLY PEA TEA

Made from the petals of *Clitoria ternatea*.

- **Other names** – blue tea, blue-pea tea
- **Flavour** – floral, sweetish, slightly earthy and spicy
- **Notable contents** – anthocyanin: a blue, antioxidant plant pigment and a flavonoid. Freshly brewed tea is blue but adding a little lemon juice turns it purple
- **Used for** – beauty aid, medicine

CALENDULA TEA

Made from the flowers and leaves of *Calendula officinalis*, a plant in the daisy family.

- **Other names** – bull's eyes; gold bloom; marigold; marybud; pot marigold
- **Flavour** – floral and sweetish, with hints of bitterness and pungency
- **Notable contents** – acids; aromatics; carotenoids; complex sugars (in mucilage); flavonoids; glycosides; resin; sterols; lupeol (a terpene)
- **Used for** – beauty aid; medicine

CHAMOMILE TEA

Made from the flowers of *Matricaria chamomilla*, an annual plant in the daisy family.

- **Other names** – German chamomile; Matricaria recutita, wild chamomile
- **Flavour** – pleasantly aromatic and slightly bittersweet, with an apple note
- **Notable contents** – aromatics; choline; coumarins; flavonoids; glycosides; acids; salicylates; terpenes (see p.85) ; tannins
- **Used for** – beauty aid; everyday drink; medicine

CHICKWEED TEA

Made from the aerial parts of *Stellaria media*, an annual wild plant in the carnation family.

- **Other names** – adder's mouth; chick wittles; clucken wort; satinflower; skirt buttons; star weed; tongue grass; winter weed
- **Flavour** – slightly salty
- **Notable contents** – acids; alkaloids; complex sugars (in mucilage); copper; coumarins; flavonoids; glycosides; quinones; saponins; sterols; tannins; vitamin C
- **Used for** – beauty aid; medicine

CORNSILK AND ROASTED-CORN TEAS

Cornsilk tea is made from the pistils of the flowers of *Zea mays*, a plant in the grass family; Roasted-corn tea is made from corn's roasted kernels (seeds).

- **Other names** – Cornsilk tea: also called maize-silk tea. Roasted-corn tea: popular in Korea (as *oksusu cha*)
- **Flavour** – Cornsilk tea: "earthy" and sweetish; roasted-corn tea: nutty and slightly sweeter than cornsilk tea
- **Notable contents** – Cornsilk tea: acids; alkaloids; allantoin; complex sugars; the phyto-oestrogen trigonelline; saponins; sterols; tannins. Roasted-corn tea: as above, plus complex flavour constituents ("Maillard-reaction compounds") created by roasting
- **Used for** – Cornsilk tea: beauty aid; medicine; roasted-corn tea: everyday drink; medicine

DANDELION AND ROASTED-DANDELION TEA

Made from the roots, or roasted roots, of *Taraxacum officinale*, a plant in the daisy family.

- **Other names** – Dandelion tea: blow-ball; dent-de-lion (lion's tooth); fairy clock; priest's crown; wet-a-bed. Roasted-dandelion tea is often called dandelion "coffee", due to its resemblance to coffee in appearance and taste
- **Flavour** – Dandelion tea: mild, pleasant, slightly bitter and slightly sweet; roasted-dandelion tea: rather like weak coffee
- **Notable contents** – Dandelion tea: acids; carotenoids; choline; complex sugars; flavonoids; glycosides; gum and resin; minerals (especially copper and iron); phyto-oestrogens; saponins; sesquiterpene lactones; sterols; tannins. Roasted-dandelion tea: as above, plus complex flavour constituents ("Maillard-reaction compounds") created by roasting
- **Used for** – beauty aid; everyday drink; medicine

DONG QUAI TEA

Made from the roots of *Angelica-sinensis*, a plant in the parsley/carrot family.

- **Other names** – angelica root; Chinese angelica; dong kwai; women's ginseng
- **Flavour** – aromatic, slightly sweet and slightly bitter
- **Notable contents** – acids; aromatics; complex sugars; coumarins; phthalides; polyacetylenes; sterols; tannins
- **Used for** – medicine

ECHINACEA TEA

Made from the roots and rhizomes of *Echinacea angustifolia* and other echinacea species, perennial plants in the echinacea family.

- **Other names** – black samson; coneflower; Kansas snakeroot; purple coneflower; rudbeckia
- **Flavour** – aromatic, earthy and sweetish, then slightly bitter. Also pungent and can cause temporary numbness and tingling of the tongue
- **Notable contents** – acids; alkylamides; aromatics; complex sugars; flavonoids; glycosides; polyacetylenes; resin; tannins
- **Used for** – beauty aid; medicine

ELDERFLOWER TEA

Made from the flowers of *Sambucus nigra*, a shrubby tree in the honeysuckle family.

- **Other names** – black elder; bore tree; elder; pipe tree.
- **Flavour** – floral, sweetish and mildly astringent. Tea made from flowers that have been fully open for some time may be slightly bitter
- **Notable contents** – acids; complex sugars; flavonoids; phyto-oestrogens; polyphenols; sterols; tannins
- **Used for** – beauty aid; everyday drink; medicine

GINSENG TEA

Made from the roots of *Panax ginseng*, a perennial plant in the ivy family.

- **Other names** – Asiatic, Chinese, Korean, oriental or true ginseng. Interestingly, *panax* means "panacea". Siberian ginseng (*Eleutherococcus senticosus*) is a different herb
- **Flavour** – pleasant; slightly sweet at first, then bitter
- **Notable contents** – acids; aromatics; choline; complex sugars; glycosides; polyacetylenes; saponins
- **Used for** – medicine

HIBISCUS TEA

Made from the sepals of the flowers of *Hibiscus sabdariffa*, a shrub in the mallow family.

- **Other names** – *bissap* or *bissop* (in West Africa, it's Senegal's national drink); *dah* (in Mali); *flor de Jamaica* (in Latin America); *karkadé* (in Jordan, Egypt and Sudan); rosemallow (in the Americas); *rosella* (in Australia); *roselle* (for example, in the Sahel, Africa); *sorrel* (in the West Indies)
- **Flavour** – sour and slightly bitter, fruity and sweet (a bit like cranberry)
- **Notable contents** – acids; an alkaloid; complex sugars; flavonoids; phascolamin; resin
- **Used for** – beauty aid; everyday drink; medicine

LAVENDER TEA

Made from the flowers of *Lavendula angustifolia*, a shrub in the mint family.

- **Flavour** – strongly aromatic, slightly sweet
- **Notable contents** – acids; aromatics; coumarins; flavonoids; tannins
- **Used for** – beauty aid; ingredient in everyday herb tea blends; medicine

LEMON BALM TEA

Made from the aerial parts of *Melissa officinalis*, a herb in the mint family.

- **Other names** – balm; bee balm; cure-all; honey plant; melissa; sweet balm
- **Flavour** – aromatic and slightly lemony
- **Notable contents** – acids; aromatics; flavonoids; glycosides; resin; selenium; tannins
- **Used for** – common ingredient of everyday herb tea blends; medicine

LINDEN BLOSSOM TEA

Made from the flowers of trees in the Tilia family.

- **Other names** – till tree blossom
- **Flavour** – notes of honey and lime; slightly pungent
- **Notable contents** – acids; aromatics; flavonoids; complex sugars; glycosides; gum; saponins; tannins
- **Used for** – beauty aid; common ingredient in everyday herb tea blends; medicine

NETTLE TEA

Made from the young tops and roots of *Urtica dioica*, a perennial wild plant in the nettle family.

- **Other names** – stinging nettle
- **Flavour** – pleasant, and slightly grassy, salty and bitter
- **Notable contents** – acids (including formic acid, responsible for stinging by fresh leaves, but inactivated in tea); amines (such as acetylcholine; histamine; and serotonin); betaine; complex sugars; coumarins; flavonoids; glycosides; minerals (for instance, calcium and iron); phyto-oestrogens; the pigment chlorophyll; a quinone; sterols; tannins; vitamin D
- **Used for** – beauty aid; medicine

PASSIONFLOWER TEA

Made from the aerial parts of *Passiflora incarnate*, a perennial climbing plant in the passionflower family.

- **Other names** – maypop; granadilla
- **Flavour** – mild and slightly floral
- **Notable contents** – acids; alkaloids; coumarins; flavonoids; glycosides; gums; sterols
- **Used for** – beauty aid; ingredient in everyday herb tea blends; medicine

PEPPERMINT TEA

Made from the aerial parts of *Mentha piperita*, a perennial plant in the mint family. *Mentha spicata* (common mint, garden mint, spearmint) contains less menthol, but is a good substitute.

- **Flavour** – minty, slightly sweet and pungent
- **Notable contents** – acids; aromatics; carotenoids; choline; flavonoids; pigments; resin; salicylates; tannins
- **Used for** – beauty aid; everyday drink; digestive; medicine

RED-CLOVER TEA

Made from the flowers of *Trifolium pretense*, a creeping biennial or perennial wild plant in the pea family.

- **Other names** – clover rose; purple clover; sugar bosses; trefoil.
- **Flavour** – slightly sweet, salty and minty
- **Notable contents** – aromatics; coumarins; flavonoids; glycosides; pectin; phyto-oestrogens; sterols; polyphenols
- **Used for** – beauty aid; medicine

ROOIBOS TEA

Made from the leaves and stems of *Aspalathus linearis*, a shrubby plant in the pea family. Green rooibos tea is made from newly picked, quickly dried leaves. Red rooibos tea is made from newly picked leaves that have been allowed to oxidize.

- **Other names** – Massai tea; redbush tea

- **Flavour** – pleasant, sweet, sour, bitter and tea-like. Red rooibos tea is sweeter than green rooibos tea
- **Notable contents** – acids; an alkaloid; aromatics; flavonoids; magnesium; phyto-oestrogens; tannins. Green rooibos tea has twice the antioxidant activity of red rooibos tea, thanks to its higher levels of the flavonoids aspalathin and nothofagin
- **Used for** – beauty aid; everyday drink; medicine; recipes

ROSEHIP TEA

Made from the fruits ("hips") of *Rosa canina*, a shrub in the rose family.

- **Other names** – dog rose
- **Flavour** – slightly fruity, sour, sweet and bitter
- **Notable contents** – organic acids; aromatics; carotenoids; complex sugars; flavonoids; tannins
- **Used for** – beauty aid; common ingredient in everyday herb tea blends; medicine

ROSEMARY TEA

Made from the aerial parts of *Rosmarinus officinalis*, a shrub in the mint family.

- **Other names** – compass plant; romero
- **Flavour** – aromatic, pleasant and slightly bitter
- **Notable contents** – acids; alkaloids; aromatics; carnosol (a diterpene, see "Terpenes", p.85); flavonoids; a quinone; resin; tannins
- **Used for** – beauty aid; medicine

THYME TEA

Made from the leaves of *Thymus vulgaris*, a small shrub in the mint family.

- **Flavour** – aromatic, pungent and slightly bitter
- **Notable contents** – acids; aromatics; flavonoids; phyto-oestrogens; saponins; tannins
- **Used for** – beauty aid; medicine

VALERIAN TEA

Made from the roots of *Valeriana officinalis*, a perennial plant in the valerian family.

- **Other names** – capon's tail; heal-all; phu; setwall; spikenard; vandal root
- **Flavour** – slightly spicy and unpleasant
- **Notable contents** – alkaloids; aromatics; choline; flavonoids; glycosides; phyto-oestrogens; tannins
- **Used for** – beauty aid; medicine

VERBENA TEA

Made from the aerial parts of *Verbena officinalis*, a perennial plant in the verbena family.

- **Other names** – vervain; holy herb; Juno's tears; pigeon's grass; simpler's joy; traveller's joy; wild hyssop
- **Flavour** – bitter and slightly sweet
- **Notable contents** – acids; aromatics; an alkaloid; complex sugars; glycosides; phyto-oestrogens; sterols; quinones; saponin; tannins
- **Used for** – beauty aid; common ingredient in everyday herb tea blends; medicine

VITEX AGNUS CASTUS TEA

Made from the berries of this shrub or small tree in the mint family.

- **Other names** – Abraham's balm; monk's pepper; chasteberry; wild lavender; tree of chastity
- **Flavour** – slightly aromatic and bitter
- **Notable contents** – alkaloids; aromatics; a "bitter" called castine; flavonoids; glycosides; iridoids; possibly phyto-oestrogens (as *Vitex agnus castus* has some oestrogenic activity); rotundifuran (a diterpene, see "Terpenes", p.85); tannins
- **Used for** – medicine

Notable contents of *Camellia-sinensis* tea and of "herb teas"

Our familiarity with these teas could make us lose sight of their very real biological activities in our bodies. Each type contains a unique blend of thousands of bioactive constituents. And whether we drink a tea to slake our thirst, give us pleasure, aid our hair or skincare or provide a healing draft, these constituents can work their magic on our mind and body. Chapter 2 explains how these bioactives work and their main groups are listed below.

- **Acids** – including amino acids, carboxylic acids and phenolic acids
- **Antioxidants** – including polyphenols
- **Aromatics** – volatile aromatic constituents of the leaves' essential oil. Green tea is richer in essential oils than other teas
- **Bitter principles** – including alkaloids (mainly caffeine), tannins and other polyphenols
- **Catechins** – polyphenols that include flavonoids and tannins. The main catechin flavonoid, epigallocatechin gallate, is a very potent antioxidant and contributes half the weight of the polyphenols in green tea; there are much lower amounts in black tea. Oxidizing tea converts 10–15 per cent of its catechin content into pigments called theaflavins; these in turn can be oxidized to become pigments called thearubigins. (See "Pigments", below)
- **Flavonoids** – polyphenols that include aluminium (see below), certain plant pigments and plant-pigment precursors called proanthocyanidins. Young-leaf and whole-leaf teas have particularly high levels
- **Lignans** – polyphenols with antioxidant and oestrogenic properties
- **Phyto-oestrogens** – certain flavonoids (flavonols and an isoflavone called formononetin: see "Pigments", below) make up 2–3 per cent of dried tea leaves' water-extractable solids
- **Pigments** – including:
    - CAROTENOIDS (orange and yellow)
    - FLAVONOIDS – these polyphenols include theaflavins (orange-red) which contribute to tea's astringency and "briskness" or

"brightness"); gallic acid (yellow-white or pale fawn); kaempferol (yellow); myricetin (yellow-brown to green-brown); and quercetin (yellow). Black tea's thearubigins (red-brown) surprisingly, form 10–20 per cent of its dry weight. Purple tea is rich in anthocyanins and anthocyanidins (blue, red or purple)

  - POLYPHENOLS – mostly astringent, bitter and antioxidant. They include anthocyanins (in purple tea), catechins, flavonoids, lignans, phenolic acids (see "Acids") and tannins. Polyphenols form 30–40 per cent of the weight of dried green tea and 3–10 per cent of that of dried black tea. Black tea also contains oxidized polyphenols. Both polyphenols and oxidized polyphenols promote good health

- **Sugars** – simple sugars such as glucose, fructose, maltose (in Assam teas), raffinose, rhamnose (in Chinese teas) and complex sugars such as pectins and stachyose. Black tea is the richest in complex sugars
- **Tannins** – polyphenols, including catechins, flavonoid-pigment precursors called proanthocyanidins, and flavonoid pigments called theaflavins and thearubigins
- **Others** – include fluoride, manganese (indeed, tea is a major dietary source), and, in unoxidized or partially oxidized tea, vitamin C.

The tea bush or tree is an "aluminium accumulator", meaning it absorbs more aluminium than do other plants. Tea and coffee contribute 5 per cent of our average daily aluminium intake. But because tannins in tea combine with aluminium, we probably absorb relatively little from the tea we drink.

CHAPTER 2
NATURAL

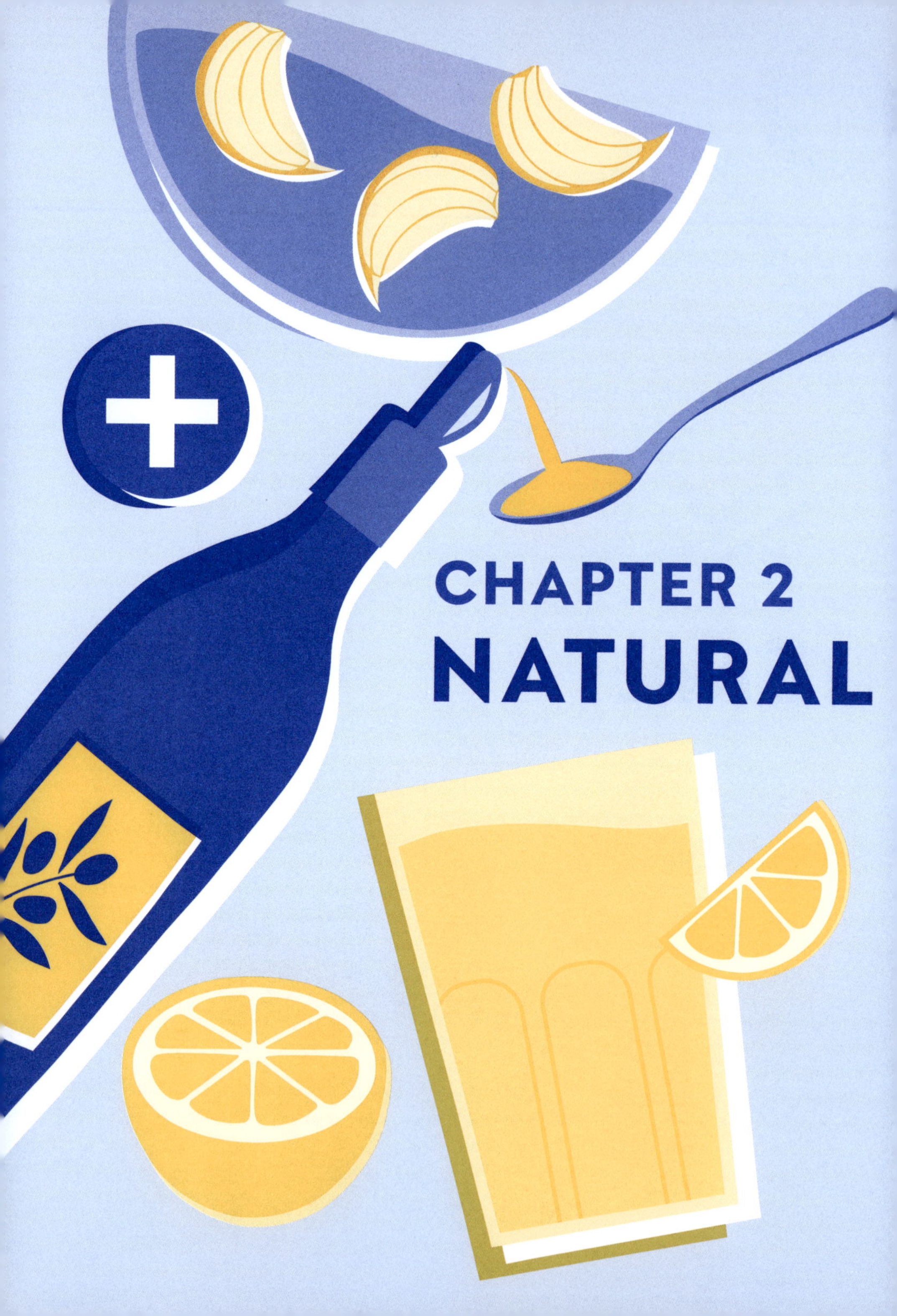

REMEDIES

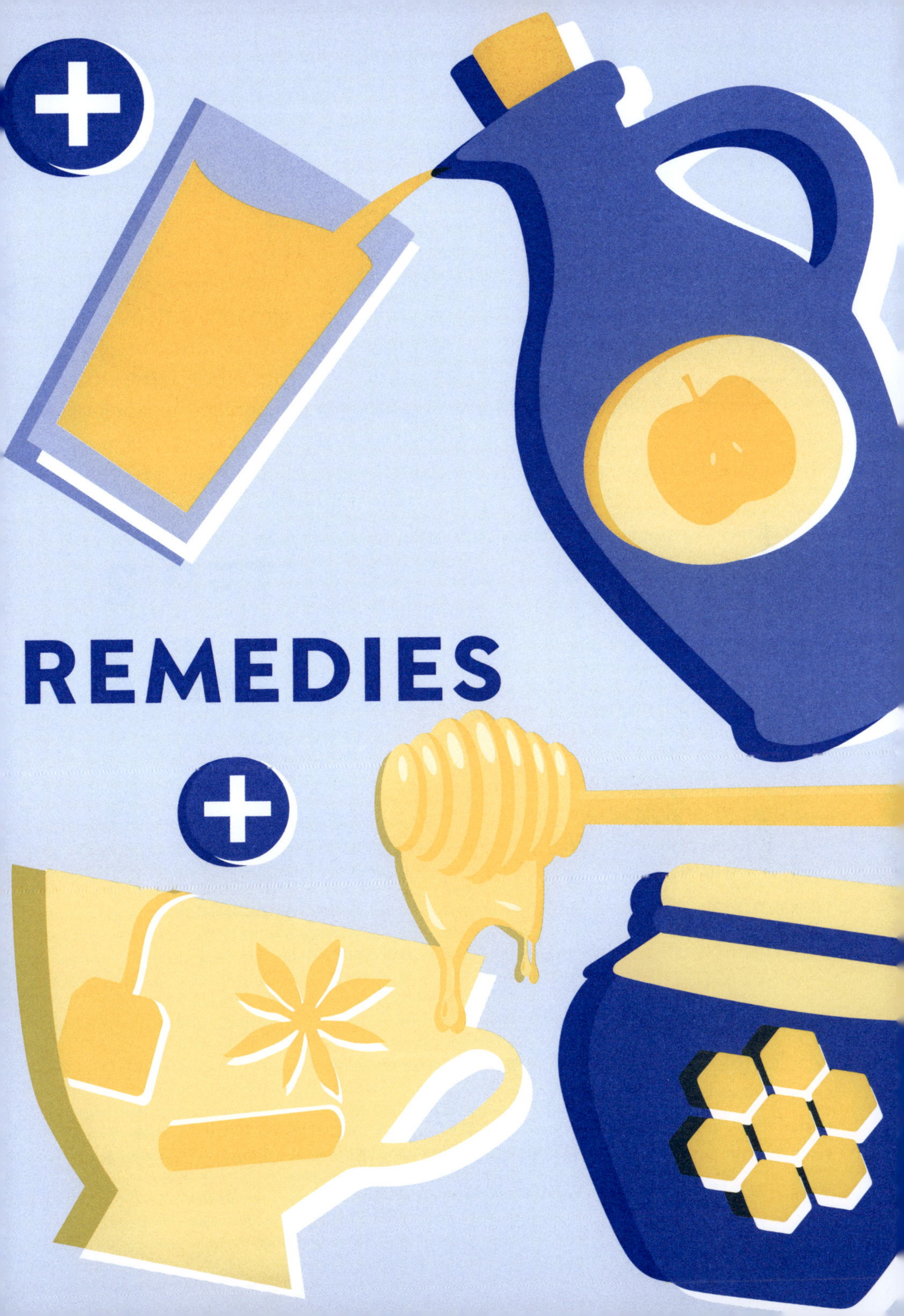

HERO INGREDIENTS FOR HEALTH

As well as their multiple benefits, our eight "cupboard heroes" – apple cider vinegar, lemons, sodium bicarbonate, olive oil, honey, garlic, spices and teas – also help prevent and treat certain common ailments. Remember you can discourage many common ailments with a healthy diet, adequate hydration, regular exercise, daily outdoor light, effective stress management and no smoking. When I mention a study, you can find out more in the reference section at the back of the book, where I will give the name of the journal reporting the study, plus the year of publication. Using these, plus some keywords about the subject of the study, you can find out more on the internet.

CAUTION: Consult a doctor about continuing, worrying, worsening, serious or unexplained symptoms and their possible causes and treatments.

The entries in the A to Z of health conditions in this chapter often mention a healthy diet, bioactives, polyphenols, plant oestrogens and progestins, gut microbiome, mild acidosis and dehydration, so read on for some information on these topics.

A healthy diet

Base your diet on a variety of vegetables (including beans), fruits, grains (preferably wholegrains), herbs, spices and sources of healthy fats – such as nuts, seeds, olive oil and oily fish. You can include dairy foods, eggs, fish and meat in moderation, though only small amounts of red meat: beef, lamb, pork, veal and venison.

- **A healthy diet** helps prevent most of the health problems highlighted in this book.

In contrast, an unhealthy diet lacks enough vegetables, fruits, wholegrains, nuts, seeds, herbs and spices but is high in sugar, ultra-processed foods (including white flour) or alcohol. It also has an unhealthy balance of fats – with too much saturated fat (in fatty meat, full-fat dairy foods, cakes and pastries) and not enough healthy fats (in nuts, seeds, avocados, fatty fish, olive oil and eggs).

- **An unhealthy diet** encourages many of the health problems highlighted in this book.

Polyphenols

These are some of the most talked about bioactive substances in our food. They have anti-cancer, anti-infective and anti-inflammatory properties. They also help keep our blood sugar at normal levels. They do this by:

- Slowing the digestion of carbohydrates and their absorption into blood
- Stimulating the secretion of insulin (a hormone that regulates sugar levels in blood, cells and the fluid around cells)
- Helping to clear sugar from blood into cells

We get polyphenols from vegetables, fruits, herbs, honey, nuts, seeds, spices, wholegrains, coffee, cocoa, certain vegetable oils (for example, olive oil), red wine and vinegars. The polyphenols in our cupboard heroes rejoice in delightful names and include:

- **Flavonoids** – apigenin, catechin, coumestans, daidzein, epicatechin, genistein, kaempferol, luteolin, myricetin, naringenin, quercetin, plant pigments (blue, purple and red anthocyanins; orange and yellow carotenoids), rutin and tannins
- **Lignans** – pinoresinol, resinol, sesamin
- **Phenolic alcohols** – tyrosol and hydroxytyrosol – found exclusively in olive oil
- **Phenolic acids** – caffeic, chlorogenic, gallic, p-coumaric and vanillic acids
- **Plant pigments other than flavonoid ones** – chlorophyll, which is the main green pigment in plants
- **Secoiridoids** – oleacein, oleocanthal, oleuropein and ligstroside
- **Stilbenes** – resveratrol
- **Others** – for example, verbascoside

Plant oestrogens (phyto-oestrogens)

These include certain polyphenols – including certain flavonoids, lignans and stilbenes. Paradoxically, plant oestrogens raise the oestrogenic activity in the body in some situations, but lower it in others. This is because:

- In someone who lacks enough of their own oestrogen to bind to all their cells' oestrogen receptors, plant oestrogens can fill empty ones, so increasing oestrogenic activity in the body. However, this does not fully restore normal oestrogenic activity in the body, as plant oestrogens are weaker than our own oestrogens.
- Plant oestrogens sometimes fill oestrogen receptors in place of a person's own oestrogen. This decreases overall oestrogenic activity in the body, as plant oestrogens are weaker than our own oestrogens.

So plant oestrogens can help problems associated with having either too much or too little oestrogen. This is why they are often described as being "oestrogen-balancing".

Plant oestrogens can also have anti-cancer, anti-inflammatory and antioxidant effects. All of our cupboard heroes, apart from sodium bicarbonate, contain plant oestrogens, for example:

- Apple cider vinegar – catechin, epicatechin
- Lemons – naringenin, rutin, quercetin
- Olive oil – pinoresinol
- Honey – chrysin, genistein, kaempferol, luteolin, naringenin, quercetin
- Garlic – ajoene
- Teas and spices – various compounds in the "oestrogen-balancing" ones (pp.102 and 92)

Plant progestins (phyto-progestins)

By binding to the body's progesterone receptors, these have some progesterone activity, though are less powerful than our own progesterone. Researchers believe their main action is to help counter overly high levels of our progesterone. However, if a person's own progesterone level is low, plant progestins exert some progesterone-like activity. They include certain flavonoids in fruits and vegetables including these cupboard heroes:

- Lemons – apigenin, luteolin, naringenin
- Olive oil – daidzein, genistein, luteolin
- Honey – apigenin, kaempferol, luteolin, naringenin
- Garlic – apigenin, luteolin, naringenin
- Spices – celery seeds have apigenin and luteolin; saffron has kaempferol
- Teas – in chamomile: apigenin; in rosemary: apigenin, kaempferol, luteolin, quercetin; in peppermint: apigenin and luteolin; in oregano: apigenin, luteolin, quercetin

The gut microbiome

Current interest in the gut microbiome echoes the proclamation about 2,500 years ago by the Greek doctor Hippocrates (460–370 BC): "All disease begins in the gut." This microbiome consists of trillions of microbes, mostly bacteria but also fungi, protozoa and viruses. Astonishingly, a healthy gut contains 1.3–1.8kg (3–4lb) of gut microbes! And researchers are fascinated by how deeply involved these are in our gut health and, indeed, our general health.

A healthy microbiome has a good diversity and balance of micro-organisms. Each person's unique balance of gut microbes helps determine their physical and mental health and perhaps even their lifespan. Having a healthy microbiome is key to good health. For example, it discourages inflammation throughout the body; it aids the body's production of neurotransmitters (nerve message carriers such as serotonin and dopamine); and it promotes a healthy body weight. In contrast, an unhealthy gut microbiome has been linked with many problems, including allergy, anxiety, asthma, colon cancer, depression, diabetes, obesity, rheumatoid arthritis and ulcerative colitis.

To encourage a good microbiome, eat a healthy diet (p.58) with at least 30 different plant foods a week, in a range of colours, for plenty of fibre and a variety of polyphenols. Gut microbes ferment fibre from our food, yielding vitally important metabolites (such as short-chain fatty acids) that are absorbed from the gut into our blood. Getting enough exercise also promotes a healthy gut microbiome, as do several of our cupboard heroes – including raw apple cider vinegar, honey, garlic and various spices and teas.

Mild acidosis

The full name of this condition is "chronic low-grade metabolic acidosis" but I will simply call it mild acidosis. It does not include more serious metabolic acidosis (for example, from diabetes, or kidney or liver disease), or any type of respiratory acidosis.

An unhealthy diet (p.58) is the commonest cause. Such a diet is high in meat, eggs, cheese and grains, which produce acids in the body; and low in vegetables, fruit, coffee and teas – which produce alkalis. Pre-diabetes (see *Diabetes*) is another common cause.

Mild acidosis implies the body is working extra hard to maintain a normal acid–alkali balance (see below). It does so by using various "buffering" systems. But the strain involved puts continued stress on the body. Mild acidosis is a cause of chronic metabolic stress (p.152).

Extraordinarily, mild acidosis can cause or contribute to so many health problems that US researchers recently dubbed its effects "a 21st-century health crisis". Yet it is almost always unrecognized![1]

Normally, the body prevents over-acidity in cells, blood and tissue fluid by using its stored bicarbonate to "buffer" (lower) threatened over-acidity. If a high need for buffering threatens to exhaust the bicarbonate stores, the kidneys buffer too, by excreting in urine more ammonia and hydrogen ions (which are acidic) and fewer citrate ions (which are alkaline). If necessary, bones buffer too, by breaking down the bone-strengthening mineral hydroxyapatite to release calcium salts (which are alkaline). And skeletal muscles can buffer in various ways, as can connective tissue (in blood vessels, corneas, joints, ligaments, skin and tendons).

If all this buffering can't maintain a normal acid–alkali balance, the result is mild acidosis. This means that the acid–alkali balance ("pH", standing for "potential of hydrogen") in each part of the body falls toward the more acidic end of its normal range.

Mild acidosis encourages a variety of health problems. For example, it:

- Increases urine volume, encouraging dehydration
- Encourages inflammation
- Encourages oxidation of fats (in turn encouraging artery disease); structural changes in proteins (as in the brain with Alzheimer's disease); and a poor oxygen supply to cells, resulting in their damage.

These damaging effects on cells and metabolism encourage anxiety, constipation, type 2 diabetes, fatty liver, heart attacks, insulin resistance, kidney stones, multiple sclerosis, muscle wasting, pain, poor circulation, poor immunity, premature ageing, pre-menstrual syndrome, strokes and weakened bones.

Eventually and at worst, kidneys function less well; bones become osteoporotic; muscles become increasingly weak; and damage to muscles and connective tissue encourages fibromyalgia. Over-55s are particularly likely to have mild acidosis; a doctor can check for it with blood and urine tests.

Four cupboard heroes can help prevent or treat mild acidosis:

1. **Apple cider vinegar** – because the body metabolizes its acetic acid to bicarbonate, our body's main buffer
2. **Lemons** – because the body metabolizes their citric and malic acids acids to bicarbonate
3. **Sodium bicarbonate itself**
4. **Honey** – because it has anti-obesity, blood fat-, blood pressure- and blood sugar-lowering actions

Dehydration

This is common – indeed, some studies suggest that three in four adults in the US are chronically dehydrated! Older adults are particularly susceptible if they forget to drink enough or find it physically difficult to keep making drinks. Some of us don't feel thirsty when dehydrated: studies show that 37 per cent of people mistake thirst for hunger!

Not drinking enough water obviously promotes dehydration. But so too does mild acidosis, described above.

A woman is generally advised to have 2.7 litres (4.7 pints) of water a day; a man 3.7 litres (6.5 pints) – more if they exercise a lot. This includes water in milk, tea, herb teas and coffee. It's a good idea to find ways of remembering to drink more. For example, keep a litre container of water in the fridge and drink it all over the course of each day.

THE EIGHT "CUPBOARD HEROES"

Now let's get to know the eight cupboard heroes – apple cider vinegar, lemons, sodium bicarbonate, olive oil, honey, garlic, spices and teas – a bit better.

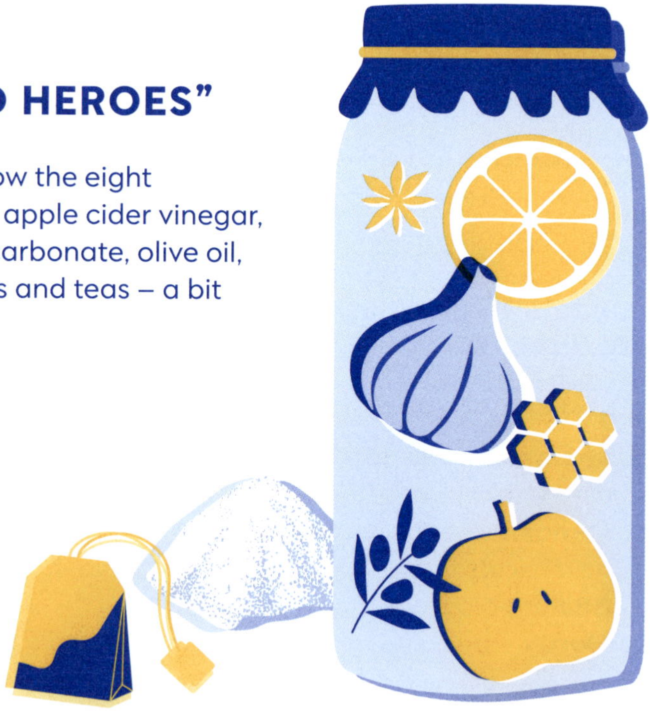

APPLE CIDER VINEGAR

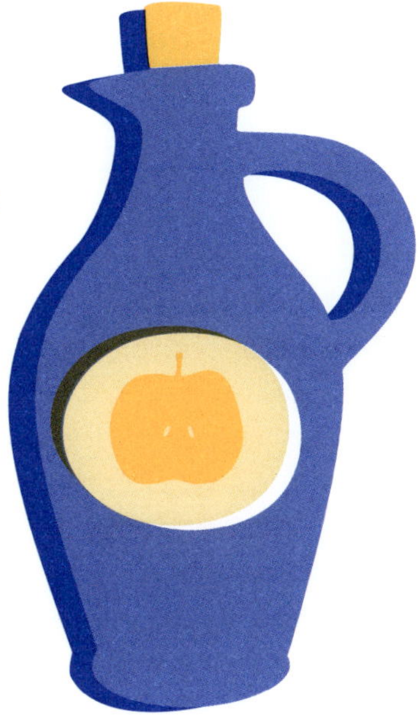

Reports of its healing properties date from thousands of years ago. In 400 BC, the Greek doctor Hippocrates recommended it to treat infections and for general health. Samurai warriors in Japan took a vinegar tonic for strength. And a vinegar solution helped prevent stomach upsets, pneumonia and scurvy in the US Civil War and wound infection in World War I.

Apple cider vinegar contains small amounts of nutrients which as part of a healthy diet (p.58) can pack a big punch healthwise. They include vitamins B and C; polyphenols, including catechin and epicatechin; organic acids (such as acetic, citric and traces of malic); phenolic acids (such as chlorogenic, caffeic, gallic, p-coumaric and acetic) and plant oestrogens. While these acids increase stomach acidity, they don't increase the body's general acidity. Indeed, they may help maintain a normal acid–alkali balance.

NOTE: It's important to be aware of certain contraindications of apple cider vinegar, so bear the following points in mind before using the ingredient as a remedy.

- If allergic to apples or any apple constituent, such as pectin, avoid apple cider vinegar.
- Its acidity may temporarily soften tooth enamel, making teeth vulnerable to damage. So before taking it on its own (as opposed to with food), dilute it, drink it with a straw and rinse your mouth with water after. Don't brush your teeth straightaway as this could cause micro-abrasions of the softened tooth enamel.
- Too much undiluted cider vinegar, or cider vinegar tablets, might damage your gullet.

- Unpasteurized cider vinegar has not been heat-treated, so may contain harmful bacteria such as *Escherichia coli* (*E. coli*). This is a red flag for pregnant women, and others with lowered immunity, who need to avoid unpasteurized products.
- Wash cider vinegar tablets down well to prevent them sticking in your throat or gullet.
- If on medical drugs, check with a doctor before consuming cider vinegar longterm, as it encourages toxicity from certain drugs, including digoxin, certain diuretics, insulin and laxatives. It also lowers blood sugar (by improving insulin sensitivity), so might have an additive effect in those on diabetes medication. It may also lower blood pressure, so might have an additive effect in those on blood pressure medication.

LEMONS

These have long been prized as a health aid. Their health-giving components include anti-cancer agents, antifungals, antihistamines, anti-inflammatories, antioxidants, antiseptics, antivirals, astringents, detoxifiers, diuretics and plant oestrogens. Lemons also contain citric acid, which can aid digestion, and hesperidin, a flavonoid that can improve blood sugar levels.

Lemons' antioxidant flavonoids, tannins and vitamin C help protect against infections and the many health problems associated with inflammation. Lemons can help prevent iron-deficiency anemia by improving iron absorption from food. Lemons' citric and malic acids help maintain a normal acid–alkali balance in the body; they also help prevent kidney stones.

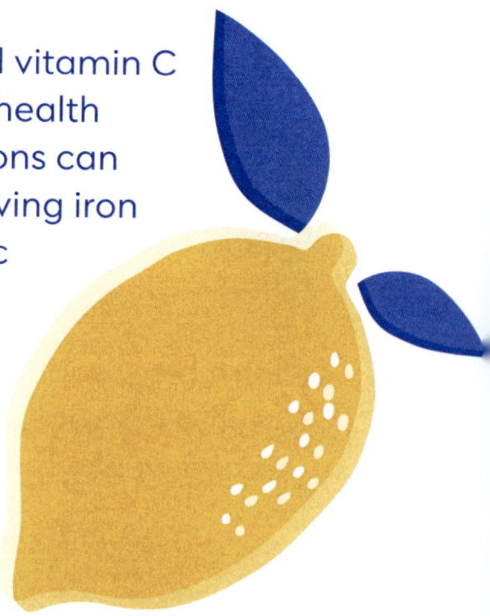

SODIUM BICARBONATE

Note that this has several other names (p.16). Taking it can help treat indigestion and aid the body's normal acid–alkali balance. Applying it can help treat certain inflammatory skin conditions.

One level teaspoon contains about about 4.6g of sodium bicarbonate. The most common reason for taking it is for indigestion, when the usual dose is ½–1 teaspoon for under-60s; ¼–½ teaspoon for over-60s. If used to make urine less acidic, it can be taken 1–4 times a day.

Sodium bicarbonate can cause belching, because it releases carbon dioxide while neutralizing stomach acid.

Tips and warnings

- Under 12s should not take it.
- One in three healthy people and 60 per cent of those with high blood pressure are "sodium-sensitive" – meaning they have a strong response to dietary sodium. This is detected by their blood pressure rising when they change from a low-salt to a high-salt diet. It is more likely in women, elderly people, those of African or East Asian descent, and those with insulin resistance or chronic kidney disease. But taking sodium bicarbonate short-term – for example, for 2 weeks – should be no problem.
- Note that its sodium contributes to your sodium intake from food. 1 tsp (4.6g) of sodium bicarbonate contains 1,260mg of sodium. The American Heart Association says an adult's daily intake should not exceed 2,300mg. The UK Department of Health recommends an upper daily limit of 2,500mg (about the same as in 1 teaspoon of table salt). So it's wise to eat a low-sodium diet if you also take sodium bicarbonate.
- Consult a doctor if you have taken sodium bicarbonate for more than two weeks and wish to continue.
- Consult a doctor before taking it if pregnant or breastfeeding, or if you have high blood pressure; heart, kidney or liver disease; or recent bleeding from your stomach or gut; or are on a sodium-

restricted diet; or are on prescription drugs, as some interact with sodium bicarbonate – for example, aspirin, benzodiazepines, calcium- or citrate-containing preparations, corticosteroids, ephedrine, fluoroquinolones, iron, ketoconazole, lithium, memantine, methenamine, certain anti-diabetes drugs, quinidine, steroids, tetracycline, urine-acidifiers, or medications with a coating to protect the stomach (enteric coating).

- Check with a doctor or sports coach before taking it to enhance exercise performance.
- Note that, in some people, toothpaste containing sodium bicarbonate irritates their gums.

Side effects

Avoid high doses as these could cause too much alkali and not enough acid ("metabolic alkalosis") in your body, and high sodium and low potassium in your blood. It makes sense to be aware of the possible side effects of excessive intake, listed below.

Possible symptoms include wind, an unpleasant taste in your mouth, fatigue, poor appetite, indigestion, nausea, vomiting, constipation, excessive urination, thirst, fluid retention, bloating, ankle swelling, high blood pressure, cramp, twitching, numbness, tingling, headache, difficulty breathing, drowsiness, weakness, dizziness, fainting, confusion, hallucinations, clumsiness, tremors, fits (seizures), irregular heartbeat, allergic swelling of the face, lips, tongue and throat, and difficulty in breathing.

Combining large amounts of sodium bicarbonate with dairy products, calcium supplements or calcium-containing antacids can cause "milk-alkali syndrome" which, if continued, can cause calcium deposits in the kidneys and other tissues, kidney stones and kidney failure.

If you have taken a large dose, or doses, and suspect a serious reaction, seek urgent medical help. If you go to a doctor or a hospital, take the container of sodium bicarbonate with you for identification purposes.

Soda water

Drinking this is a pleasant way of taking sodium bicarbonate.

Make it using a 35fl oz (1-litre/4-cup) rechargeable soda siphon and a disposable one-shot screw-in cartridge of pressurized carbon dioxide. Put 1 litre (35fl oz/4 cups) of water into the siphon and add ¼–½ teaspoon of sodium bicarbonate. Flavour soda water with plain or fruit syrup if desired.

Skin paste

Mix a tablespoon of sodium bicarbonate with a teaspoon of water to form a paste. This can help relieve itching or redness.

In the bath

Add 100–200g (3½–7oz/½–1 cup) of sodium bicarbonate to your bathwater. Add a few drops of lavender or other essential oil for fragrance. If bathing your baby, add 1–2 tablespoons of sodium bicarbonate to a baby-sized bath of water. Used in this way, it can help alleviate skin irritations.

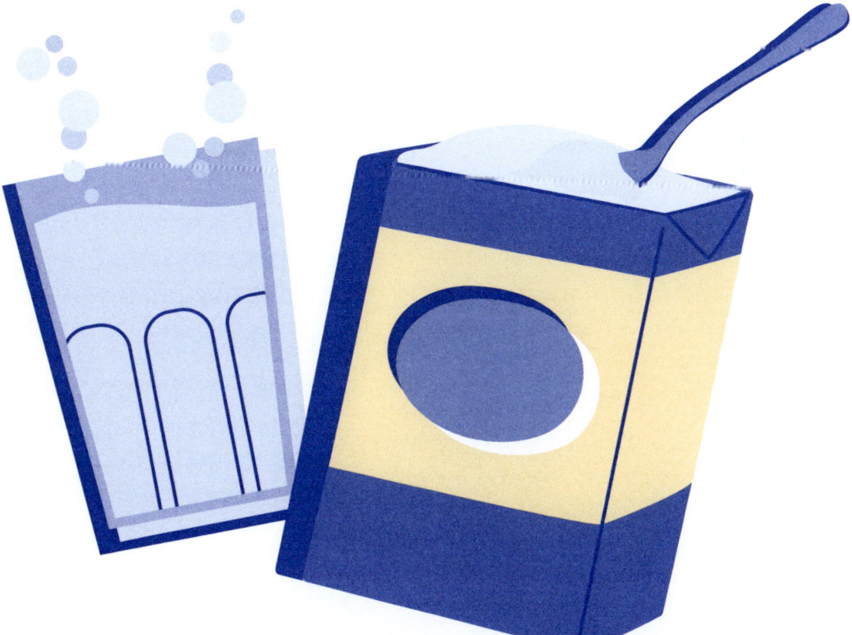

OLIVE OIL

Choose extra-virgin olive oil (EVOO) as this has been pressed from olives mechanically, not by using heat or chemical solvents. This maintains its polyphenols.

Polyphenols are responsible for olive oil's scent, flavour and green colour. They include hydroxytyrosol, oleocanthal, oleuropein phenolic alcohols, secoiridoids and tyrosol. They also contribute to its health benefits. Oleocanthal, for example, inhibits two of our enzymes (COX-1 and COX-2) that help make prostaglandin that enables inflammation. This means it acts as an anti-inflammatory agent and a painkiller.

Olive oil is rich in monounsaturated fats and low in saturated fat.

Health benefits

Traditional use, common sense and anecdotal evidence suggest that olive oil as part of a healthy diet (p.58) can help to prevent or treat many ailments. Scientific research Increasingly backs this claim.

Each year, the US News & World Report publishes its "Best Diet Rankings", created by experts assessing 30 diets that aid health. In 2025, they again chose the Mediterranean diet as the "Best Diet Overall". Olive oil is a star of this diet, partly because its balance of fats and its high content of antioxidant and therefore anti-inflammatory polyphenols promote good health.

You can incorporate olive oil into salad dressings, add it to cooked foods (such as soups) and use it instead of butter or other fat or oil in almost any recipe. Avoid heating it to high temperatures, as heat degrades its polyphenols.

One study found that frying with extra-virgin olive oil decreased its polyphenol content by 40 per cent at 120°C (248°F) and by 75 per cent at 170°C (338°F).[2]

CAUTION: Use olive oil within a year of buying it as its polyphenols will fall over time.

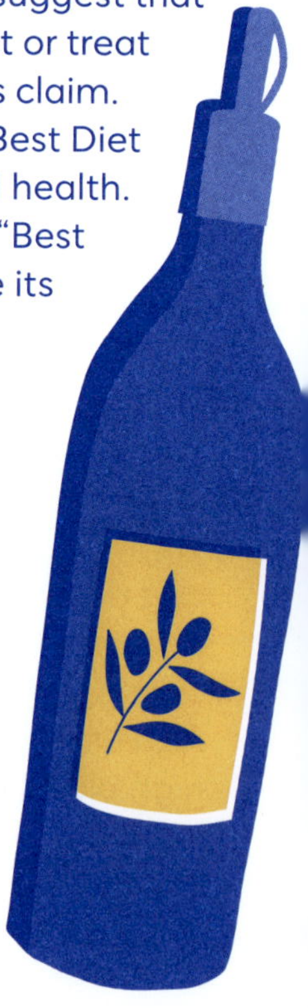

HONEY

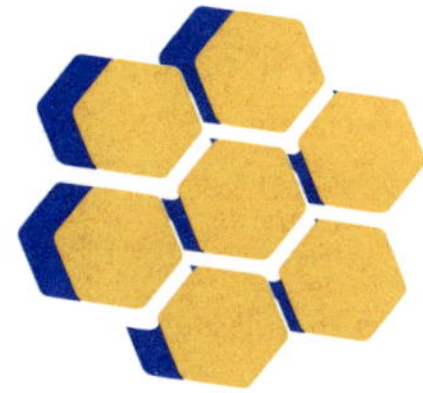

Recent studies show that the properties of this amber elixir can be: alkalinizing, anti-cancer, anti-inflammatory, antimicrobial, anti-obesity, antioxidant, capillary-strengthening, cholesterol-lowering, detoxifying, digestion-enhancing, immunity-boosting, nerve message-carrying and smooth muscle-relaxing.

Honeys originating from medicinal plants may contain healing compounds from the plants' roots, stems, leaves, flowers, seeds or fruits. So, in a way, honeys are herbal remedies.

Honey's main bioactives are polyphenol antioxidants called flavonoids.[3]

Choice of sweetener

Refined white sugar is the commonest sweetener in the average Western diet. High-fructose corn syrup is widely used in the US and Japan. Both these sweeteners provide "empty calories", having no nutritional benefit other than providing energy.

HONEY – AN EXCELLENT CHOICE

In contrast, honey provides not only sweetness and energy but also many health-enhancing compounds. We tend to consume less of it than we would of sugar, as it is sweeter and tastes more characterful. It also behaves differently from sugar in the body because of its acidity, polyphenols, vitamins, copper and zinc.

Compared with sugar, the average honey makes blood sugar and insulin (a hormone that helps control blood sugar) rise more slowly and climb less high. Certain honeys, including acacia and yellow-box, and raw honey in general, make blood sugar rise even less.

This is good, because many health problems (including Alzheimer's disease, anxiety, artery disease, diabetes, eye disease, high blood pressure and inflammation) are encouraged by an unhealthy diet causing repeated episodes of high blood sugar ("blood sugar spikes").

Abnormally high blood sugar encourages:

- Damage to artery linings by oxidation
- Damage to body proteins (such as collagen and certain brain proteins) by sugar binding to them: this is called "glycation"
- Resistance of body cells to insulin. This hormone is the "key" that lets cells take sugar from the blood. Without enough insulin, cells don't get enough sugar to burn for energy, yet at the same time the blood sugar level rises

The **glycaemic index** (GI) is a ranking of foods from 1–100, or more, according to their ability to raise blood sugar. It compares a food's ability to raise blood sugar with that of a reference food – usually glucose, whose GI is 100. High-GI foods are mostly high-carbohydrate and low-fibre. Fats don't raise blood sugar; proteins do if you eat a lot of them or have low insulin.

A honey's GI depends on its proportions and amounts of sugars, and on its acids, polyphenols and other contents that influence blood sugar.

Glycaemic index of honeys, sugars and corn syrups

	GLYCAEMIC INDEX	FOOD
Low	55 or less	Fructose ("fruit sugar") 19 Black locust honey 32 Yellow box honey 35 Raw honey 30–40 Acacia, chestnut, heather and linden honeys 49–55
Medium	56–69	"Average" honey 58 Oilseed rape honey 64 Raw sugar 65 Sucrose 68 High-fructose corn syrup (42g fructose/100g) 68 Clover honey 69
High	70 or more	Corn syrup 75 High-fructose corn syrup (55g fructose/100g) 87 Honeydew honey 89 Glucose 100 Maltose 105

Which honey to use medicinally?

The options include any honey, raw honey and a monofloral honey (p.26) with particular healing potential. Note that certain honeys are rated for their antibacterial, antioxidant or oligosaccharide activity.

- **To improve gut health** – and therefore general health – choose a honey rich in oligosaccharides. These sugars are prebiotic, promoting the growth of beneficial gut bacteria. Some honeys, including manuka (made from nectar from the manuka bush or tree) are particularly rich in oligosaccharides.
- **To combat infection** – note that manuka honey is powerfully antibacterial as it is rich in a compound called methylgloxal. If

choosing a manuka honey, be guided by its UMF (Unique Manuka Factor) number. This is assigned by The UMF Honey Association after testing a honey. The higher a honey's UMF number, the greater its antibacterial power. Honey with a UMF of 15+ or 20+ is better at killing bacteria than honey with a lower UMF. Several other honeys are also powerfully antibacterial – see the chart below.

- **For wound care** – ideally choose "medical-grade" honey, meaning honey that has been sterilized by gamma irradiation.

Honey-containing lozenges, eyedrops, dressings, creams, ointments, gels and patches are available from certain pharmacies, or on the internet, as are supplements containing concentrated honey extract. Honey is generally very safe and often cheaper than other treatments.

Health benefits of monofloral honeys

Honeys vary in their healing potential. This table explains known health benefits, as well as historic uses in folk medicine (remedies based on traditional beliefs) for particular ailments.

	PARTICULAR HEALTH BENEFITS	USES IN FOLK MEDICINE
Acacia	Antioxidant-rich, fructose-rich	Headache, heart, kidney and respiratory diseases, insomnia
Arbutus	None in particular	Asthma
Avocado	Rich in vitamins and minerals	None in particular
Blueberry	Powerfully antimicrobial	None in particular
Buckwheat	Powerfully antimicrobial; rich in antioxidants (more than eight times the anti-oxidant power of clover honey, for example), iron and other minerals, and amylase	High blood pressure, rheumatism, streptococcal throat infections

Darker honeys	The richest in antioxidants of all honeys; also rich in minerals	Infections
Echium	None in particular	Brain and nerve disorders, including epilepsy and phlegm
Eucalyptus	Rich in pinocembrin	Colds, coughs, headaches, other pain
Hawthorn	None in particular	Abnormal heartbeat, artery disease, high blood pressure, insomnia, overactive thyroid
Heather (bell)	Powerfully antimicrobial; antioxidant-rich; fructose-rich	Cancer, digestive problems
Honeydew	Powerfully antimicrobial; antioxidant-rich – more than twice the antioxidant capacity of honey made only from nectar; rich in oligosaccharides	Sore throat, weakness
Jellybush	Powerfully antimicrobial	Infection, inflammation, wound healing
Linden	Fructose-rich	Anxiety, bronchitis, colds, coughs, insomnia
Manuka	Anti-inflammatory and powerfully antimicrobial	Infection and wound healing
Motherwort	None in particular	Heart disease, insomnia, wound healing
Neem	Allergies, diabetes, gum infection, high blood pressure, skin problems, sore throat	Allergy, gingivitis, high blood pressure, skin conditions, sore throat
Pine	Powerfully antimicrobial	Infections
Raspberry	None in particular	Gastroenteritis, inflamed mouth, upper respiratory disease

Red box gum	Antioxidant-rich	Colds, coughs, headaches, pain
Rewarewa	Powerfully antimicrobial	Infections
Rosebay willowherb (fireweed)	Antioxidant-rich	Constipation, gastritis, headache, insomnia, peptic ulcer, skin disease, throat infection
Rosemary	Powerfully antimicrobial	Bacterial infections
Sage	Powerfully antimicrobial; antioxidant-rich	Coughs, kidney and heart disease, weakness
Sainfoin	Rich in vitamins (especially vitamin C and beta-carotene)	Headache, heavy periods, impotence, upper respiratory infections
Sidr	Powerfully antimicrobial	Constipation, eye disease, liver disorders, peptic ulcer
Sunflower	Antioxidant-rich	Asthma, catarrh, colic, flu, malaria, heart disease
Sweet chestnut	Powerfully antimicrobial; fructose-rich	Fluid retention, malaria, respiratory, gut and kidney disorders, rheumatism
Thyme	Powerfully antimicrobial; very antioxidant-rich: the most antioxidant thyme honey has antioxidant power 10 times as high as clover honey and, weight for weight, fructose-rich	Digestive problems, wound infection
Tupelo	Antioxidant-rich; fructose-rich	Health problems related to inflammation
Ulmo	Powerfully antimicrobial; antioxidant-rich	Bacterial infections, health problems related to inflammation

Adverse effects of honey

- Experts advise against honey for babies under one year old, to protect against the risk of botulism – an illness caused by a toxin made by the *Clostridium botulinum* bacteria in a very small proportion of honeys.
- Mouth bacteria use honey's sugars to make acid which temporarily softens enamel, making it vulnerable to damage. Brushing teeth after having honey could cause micro-abrasions of the softened enamel. So rinse your mouth with water instead.
- Honey can raise blood sugar, so consume it only in moderation, especially if you have pre-diabetes or diabetes. Note, though, that honey has a lower glycaemic (blood sugar-raising) effect than table sugar.
- Honey slightly stings broken skin in 1 in 20 people.
- One very rare possibility is an allergic reaction to pollen or bee proteins in honey. Get urgent medical help if you experience itching or swelling of the lips, swelling in the mouth or throat, breathing difficulty or faintness after consuming honey.

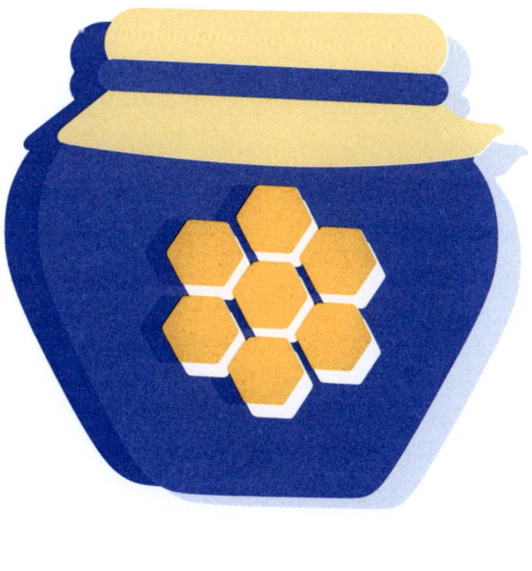

GARLIC

This popular cooking ingredient has long been prized as an aid to health. Both raw and cooked garlic can be useful. Its positive effects include:

- Boosting the body's level of the neurotransmitter (nerve message carrier) acetylcholine, needed for brain function and for the body's metabolism in general
- Countering infection
- Countering inflammation and the many health problems that a general tendency toward inflammation in the body may cause
- Helping balance high or low oestrogen
- Improving blood sugar and insulin levels
- Improving liver function
- Lowering high blood fats, including cholesterol
- Promoting a healthy gut microbiome (the populations of bacteria, viruses and fungi in the gut, p.61)
- Reducing high blood pressure
- Thinning overly thick blood

To include garlic in a healthy diet, some people chew a fresh raw clove of garlic each day, though the release of sulphenic acid and allicin when chewing may not be to your taste! Others add raw garlic to foods such as salad dressings. You could drink hot water to which you have added a crushed clove, 1–2 teaspoons of honey and a squeeze of lemon juice. Or you can add garlic to salad dressings, spread it on bread or incorporate it into soups, stews and stir-fries.

How to prepare garlic for remedies

The nature and extent of garlic's bioactivity – action in the body that may promote good health – depend on its preparation:

Garlic's **water-soluble bioactive** compounds, for example, S-allylmercaptocysteine, are its main bioactives; they have less odour than its oil-soluble compounds. They have antioxidant and bioactive effects, and may help prevent cancer and treat Alzheimer's

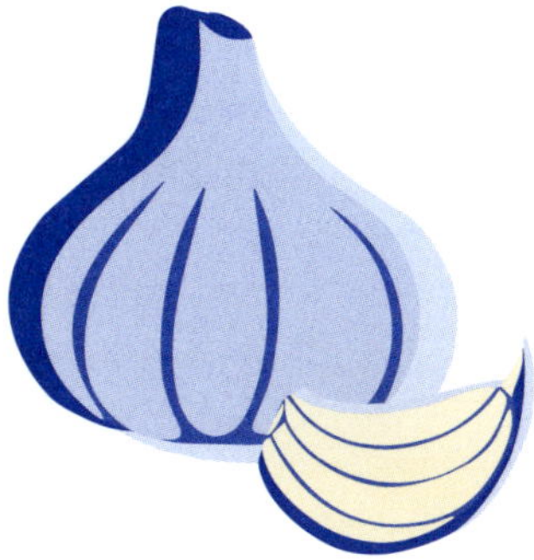

disease. S-allyl cysteine may also reduce the bioactivity of certain carcinogens (substances that can cause cancer).

Garlic's **oil-soluble bioactive compounds** include allicin, diallyl disulphide, diallyl sulphide, diallyl trisulphide, vinyl dithiin and ajoene. Allicin is responsible for garlic's pungent flavour, has antibacterial properties and may suppress cancer-cell multiplication.

How you prepare garlic influences the amounts and proportions of these bioactives. Allicin release occurs when crushing or chopping garlic and peaks after 90 minutes. You get a good balance of garlic's water- and oil-soluble sulphur compounds if you leave chopped or crushed garlic to stand for 30–60 minutes before use. See the chart below for efficacy of water-soluble vs oil-soluble garlic compounds in bioactive reactions.

The bioactivity of garlic's sulphur compounds

BIOACTIVITY	WATER-SOLUBLE COMPOUNDS	OIL-SOLUBLE COMPOUNDS
Anti-clotting	No	Yes
Anti-diabetic	No	Yes
Anti-obesity	Yes	Yes
Antimicrobial	No	Yes
Antioxidant and therefore anti-inflammatory	Yes	Yes
Detoxifying	No	Yes
Immunity-enhancing	No	Yes

To maximize garlic's water-soluble and oil-soluble compounds, consume:

- Crushed or chopped garlic that has been left to stand for 30–60 minutes
- A garlic powder supplement with a high yield of allicin: this is one of garlic's main "active" compounds and has antioxidant and anti-inflammatory properties

To maximize mainly its oil-soluble compounds, consume:

- Crushed or chopped garlic that has been left to stand for 90 minutes

There are several ways of consuming garlic as a remedy other than in food.

GARLIC JUICE

Crush or blend peeled garlic cloves into a paste, then sieve this to separate the juice and pulp.

GARLIC OIL

This is available in capsules from health-food stores and pharmacies. Garlic oil capsules are also called "garlic perles". While garlic oil lacks garlic's irritating agents (sulphenic acids and allicin), it also lacks the bioactivity of allicin and its derivatives. Garlic supplements vary in the amounts and proportions of their bioactives (p.59).

When garlic, garlic oil, garlic oil macerate or garlic water are applied to skin, their sulphur compounds act on local skin cells and are also absorbed into the tissue fluid and hence into the capillaries (tiny blood vessels) and tiny lymph vessels around the body.

GARLIC OIL MACERATE

Crush some garlic cloves, let them stand for 90 minutes to maximize their allicin, then mix with olive oil.

GARLIC POWDER CAPSULES

Buy empty animal- or vegetable-gelatine capsules from a health-food store or on the internet. Dry out the cloves of several garlic bulbs then crush with a pestle and mortar or in a spice mill. Fill the capsules with the resulting powder. Keep in an airtight container.

GARLIC TEA

For alliin-rich tea, add a peeled garlic clove to a cup of just-boiled water and steep for 5 minutes. Sweeten with honey if desired.

For tea rich in allicin and its derivatives, leave a crushed garlic clove for 60–90 minutes. Add it to a cup of just-boiled water and steep for 5 minutes. Sweeten with honey or sugar if desired.

GARLIC SYRUP

- 100ml (3½fl oz/scant ½ cup) water
- 100g (3½oz/½ cup) caster sugar
- 100g (3½oz) garlic cloves, peeled
- OPTIONAL: a few drops of orange, lemon or cinnamon oil

Put the water, sugar and garlic in a pan. Heat gently to dissolve the sugar. Bring the syrup to the boil, then remove from the heat. Cool, then strain. Flavour with orange or lemon juice, or cinnamon oil.

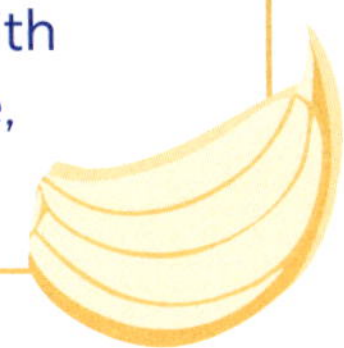

GARLIC WATER

This is less likely to irritate skin than is crushed garlic. To make it, mix 1 part of garlic juice with 3–4 parts of water. Or stir a peeled, crushed clove into half a glass of water and wait 30–60 minutes (for allicin to develop).

To treat a large area of skin (for example, for widespread psoriasis), let six crushed cloves stand for 30–60 minutes then add them to your bath water – perhaps with some mint leaves to freshen the smell.

How much garlic should I take?

The World Health Organization says adults can promote health by taking one of these daily:

- ½–1 medium clove of garlic, eaten with food – for example, crushed in a salad dressing; in warm water with honey; or added to other food towards the end of the cooking time

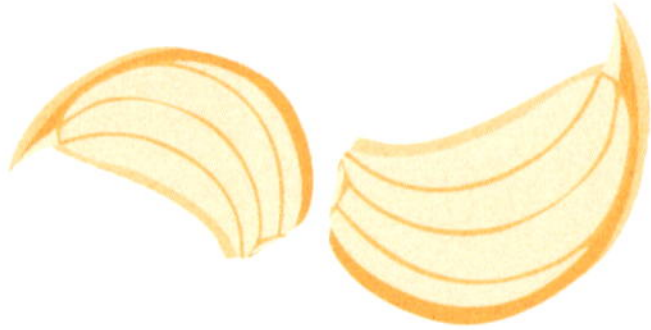

- 0.4–1.2g garlic-powder product
- 300–1,000mg garlic extract
- 2–5mg garlic oil
- Any garlic product supplying 2–5mg allicin

Studies have found no adverse effects from eating 3–5 medium cloves a day. One study found no serious adverse effects from up to 15 cloves a day for 3 months.

CAUTION: Garlic has powerful biological effects, so read the following warnings carefully before embarking on garlic consumption.

Contraindications of garlic

Avoid garlic or talk to a healthcare professional if you:

- **Are awaiting surgery** – it can prolong bleeding, so avoid garlic for 2 weeks before
- **Have a bleeding disorder** (such as bleeding gums, easy bruising, heavy menstrual periods or unexplained nosebleeds), as garlic can encourage bleeding
- **Are pregnant** – while normal amounts of garlic are likely to be safe for an unborn baby, avoid consuming large amounts and don't apply garlic to your skin. If due to give birth within 2 weeks, large intakes might encourage bleeding during childbirth or associated surgical procedures
- **Are breastfeeding** – avoid consuming, or applying to your skin, large amounts of garlic, as there is insufficient data to confirm its safety for your baby
- **Are a heavy drinker** – avoid consuming large amounts of garlic, as this could slow the breakdown of the liver's P450 2E1 enzyme, which helps to break down alcohol
- **Have a skin problem** – if you try garlic, check it is safe for your skin: apply garlic to a small, inconspicuous area of the affected skin and after several hours check it has not caused irritation. If it has, don't apply it again. Consider applying garlic oil instead of garlic itself, as the oil lacks garlic's irritating agents (sulphenic acids and allicin). Be very wary of applying garlic to a child's skin

- **Have a stomach or digestive problem** – note that large amounts of garlic can irritate the stomach and gut
- **Are on anticoagulant (anti-clotting or "blood-thinning' medication, including aspirin and warfarin)** – this is because garlic could further reduce clotting, thus encouraging bruising and bleeding; though small amounts of garlic are unlikely to be a problem. If on warfarin, be sure to have regular blood tests
- **Are on blood sugar-lowering medication** – as garlic may further lower blood sugar, though normal amounts are unlikely to be a problem
- **Are on cyclosporine (an immunity-suppressor)** – as allicin-containing garlic products can decrease its efficacy
- **Are on high blood pressure medication** with a calcium channel blocker (such as amlodipine) – as garlic's mild blood pressure-lowering effects might increase its action. Be sure to have regular blood pressure checks
- **Are on HIV/AIDS medications** – discuss with your doctor whether you should avoid garlic
- **Are on medications affected by cytochrome P450 enzymes**, such as paracetamol (acetaminophen); calcium channel blockers for high blood pressure (such as nicardipine), losartan (for high blood pressure), certain anti-cancer drugs (such as paclitaxel), certain antifungals (such as ketoconazole), cortisol and other glucocorticoids (for allergy and autoimmune disease), chlorzoxazone (a muscle-relaxant), theophylline (for certain respiratory disorders), fentanyl (a pain-reliever), midazolam (for epilepsy), lidocaine (a local anaesthetic and a heart medication) and certain anaesthetics (such as halothane) – note that garlic can slow their breakdown, thus increasing their effects. Discuss with your doctor whether to avoid or cut back on garlic
- **Are taking oral contraception** containing oestrogen – note that garlic could speed its breakdown and endanger birth control. If you consume a lot of garlic, consider using additional

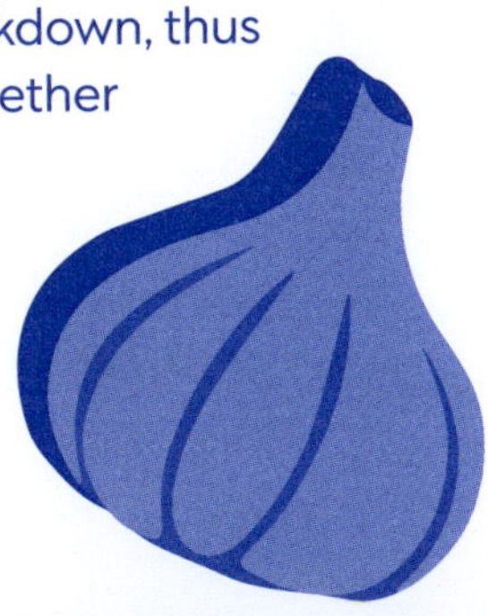

birth control (such as a condom)

- **Are on the TB drug isoniazid** – avoid garlic as it could reduce the drug's absorption
- **Have a vaginal, anal or rectal problem** – don't use garlic locally, as it could irritate or burn

Adverse reactions

Note that garlic's oil-soluble sulphur compounds can cause problems, for example:

- Burning mouth, heartburn, nausea, vomiting, wind, diarrhoea and appetite loss if you consume raw garlic or garlic oil on an empty stomach
- Faintness, flushing, headache, dizziness, sweating, rapid pulse, insomnia
- Haemolytic anaemia if you eat a large amount of raw garlic
- Redness, burning and blisters if you leave garlic or a garlic remedy rich in oil-soluble compounds on the skin for a long time

Garlic can also cause allergic reactions in certain people. These are most likely in those who work with garlic without wearing protective gloves. Garlic's oil-soluble compound iallyl disulphide is often to blame. The garlic enzyme alliinase is another possible culprit. Someone sensitive to garlic may have a cross-sensitivity – meaning they are also sensitive – to other alliums, or to *Liliaceae* plants (such as lilies, ginger, bananas). Possible allergic reactions include allergic contact dermatitis, allergic rhinitis ("hay fever"), asthma and anaphylaxis (a rare and potentially fatal condition, possibly including mouth and throat swelling, breathing difficulty and shock, which require urgent treatment with medically prescribed adrenaline).

Is garlic an effective remedy?

Scientists have investigated garlic more than almost any other medicinal plant. The number of volunteers in a study is often small and the duration of many studies short. But there are tantalizing clues that garlic is very useful.

SPICES

These are popular folk remedies and are recommended in various healing systems. Researchers agree they encourage good health and studies associate a high intake with a reduced risk of chronic illness in general.

Each spice has a particular profile of bioactives. These include:

- Polyphenols (such as flavonoids, catechins, epicatechin, eugenol, gingerol, rutin, plant oestrogens, phenolic compounds, coumestans, curcumin, lignans, stilbenes, tannins) – in many spices
- Glycosides – for example, in aniseed, coriander and cumin
- Phyto-progestins – for example, in saffron and turmeric
- Terpenes – for example, in caraway, cinnamon, cloves, coriander, cumin, pepper and saffron

How to prepare spices for remedies

There are several ways of using spices:

Add spices to food; chew them (for example, ajowan, aniseed, caraway, cardamom, cinnamon pieces, dill seeds, fennel seeds, juniper, liquorice, mahlab, mastic drops, star anise); put them into coffee or cocoa (allspice, cardamom, cinnamon or cloves with coffee, cinnamon, ginger or vanilla with cocoa); or drink a spice tea.

- **To make spice tea** – pour just-boiled water into a cup or mug containing a teaspoon of crushed, dried spice; steep for two minutes, then flavour with heated (but not boiled) orange or lemon juice, and honey.

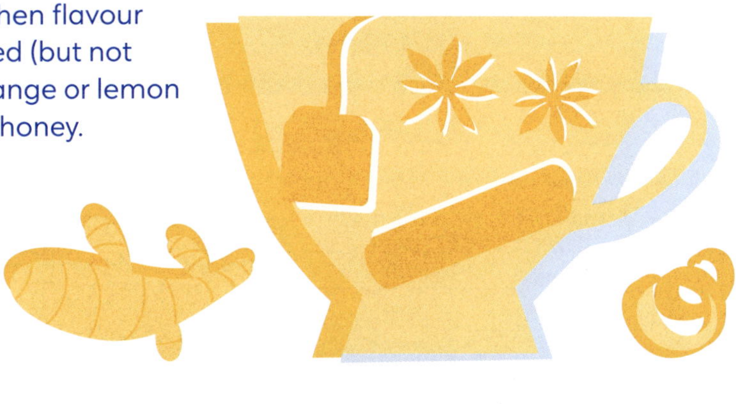

For upper respiratory infections, gargle with spice tea, or use a spice essential oil in a steam inhalation.

- **To prepare a spiced steam inhalation** – add a teaspoon of your chosen crushed spices, or a few drops of spice oil, to a bowl of just-boiled water. Sit and inhale the steam while leaning over the bowl with a towel draped over your head and the bowl.

For skin conditions, add 1–2 cupfuls of spice tea, or a few drops of spice essential oil, to your bathtub, use spice essential oil in a massage oil or apply a spice compress or poultice.

- **To make spice-infused oil** – crush your chosen spices; put them in a clean, dry, glass jar; then half-fill the jar with warmed carrier oil (sweet almond, jojoba or safflower) and add a lid. Keep the labelled jar in a cool, dark place for two weeks, shaking it every day or two. Finally, strain the oil through a fine sieve into a clean jar or bottle and store in a cool, dark place.
- **To make a spice compress** – shake 1–2 drops of your chosen spice oil into a shallow pan of water and stir gently. Lay a piece of muslin or other cotton cloth on the water so it absorbs a film of oil. Lift it off, letting excess water drip away. Lay it, oily-side down, on the area being treated.
- **To make a spice poultice** – make a paste by stirring ground ajowan, cloves or mustard, or grated horseradish, into water. Apply this to the aching or sprained or otherwise inflamed area; cover with a piece of gauze or other cotton fabric, and secure with a crêpe bandage. A poultice dilates the skin's blood vessels, increasing the blood supply to underlying tissues; it also reduces inflammation and aids recovery.

Alternatively, take a medication containing the whole of a spice, or one or more of its important constituents. Examples include tablets of powdered spice, capsules of a spice constituent, an extract of a spice (such as a tincture), and cream or patches containing a spice. Use as recommended on the pack or by a doctor or herbal-medicine practitioner.

CAUTION: If considering using a spice oil on your skin:
• Apply it to a small area to see if it causes irritation in the next 24 hours; if not, you can use it more extensively.
• Cassia, celery seed, cumin and ginger oils can cause a photosensitive rash in skin exposed to sunlight. So after use and before going out in sunlight, wash off the oil with soap and water, or cover your treated skin.
• Certain oils can irritate the skin. Avoid frequent use of aniseed, cassia, cinnamon, coriander, juniper, nutmeg, black pepper or turmeric oil.
• Never use fennel, mustard or horseradish oil on your skin.

Some medicinal actions of spices

Spices can come from any part of a plant, including its roots, stems, leaves, bark, flowers, fruits and seeds. Each spice has a unique blend of bioactive ingredients. Traditional use and/or scientific studies indicate the possible healing properties of these bioactives, which are listed below alphabetically according their actions on various ailments.

Anti-adrenaline – ginger, saffron, turmeric.
Antibacterial – ajowan, allspice, aniseed, caraway, cardamom, cassia, cayenne, chilli, cinnamon, cloves, coriander, cumin, dill seeds, fenugreek, ginger, grains of paradise, horseradish, juniper, kokum, mastic, mustard, nigella, nutmeg, pepper, star anise, tamarind, turmeric, vanilla.
Anti-cancer – allspice, ginger, cinnamon, curcumin, turmeric, black pepper, fenugreek, nigella, saffron, chilli, cocoa (technically a spice).
Anticoagulant (thins blood) – asafoetida, cardamom, cassia, cayenne, chilli, cloves, curcumin, fennel seeds, ginger, nutmeg, turmeric, wasabi.
Antidepressant – cardamom, liquorice, pepper, saffron, turmeric
Antifungal – allspice, aniseed, cardamom, celery seeds, cinnamon, cloves, coriander, cumin, dill seeds, grains of paradise, lemongrass, mace, mastic, pepper, star anise, tamarind, turmeric.
Antihistamine – allspice, aniseed, cayenne, chilli, cloves, coriander, dill seeds, fenugreek, ginger, kokum, liquorice, nigella.

Anti-inflammatory – ajowan, annatto, aniseed, black pepper, caraway, cardamom, cayenne, celery seeds, chilli, cinnamon, cloves, cocoa, coriander, dill seeds, fennel seeds, fenugreek, ginger, juniper, kokum, liquorice, nigella, nutmeg, pepper, saffron, sesame seeds, star anise, turmeric.
Anti-nausea – cinnamon, ginger, peppermint.
Antioxidant (reduces damage in the body caused by over-active oxygen particles, so discouraging, for example, Alzheimer's disease, artery disease, arthritis, asthma, blood clots, cancer, inflammation and kidney disease) – allspice, cayenne, chilli, cinnamon, cloves, cocoa, cumin, fennel seeds, galangal, ginger, ginkgo, grains of paradise, juniper, kokum, lemongrass, liquorice, mastic, mustard, nigella, nutmeg, saffron, sesame seeds, turmeric.
Antispasmodic (relaxes muscles in the gut, womb, breathing passages and bile ducts) – ajowan, aniseed, asafoetida, caraway, cardamom, cassia, cayenne, celery seeds, cinnamon, cloves, coriander, cumin, dill seeds, fennel seeds, fenugreek, ginger, juniper, lemongrass, liquorice, nutmeg, poppyseeds, saffron, sumac, vanilla.
Antiviral – allspice, asafoetida, cinnamon, cloves, ginger, liquorice, nigella, black pepper, star anise.
Aphrodisiac (boosts sex drive) – celery seeds, cinnamon, cloves, coriander, ginger, vanilla.
Astringent ("shrinks" tissues and hardens skin, so reducing mucus and/or bleeding, thanks to its tannins and/or polyphenols) – allspice, annatto, cassia, cinnamon, cloves, cocoa, coriander, cumin, fenugreek, ginger, juniper, kokum, liquorice, mace, mustard, nigella, nutmeg, star anise, sumac, vanilla.
Aromatase-inhibiting (inhibit the conversion of testosterone to oestrogen) – chili, cocoa, ginger, liquorice.
Bitter-tasting (stimulates the production of bile) – ajowan, asafoetida, cassia, cayenne, celery seeds seed, chilli, cocoa, cumin, dill seeds, fennel seeds, fenugreek, horseradish, juniper, liquorice, mace, mahlab, mastic, mustard, nigella, nutmeg, saffron, star anise, turmeric.

Blood pressure-lowering (including calming spices, see "Calming" below) – ajowan, allspice, asafoetida, cardamom, cassia, cayenne, celery seeds, chilli, cinnamon, cocoa, coriander, fennel seeds, fenugreek, ginger, mastic, nigella, pepper, sesame seeds, sumac, tamarind, turmeric.

Blood sugar-lowering (helps prevent diabetes, and inflammation from sugar-damage – "glycation" – of proteins) – caraway, cloves, cocoa, coriander, cumin, fenugreek, ginger, lemongrass, mustard, nigella, sesame seeds, tamarind, turmeric, and perhaps (though studies have mixed results) cassia and cinnamon.

Blood vessel-relaxing ("vasodilatory", including calming spices, and cholinergic spices, see below; also certain antioxidant spices, such as juniper, which make blood vessels healthier, and horseradish, whose peroxidase boosts nitric oxide in blood vessels. Applied externally they warm the skin and aid its healing as well as that of underlying muscles and joints) – ajowan, allspice, cassia, cayenne, celery seeds, chilli, cinnamon, cloves, cocoa, galangal, ginger, juniper, horseradish, Sichuan pepper.

Calming – aniseed, asafoetida, cayenne, cassia, celery seeds, chilli, cinnamon, cloves, cocoa, coriander, ginger, lemongrass, nigella, nutmeg, poppyseeds, saffron, turmeric, vanilla.

Carminative (expels wind) – ajowan, allspice, aniseed, asafoetida, caraway, cardamom, cassia, cayenne, celery seeds, chilli, cinnamon, cloves, coriander, cumin, dill seeds, fennel seeds, galangal, ginger, juniper, mace, nutmeg, saffron, star anise.

Cholesterol-lowering – annatto, caraway, cardamom, cassia, cayenne, celery seeds, chilli, cinnamon, cocoa, coriander, cumin, fenugreek, ginger, horseradish, kokum, lemongrass, liquorice, mastic, nigella, nutmeg, saffron, tamarind, turmeric, wasabi.

Cholinergic (provides or helps the body make the "rest and digest" neurotransmitter (nerve message carrier) acetylcholine, p.91) – ajowan, aniseeds, cardamom, cassia, cayenne, chilli, cinnamon, cloves, coriander, cumin, fennel seeds, fenugreek, ginger, mustard, nigella, paprika, pepper, saffron, turmeric.

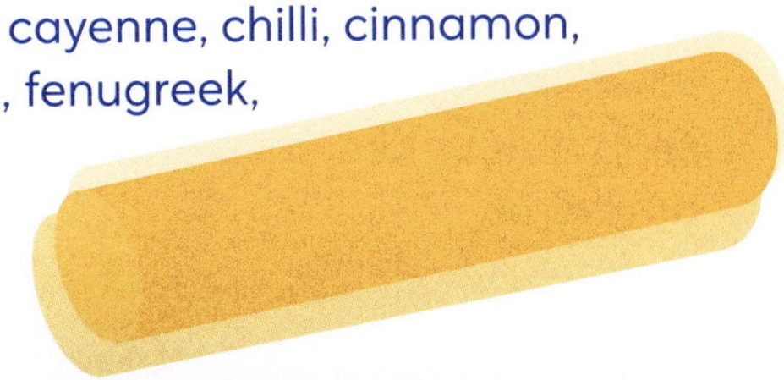

Circulation-boosting – cassia, cayenne, chilli, cinnamon, cloves, cocoa, ginger, horseradish, mustard, pepper, wasabi.
Coumarin-containing – cinnamon, nutmeg, cloves.
Counter-irritant (causes local "heat" or irritation that reduces underlying pain) – cayenne, chilli, horseradish, mustard.
Decongestant – cayenne, chilli, pepper.
Demulcent (soothes skin and mucous membranes, thanks to their gums, saponins or tannins it contains) – fenugreek, kokum, liquorice, sesame seeds.
Diaphoretic (causes sweating, so cooling the body) – ajowan, anise, caraway, cardamom, cassia, cayenne, chilli, cinnamon, coriander, cumin, fennel seeds, galangal, ginger, horseradish, juniper, lemongrass, mustard, nigella, pepper, saffron.
Digestive (aids appetite and digestion by boosting saliva and digestive enzymes) – ajowan, allspice, aniseed, asafoetida, caraway, cardamom, cassia, cayenne, celery seeds, chilli, cinnamon, cloves, coriander, cumin, dill seeds, fennel seeds, fenugreek, galangal, ginger, grains of paradise, horseradish, juniper, kokum, mustard, nutmeg, pepper, turmeric.
Diuretic (increases urine output) – aniseed, caraway, cardamom, celery seeds, cocoa, coriander, cumin, dill seeds, fennel seeds, horseradish, juniper (**Caution:** not with kidney disease), mastic, mustard, nigella, star anise, sumac.
Expectorant (constituents such as diosgenin and saponins thin and break up bronchial mucus, making it easier to cough it up) – aniseed, asafoetida, butterfly pea, caraway, cardamom, cayenne, chilli, cinnamon, fenugreek, ginger, liquorice, nigella, pepper.
Gut microbiome-enhancing – cinnamon, cloves, cumin, ginger, turmeric.
Immunity-enhancing (boosts white cell production) – nigella, pepper.
Laxative (encourages bowel-opening) – ajowan, aniseed, asafoetida, caraway, coriander, fennel seeds, fenugreek, grains of paradise, juniper, liquorice, mustard, nigella, black pepper, sesame seeds, tamarind.

Local anaesthetic – allspice, cloves.
Memory-boosting – ginkgo.
Muscle-relaxing – chamomile, cinnamon, cumin, ginger.
Neurotransmitter action-boosting: this may result from the reduced breakdown in the body of one of these neurotransmitters ("nerve message carriers"), or activation of their cell receptors:

- Acetylcholine – this "rest-and-digest" neurotransmitter slows the heart; encourages stomach and bowel movements; dilates blood vessels (lowering blood pressure the same way as calcium channel-blocker drugs do); improves memory and concentration and therefore the speed and accuracy of learning; and affects mood and skeletal-muscle movement. Cholinergic spices (p.89) boost acetylcholine.
- Adrenaline and noradrenaline (norepinephrine) – are neurotransmitters and hormones. Adrenaline increases heart rate, breathing rate, blood sugar, blood pressure and blood flow to muscles, and sharpens senses. Chilli increases these actions. Noradrenaline increases heart rate and blood pressure, widens airways and directs more blood to essential organs. Ginger and turmeric increase these actions.
- Cannabinoids – reduce inflammation and pain and, perhaps, prostate cancer and osteoporosis, They include alkylamides (in black pepper), anandamide (in cocoa, which is technically a spice) and beta-caryophyllene (in black pepper, cinnamon, cloves).
- Dopamine – this produces satisfaction and aids fine-movement control; its actions are increased by ginger and turmeric.
- Gamma-aminobutyric acid (GABA) – the action of this calming and relaxing neurotransmitter is increased by aniseed and cumin. (Benzodiazepine tranquillizers also work this way.)
- Monoamine-oxidase inhibitors (MAOIs) – these inhibit monoamine oxidase, the enzyme that breaks down adrenaline, dopamine, melatonin, noradrenaline and serotonin, thereby increasing their action. This could reduce depression or otherwise stabilize mood. (MAOI medications work in the same way.) There are small

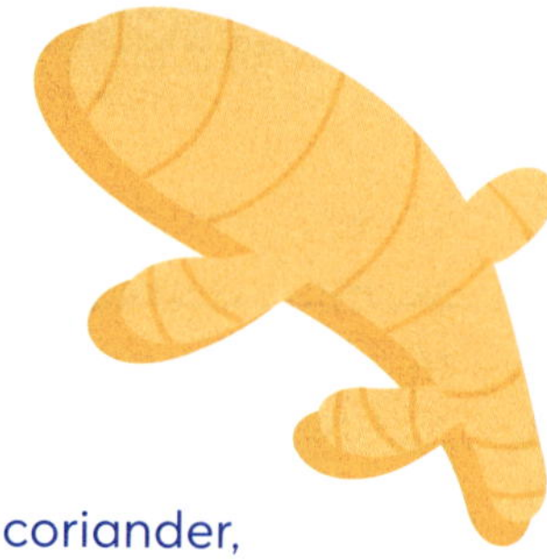

amounts of MAOIs in certain spices, including black pepper, ginger, liquorice, nutmeg.
- Serotonin – the actions of this "feel-good" neurotransmitter are boosted by turmeric.

Oestrogen-balancing – aniseed, caraway, cloves, coriander, cumin, dill seeds, fennel, fenugreek, ginger, juniper, liquorice, nigella, sesame, turmeric.
Pain-relieving (analgesic) – ajowan, allspice, cayenne, chilli, cinnamon, cloves, cumin, ginger, juniper, nigella, paprika, tamarind, turmeric.
Progesterone-balancing – celery seeds, cinnamon, ginger, liquorice, saffron, turmeric.
Rutin-containing – coriander.
Sedative (relax body and mind) – cinnamon, cloves, cocoa, coriander, ginger, lemongrass, nigella, nutmeg.
Testosterone-boosting – fenugreek, ginger
Warming ("thermogenic": warm the body) – boost metabolism by:

- Activating brown fat (a type of fat found between the shoulder-blades and particularly active metabolically) – for example, cayenne, chilli, mustard, wasabi
- Attaching to capsaicin or "spiciness" receptors in the mouth and gut, so triggering the brain to boost the heart rate and thus the circulation – for example, cayenne, chilli, cinnamon, ginger, horseradish, mustard, pepper, wasabi
- Acting in other ways – for example, aniseed, caraway, cardamom, cloves, cocoa, cumin, fennel seeds, grains of paradise, nutmeg, turmeric

Traditional uses and research evidence

Scientific studies confirm some of the many traditional uses of spices for preventing and treating common ailments. They also suggest certain new ones. Although much of the research is in laboratories, or with animals, or involves only small numbers of people, and although we tend to consume only small quantities of spices and therefore of their bioactive constituents, the findings are exciting.

CAUTION: Spices can have adverse effects if consumed in large amounts, so read the following warnings carefully before using them to remedy ailments.

Contraindications of spices

Ajowan – may lower blood pressure and slow the heart rate.
Aniseed – large amounts can be toxic because of its estragole.
Annatto – has been linked with allergic reactions.
Chilli – large amounts can cause gastritis (though normal amounts protect the stomach).
Fennel seeds – in remedies for infant wind or colic can temporarily enlarge a baby's breasts.
Fenugreek – is related to peanuts, so avoid if allergic to these.
Juniper – prolonged use can irritate kidneys, so avoid taking it frequently for more than six weeks, or at all if you have cystitis or kidney disease. Large amounts could irritate the stomach, especially if you have "acid indigestion" or a peptic ulcer. Large amounts in pregnancy could encourage womb contractions.
Kokum – is unsuitable for anyone who is pregnant or breastfeeding, has diabetes or a heart disorder, or is on high blood pressure medication.
Lemongrass – avoid if pregnant or breastfeeding.
Liquorice – large amounts contain enough glycyrrhizin to lower the body's potassium and cause, for example, confusion; diarrhoea; faintness; fatigue; fluid retention (which can raise blood pressure); headache; a fast, slow or uneven heartbeat; nausea; a rash; sight problems (double vision, or seeing haloes around things); and weakness. Men may develop enlarged breasts and erectile dysfunction. Large amounts can interfere with the action of blood pressure medication, digoxin, diuretics ("water tablets"), oestrogen, steroids and warfarin (a blood thinner).

- A 250ml (8.5fl oz) cup of liquorice tea contains about 31.5mg of glycyrrhizin. The European Scientific Committee on Food recommends no more than 100mg daily for the average adult. A safe daily amount is generally considered to be half a cupful of the tea.

- Look out for certain liquorice teas that contain "deglycyrrhinized liquorice".
- Speak to a doctor before drinking liquorice tea if you have a heart problem or high blood pressure. Don't give it to children under the age of two and give to older children only with a doctor's approval. Some people are more sensitive to glycyrrhizin than others.

Nigella – use in moderation as large amounts can be toxic (because of the bitter glycoside melanthin) or even paralyzing (because of the alkaloid nigellin).
Nutmeg – use in moderation as large amounts can be intoxicating and sleep-inducing and cause nausea, vomiting, flushing, dry mouth, rapid heartrate, double vision, hallucinations, convulsions and delirium. The main culprit, myristicin, is related to mescalen, a psychoactive substance from the peyote cactus.
Sesame – can trigger allergy in susceptible people.

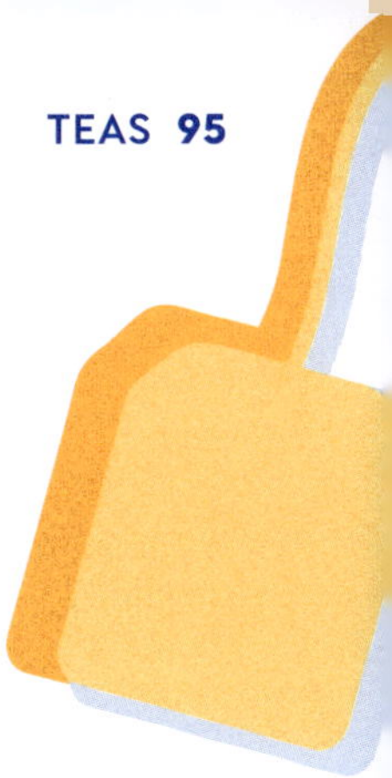

TEAS

Black, green, white, purple, oolong and *puerh* (pronounced "poo-er") teas are infusions in water of the leaves of *Camellia-sinensis* tea bushes and trees (p.39). Black tea is the type most often enjoyed in the US, Europe, Australia and India. It is made by infusing leaves of black tea in water. Green tea is the type most often enjoyed in China.

"Herb tea" is the traditional term for tea made from the leaves of certain other plants, bushes or trees; infusions made from these are naturally caffeine-free.

Whole-leaf tea is richer in bioactives than is chopped, fragmented or powdered tea. Surprisingly, phenolic compounds make up 30 per cent of the weight of dried tea leaves. Teas are popular folk remedies and are used in various healing systems, including herbal medicine. Scientific research increasingly supports their use.

How to prepare teas for remedies

Steep your chosen leaves in water that is hot but not boiling. (Boiling water can scald the leaves, so extracting more of their bitter compounds and perhaps destroying some of their flavour notes.) The ideal temperature depends on the type of tea. For example, steep black and herbal teas in water at 194–208°F (90–98°C), and green tea in water at 176°F (80°C). (Note that boiling water's temperature is 212°F (100°C). Drink one or two cups of your chosen tea; elderly people may need less. Children should also have less – for example, half the adult dose for a 12 year old; a quarter for a 4 year old.

You can also use a tea in the following ways:

BATH – add 570ml (1 pint) of the tea to bathwater.

COMPRESS – a hot compress can help arthritis, backache, boils and muscle aching. Tension headaches and sprains do better with a cold compress. After a few days, you may speed healing by alternating hot and cold compresses several times during a treatment, ending with a cold one.

- **For a hot compress**: soak a cotton pad in your chosen hot tea. When cool enough, squeeze out and apply to the affected area. To keep it warm, cover it with cling film, then a towel or hot-water bottle; re-soak it in hot tea as necessary.
- **For a cold compress:** cool the tea first. Secure it with a crêpe bandage if necessary.

EYEBATH (eyecup) – these specially shaped containers are available from pharmacies. Sterilize an eyebath by washing it in a dishwasher with a heated drying cycle, or pouring just-boiled water into it and letting it stand for 1 minute.

- Strain your chosen tea; simmer it for 10 minutes to sterilize it; cool it to body temperature, then pour it into the eyebath. Leaning slightly backwards, pour a little into your affected eye.
- Cover the remaining tea with cling film and refrigerate for later use. Next day, make a fresh supply.

FACIAL STEAMING – put 570ml (1 pint) of a just-made tea into a bowl. Put this on a table. Sit, leaning over the bowl, with a towel over your head and the bowl, for 5 minutes.

FOOTBATH – fill a large bowl ¾ full of water then add 570ml (1 pint) of your chosen tea. Use hot or cold. A folk remedy for soothing a feverish cold, cough or sore throat is to put a cold compress on your forehead, while soaking your feet in a hot footbath. Another option is to soak your feet first in a bowl of a hot tea for 2 minutes, then in a bowl of cold tea for 2 minutes. Repeat several times.

GARGLE – continue for at least 20 seconds and repeat 2–3 times a day.

HAIR RINSE – pour a tea over your hair after shampooing.

MOUTHWASH – swill a tea around your mouth then spit it out.

POULTICE – discard the liquid from your chosen brew, let the wet leaves cool enough to be comfortable, then put them on the affected area. Cover with a cotton pad followed by cling film.

STEAM INHALATION – as for "Facial steaming", but inhale deeply.

Some medicinal actions of teas

The herbs in herb teas typically come from the leaves and stems of non-woody plants. Note that dong quai is the root of *Angelica sinensis*, and *Vitex agnus castus* is also called "female ginseng". Traditional uses and/or scientific studies indicate various actions of different teas:

Adaptogenic (a nervous system "tonic" that increases resistance to stress, probably by boosting or reducing – depending on need – adrenal hormones such as adrenaline) – ginseng, rooibos.
Anti-allergic – *Camellia-sinensis* tea (especially green tea), chamomile, echinacea, lemon balm, nettle.
Antibacterial – barley, calendula, *Camellia-sinensis* tea (especially green tea), chamomile, chickweed, dandelion, dong quai, echinacea, elderflower, hibiscus, lavender, lemon balm, linden, nettle, peppermint, red clover, rosehip, rosemary, thyme, valerian.
Anti-cancer – barley, black cohosh, butterfly pea, calendula, *Camellia-sinensis* tea (especially green tea), chamomile, chickweed, corn, dandelion, dong quai, echinacea, elderflower, ginseng, hibiscus, lavender, peppermint, red clover, rooibos, rosehip, rosemary, valerian. (See also "Aromatase-inhibiting".)
Anticoagulant (thins blood) – roasted-barley, *Camellia sinensis* tea (especially green tea), chamomile, dong quai, ginseng, nettle, red clover.
Anticonvulsant – chamomile, lavender, linden, passionflower, rosemary, valerian (if convulsions are provoked by poor sleep), verbena.
Antidepressant – black cohosh, calendula, *Camellia-sinensis* tea (especially green tea), chamomile, dandelion, dong quai, elderflower, ginseng, lavender, lemon balm, linden, nettle, passionflower, peppermint, red clover, rooibos, rosehip, rosemary, valerian.
Antifungal – calendula, *Camellia-sinensis* tea, chamomile, dandelion, dong quai, echinacea, hibiscus, lavender, peppermint, rosemary, thyme.
Antihistamine – chamomile, dong quai, lemon balm, nettle.

Anti-inflammatory – black cohosh, calendula, *Camellia-sinensis* tea (especially green tea), chamomile, chickweed, cornsilk, dandelion, dong quai, echinacea, elderflower, ginseng, hibiscus, lavender, lemon balm, linden, nettle, peppermint, red clover, rooibos, rosehip, rosemary, red clover, sage, *Vitex agnus castus.*

Antioxidant – barley, butterfly pea, calendula, *Camellia-sinensis* tea (especially green tea), chickweed, dandelion, echinacea, ginkgo, lavender, lemon balm, linden, nettle, peppermint, rooibos, rosehip, rosemary, sage, thyme, verbena.

Antispasmodic (relaxes "smooth" muscle in blood vessels, breathing passages, gut or womb) – black cohosh, calendula, chamomile, dong quai, echinacea, elderflower, hibiscus, lavender, lemon balm, linden, nettle, passionflower, peppermint, red clover, rooibos, rosemary, thyme, valerian, verbena, *Vitex agnus castus.*

Antiviral – calendula, *Camellia-sinensis* tea (especially green tea), chamomile, dandelion, dong quai, echinacea, lemon balm, peppermint, rooibos, rosehip, thyme.

Aromatase-inhibiting (inhibit the conversion of testosterone to oestrogen) – bergamot, chamomile, clover, dandelion, mint, oregano, parsley, passionflower, peppermint, rosemary, thyme

Astringent (reduces bleeding and inflammation of skin and mucus production by mucous membrane) – calendula, *Camellia-sinensis* tea, chickweed, dandelion, echinacea, elderflower, hibiscus, linden, nettle, peppermint, rooibos, rosehip, rosemary, thyme, verbena.

Bile-stimulating (boosts bile production or flow): the "bitters" – calendula, dandelion, dong quai, lavender, lemon balm, linden, peppermint, nettle, rosemary, verbena.

Bitter-tasting – barley, black cohosh, calendula, chamomile, dandelion, dong quai, ginseng, hibiscus, nettle, rooibos, rosehip, rosemary, thyme, verbena.

Blood cell-boosting – dong quai, echinacea.

Blood fat-lowering – cornsilk, dandelion, elderflower, ginseng, rooibos, tea.

Blood pressure-lowering – (see also "Antispasmodic", "Calming" and

"Diuretic") – black cohosh, *Camellia-sinensis* tea (especially green tea), dong quai, ginseng, hibiscus, lemon balm, linden, nettle, passionflower, valerian, verbena.

Blood sugar-lowering – black cohosh, butterfly pea, calendula, *Camellia-sinensis* tea (especially green tea), chamomile, cornsilk, dandelion, dong quai, elderflower, ginger, ginkgo, ginseng, hibiscus, nettle, rosemary.

Calming – black cohosh, butterfly pea, *Camellia-sinensis* tea (especially green tea), chamomile, lavender, lemon balm, linden, passionflower, peppermint, thyme, valerian, verbena, *Vitex agnus castus.*

Carminative (expels wind) – chamomile, fennel, ginger, lavender, peppermint.

Cholesterol-lowering – roasted-barley, black cohosh, cornsilk, dandelion, dong quai, elderflower, ginseng, hibiscus, lavender, linden, rosehip, *Camellia-sinensis* tea, thyme.

Cholinergic (boosts the "rest and digest" neurotransmitter acetylcholine; see "Neurotransmitter") – basil, butterfly pea, *Camellia-sinensis* tea, chamomile, dill, dong quai, ginkgo, ginseng, lemon balm, marjoram, nettle, oregano, peppermint, saffron, sage, rosemary, thyme, valerian.

Decongestant – dandelion, elderflower, nettle, peppermint, tea, thyme.

Demulcent (soothes and protects mucous membranes, reducing colic, coughs and diarrhoea, for example) – barley, calendula, chickweed, cornsilk.

Digestive (aids appetite and aids digestion – possibly by boosting saliva and digestive enzymes) – butterfly pea, calendula, *Camellia-sinensis* tea, chamomile, cinnamon (boosts trypsin), dandelion (leaf/root), dong quai, echinacea, elderflower, lavender, lemon balm, linden, passionflower, peppermint, rosehip, rosemary, thyme, verbena (see also "Bile-stimulating").

Diuretic (increases urine production, so reducing blood pressure and weight) – black cohosh, butterfly pea tea, calendula, *Camellia-sinensis* tea, chamomile, chickweed, cornsilk, dandelion, dong quai, elderflower, hibiscus, linden, nettle, peppermint, red clover, rooibos, rosehip, rosemary, thyme, valerian.

Emollient (soothes and protects inflamed skin) – barley, calendula, chickweed, cornsilk.

Expectorant (increases and dilutes bronchial secretions, making them easier to cough up) – butterfly pea, chickweed, dong quai, elderflower, hibiscus, linden, nettle, peppermint, red clover, thyme, valerian, verbena.

Immunity-boosting – calendula, *Camellia-sinensis* tea (especially green tea), dandelion, dong quai, echinacea, elderflower, ginseng, hibiscus, peppermint, rosehip.

Laxative (bowel-stimulating) – chickweed, dandelion, dong quai, elderflower, linden, rosehip, verbena.

Memory-enhancing – butterfly pea, *Camellia-sinensis* tea (especially green tea), peppermint, rosemary.

Muscle-relaxing – black cohosh, chamomile, hibiscus, lavender, lemon balm, nettle, peppermint, red clover, rosemary, thyme, valerian, verbena.

Nerve-protecting ("neuroprotective") – *Camellia-sinensis* tea.

Neurotransmitter (nerve message carrier) – action-boosting: this may result from reduced breakdown, or activation of their cell receptors.

- Acetylcholine – this "rest-and-digest" neurotransmitter slows the heart; encourages stomach and bowel movements; dilates blood vessels (lowering blood pressure the same way as calcium channel-blocker drugs do); improves memory and concentration and therefore the speed and accuracy of learning; and affects mood and musculoskeletal movement. These actions are increased by cholinergic teas (p.99).
- Adrenaline and noradrenaline – are also hormones. Adrenaline increases heart rate, breathing rate, blood sugar, blood pressure and blood flow to muscles; and sharpens senses. *Camellia-sinensis* tea and ginseng increase these actions. Noradrenaline increases heart rate and blood pressure, widens airways and

directs more blood to essential organs – and *Camellia-sinensis* tea increases these actions.

- Cannabinoids – the actions of those that reduce inflammation and pain and, perhaps, prostate cancer and osteoporosis, are increased by alkylamides (in echinacea), cannabinoids (in *Camellia-sinensis* tea, especially green tea) and beta-caryophyllene (in dong quai, echinacea, lavender, lemon balm, rosemary and *Vitex agnus castus*).
- Dopamine – this produces satisfaction and aids fine-movement control; its actions are increased by *Camellia-sinensis* tea and *Vitex agnus castus*.
- Gamma-aminobutyric acid (GABA) – the action of this calming and relaxing neurotransmitter is increased by *Camellia-sinensis* tea, lavender, lemon balm, passionflower, thyme and valerian. (Benzodiazepine tranquillizers also work this way.)

Monoamine-oxidase inhibitors (MAOIs) – these compounds inhibit monoamine oxidase, the enzyme that breaks down adrenaline, dopamine, melatonin, noradrenaline and serotonin in the brain, so increasing their action. This could reduce depression or otherwise stabilize mood. Note that MAOI medications (prescribed for depression and Parkinson's disease) work this way. MAOIs are present in small amounts in certain teas including:

- Anthocyanins (in rosehip)
- Epigallocatechin gallate (in *Camellia-sinensis* tea)
- Certain flavonoids: apigenin (in chickweed, lemon balm, passionflower, rosemary and thyme); kaempferol (in calendula, chickweed, elderflower, lemon balm, linden, nettle, passionflower, rosemary, tea and *Vitex agnus castus*); and quercetin (in calendula, *Camellia-sinensis* tea, chamomile, elderflower, lemon balm, linden, nettle, passionflower, rooibos, rosehip, rosemary, valerian)
- Harman-group alkaloids (in barley, cornsilk and passionflower)
- Quercetin (in calendula, *Camellia-sinensis* tea, chamomile,

elderflower, lemon balm, linden, nettle, passionflower, rooibos, rosehip, rosemary, valerian) which can be an antidepressant

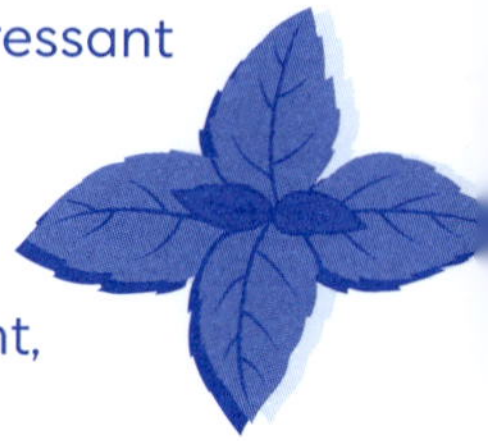

- Scopoletin (in dong quai)
- Serotonin – the actions of this "feel-good" neurotransmitter are boosted by black cohosh, *Camellia-sinensis* tea, dandelion, ginseng, peppermint, red clover, valerian

Oestrogen-balancing – chamomile, fennel, ginger, ginseng, green tea, nettle, red clover, rooibos, thyme, valerian, verbena.
Pain-relieving (analgesic) – black cohosh, calendula, chamomile, chickweed, dandelion, dong quai, echinacea, elderflower, lavender, passionflower, peppermint, rosemary, *Camellia-sinensis* tea, thyme, valerian.
Progesterone-balancing – chamomile, ginger, oregano, peppermint, red clover, rosemary, *Vitex agnus castus.*
Rutin-containing – basil, elderflower, green tea, lemon balm, oregano, passionflower.
Testosterone-boosting – ginseng.
Sedative (calms body and mind) – black cohosh, chamomile, dandelion, dong quai, ginseng (which, because of its adaptogenic properties, can instead be stimulating, if necessary), lavender, lemon balm, linden, peppermint, red clover, rooibos, thyme, valerian, verbena.
Sleep-inducing (hypnotic) – chamomile, dandelion, lavender, linden, passionflower, valerian, verbena.
Stimulating (stimulates nerves) – *Camellia-sinensis* tea, dong quai, echinacea, elderflower, ginseng (which, because of its adaptogenic properties, can instead be sedating, if necessary), linden, peppermint, rosehip, rosemary, thyme.
Thyroid hormone-balancing – lemon balm may lower high levels. But it may also improve mild thyroid underactivity from an autoimmune disorder (possibly thanks to its selenium).

Tonic (herbs traditionally called "alteratives" aid healing) – chickweed, rooibos and, for the following systems:

- Cardiovascular: linden
- Digestive: chamomile, dandelion, nettle
- Hormonal: plant oestrogens, including chamomile, ginger, ginseng, green tea, nettle, red clover, rooibos, thyme, valerian, verbena
- Liver: bitter-tasting herbs
- Urinary: cornsilk, nettle
- Nervous system: ginseng, red clover, verbena
- Musculoskeletal: black cohosh, nettle
- Reproductive: black cohosh
- Respiratory: echinacea
- Skin: echinacea, nettle, red clover

Warming ("thermogenic": warm the body) – contain substances that:

- Boost metabolism, so increase heat production. This is partly thanks to certain alkaloids and aromatics in, for example, *Camellia-sinensis* tea, chickweed, dandelion, hibiscus
- Speed the heart rate and therefore boost the circulation. This is mostly thanks to certain alkaloids, glycosides and phenolic compounds, for example, in nettle, rosemary, thyme
- Dilate small arteries and veins

Wind-expelling (carminative) – chamomile, echinacea, dong quai, elderflower, lavender, lemon balm, linden, nettle, peppermint, rooibos, rosemary, thyme, valerian.

Wound healing (vulnerary, stimulating new cell growth) – calendula, chamomile, echinacea, linden, red clover, rosemary, thyme.

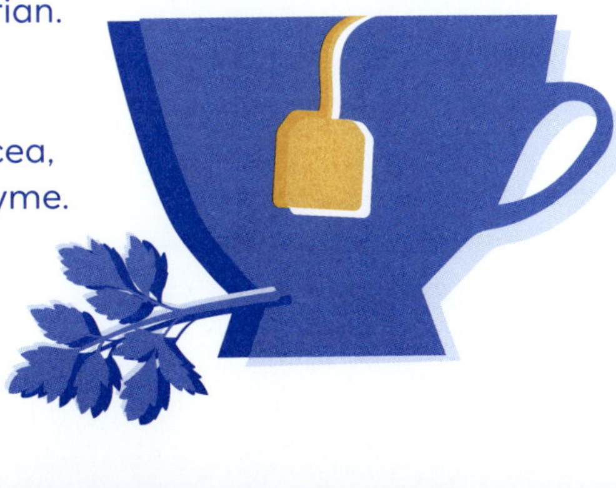

Using *Camellia-sinensis* teas and herb teas for health

Studies back up many of the traditional medicinal uses of tea and herb teas. Much of the research is early but the findings are exciting.

Studies show or suggest *Camellia-sinensis* tea is a potent antioxidant; discourages allergy; improves atopic eczema; reduces high cholesterol, fats and blood pressure; discourages flu and herpes (5 cups a day raise virus-fighting interferon tenfold); protects against heart attacks (3 cups a day reduce the risk by 11 per cent) and strokes; slows memory loss and cognitive decline; discourages certain cancers and type 2 diabetes; and may improve bone strength. In particular, its:

- **Caffeine and theanine** boost concentration and mental relaxation; caffeine may discourage Parkinson's disease.
- **Caffeine, catechins and theanine** promote fat loss (by inhibiting enzymes that digest fats), specifically, the loss of visceral fat, the "belly fat" highly associated with an increased risk of diabetes and metabolic syndrome (p.152).
- **Catechins** may discourage Alzheimer's disease, eye diseases (such as glaucoma), candida and, perhaps, osteoporosis.
- **Epigallocatechin gallate's** anti-inflammatory effects inhibit the excessive production of the COX-2 enzyme that encourages arthritis and cancer. It may also reduce weight by helping to convert calories into muscle, not fat, by prolonging the metabolism-boosting action of noradrenaline (norepinephrine), and by reducing appetite. It also reduces brain damage after a stroke.
- **Fluroride** discourages tooth decay.
- **Tannins** might help diarrhoea and heavy periods.
- **Theophylline** widens airways and arteries and reduces cholesterol.

Green tea can be used to treat arthritis, bad breath, diabetes, infection, inflammatory bowel disease, obesity, poor immunity and, externally, for conjunctivitis and styes. It is also used to aid longevity. One cup has greater antioxidant power than a serving of broccoli, carrots, spinach or strawberries. It also helps prevent abnormal blood clots. And drinking it regularly may discourage "all-cause death".

CAUTION: Certain bioactives in particular teas can have side effects, most short-lived and not serious, as described below. Consult the list to make sure the tea you choose as a remedy will not pose a problem for you.

Contraindications of teas

Certain bioactives contained in certain teas can have side effects, though most are short-lived and not serious. If you:

- Are pregnant or breastfeeding, on medication, or have a chronic ailment, consult the list below
- Develop potentially serious allergic symptoms (such as mouth swelling or breathing difficulty), get urgent medical help
- Get dermatitis for the first time, consult a doctor
- Have kidney stones, gallstones or period pain, avoid bitter-tasting teas
- Have an inflamed gallbladder, painful gallstones, "obstructive" jaundice, or viral hepatitis (liver inflammation), avoid bile-stimulating teas

Barley or roasted-barley – can trigger an allergic reaction in a susceptible person. Avoid if gluten-sensitive. If on prescription medication, take this 1 hour before or 2 hours after drinking the tea, as barley reduces the efficacy or increases the adverse effects of certain drugs. Consult a doctor first if on anti-diabetes, blood pressure-lowering, or heart medication.

Black cohosh – long-term safety data is lacking, so avoid regular consumption for more than 6 months. It's probably better avoided during pregnancy or breastfeeding.

Calendula – can trigger an allergic reaction in someone sensitive to ragweed. Avoid it during pregnancy or breastfeeding.

Chamomile – can trigger an allergic reaction in a susceptible person. It's probably better avoided in pregnancy, as it can stimulate the womb.

Chickweed – is best avoided during pregnancy or breastfeeding, as safety data is lacking.

Cornsilk – aids fluid retention but also flushes potassium from the body. Consult your doctor first if taking diuretic medication.
Dandelion root – can trigger an allergic reaction in a susceptible person. Consult a doctor first if you have gallstones. It's better avoided during pregnancy or breastfeeding, as safety data is unreliable.
Dong quai – can make skin more sensitive to sunlight, so use sunscreen. Consult a doctor first if on anticoagulants (blood thinners), medication for high blood pressure or an abnormal heart rhythm, selective-serotonin-reuptake-inhibitor antidepressants, or L-dopa medication (for Parkinson's disease), or if you have heavy periods or a hormone-sensitive cancer. Consult a doctor before taking it in high doses or for more than six months as long-term safety data is lacking. Avoid it during pregnancy or breastfeeding.
Echinacea – any immunity-boosting effect may gradually become less effective, so take a break every few weeks. Stop it before planned surgery, as it can suppress immunity. Consult a doctor first if you have an autoimmune disorder. It's thought to be safe when pregnant or breastfeeding.
Elderflower – consult a doctor first if on anti-cancer chemotherapy or anti-diabetes drugs. It's probably better avoided during pregnancy or breastfeeding, as safety data is lacking.
Fennel – limit this to a cup a day if pregnant or breastfeeding.
Ginseng – is often recommended for the over-40s – men in particular. Some experts suggest young people should take it for only up to 3 weeks in each month. Avoid other stimulants, such as coffee and tea. Also avoid if you are anxious or depressed, or have an infection, inflammatory condition, or acute asthma, or are pregnant or breastfeeding. It can provoke unwanted oestrogenic effects. Consult your doctor if on anticoagulants, antipsychotics, blood pressure-lowering medication, or steroids. Stop it at least 7 days before planned surgery, to prevent low blood sugar and bleeding during or after.
Green tea – see "Tea", below.

Hibiscus – is relatively acidic, so avoid if prone to acid reflux ("heartburn"). Avoid it if taking the painkiller paracetamol (acetaminophen), as it can encourage adverse effects. It can trigger an allergic reaction in someone sensitive to the mallow plant family. It's best avoided during pregnancy or breastfeeding. Avoid if trying to conceive, as it can reduce fertility.

Hops – avoid if pregnant or breastfeeding.

Lavender – safety information is incomplete, so drink only 1–2 cups a day to prevent ailments or treat chronic ones; and only 3 cups a day to treat an acute ailment. Avoid it during pregnancy or breastfeeding. It can trigger an allergic reaction in a susceptible person. It can increase both wanted and unwanted effects of antidepressant and sedative medications: consult a doctor first if taking diazepam or lorazepam. Avoid it for two weeks before planned surgery as it can magnify the nervous-system-dampening effect of anaesthesia or medication.

Lemon balm – daily use over a long period of time can depress thyroid function. Avoid if on barbiturates, as it can prolong their action. It's generally considered safe when pregnant or breastfeeding.

Linden – consult a doctor first if on anticoagulants, medication for high blood pressure or heart disease, or lithium (for bipolar disease), as it can increase their effects. It's probably better avoided when pregnant or breastfeeding as safety data is scanty.

Nettle – consult a doctor if on anticoagulants, or medication for diabetes or high blood pressure, as it can interact with certain of these. Avoid during pregnancy or breastfeeding.

Oregano – avoid if pregnant or breastfeeding.

Passionflower – may trigger dizziness or sleepiness, or, in a susceptible person, an allergic reaction. It can interact with certain drugs, including anticoagulants and benzodiazepine tranquillizers. Avoid during pregnancy or breastfeeding.

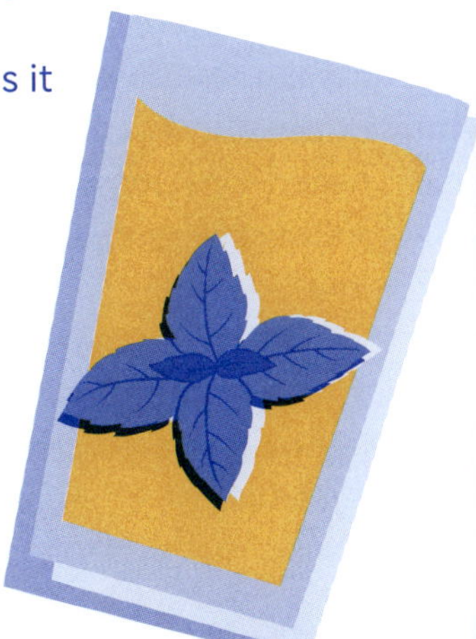

Peppermint – avoid if you have gallstone pain. It's generally considered safe during pregnancy and breastfeeding.
Red clover – avoid during pregnancy or breastfeeding, and for at least a week before planned surgery.
Rooibos – consult a doctor if on anti-cancer chemotherapy.
Rosehip – is generally considered safe during pregnancy or breastfeeding, though confirmatory data is lacking.
Rosemary – is probably best avoided during pregnancy or breastfeeding.
Sage – avoid if pregnant or breastfeeding.
Tea – the common name for black *Camellia-sinensis* tea: experts suggest the average adult's all-source caffeine consumption should be no more than 300mg a day, or 200mg if pregnant or breastfeeding. Drinking seven to eight cups of average-strength tea, or five cups of very strong tea, provides 300mg of caffeine. But studies show no adverse effects from consuming six to nine average-strength cups a day. Too much caffeine can irritate the stomach, and cause anxiety, twitchy muscles, raised heart rate, palpitations, insomnia (from tea drunk within four hours of trying to sleep) and, later, fatigue. If unusually caffeine-sensitive, you may have insomnia or a faster heartbeat after smaller amounts. At least 250mg of caffeine is needed for a diuretic effect. Caffeine temporarily raises blood pressure in those unused to it. Suddenly stopping regular consumption can cause headaches.

This tea reduces iron absorption by 60 per cent but an intake of fewer than eight cups a day is unlikely to harm iron status in healthy people whose diet is varied and balanced. If you have iron-deficiency anaemia, abstain from drinking tea during a meal and for the hour afterwards.

Tea's caffeine and tannins can change the absorption or alter the effects of certain drugs. If on medication, check the patient information leaflet, or consult your doctor, to see if yours is one of these.

This tea contains oxalates that encourage oxalate kidney stones in certain people. Longer steeping produces higher oxalate levels. Adding milk to tea discourages stones.

NOTE: Green tea, also made from *Camellia sinensis*, makes the anticoagulant drug warfarin less effective. It also reduces iron absorption by 30 per cent.

Thyme – can trigger an allergic reaction in someone sensitive to mint-family plants. Consult a doctor if on anticoagulants as thyme can increase their action. Avoid if you have epilepsy or heart disease. More than an occasional cup is probably best avoided in pregnancy, as it can stimulate the womb.

Valerian – can add to the sedative effects of alcohol or drugs such as barbiturates and benzodiazepine tranquillizers. Consult a doctor first if on these drugs or anticonvulsant drugs. Avoid during pregnancy or breastfeeding.

Verbena – avoid regular large or therapeutic amounts. Avoid during pregnancy (though it can be taken in labour to stimulate contractions) and breastfeeding.

Vitex agnus castus – avoid if using oral contraception or hormone replacement therapy, or if pregnant or breastfeeding.

Yarrow – can trigger an allergic reaction (such as contact dermatitis, and photosensitive dermatitis triggered by sunlight), dizziness and headaches. Avoid during pregnancy or breastfeeding.

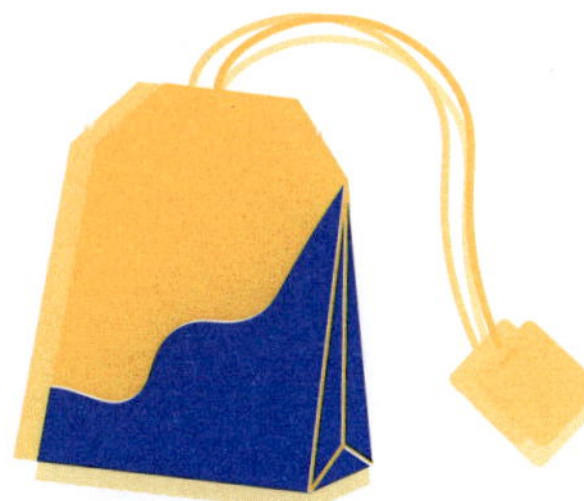

TEAS FOR CHILDREN: Chamomile tea is considered generally safe in small amounts for babies over six months old. For children over one year old, elderflower, peppermint and *Camellia-sinensis* tea are considered generally safe in small amounts as everyday drinks.

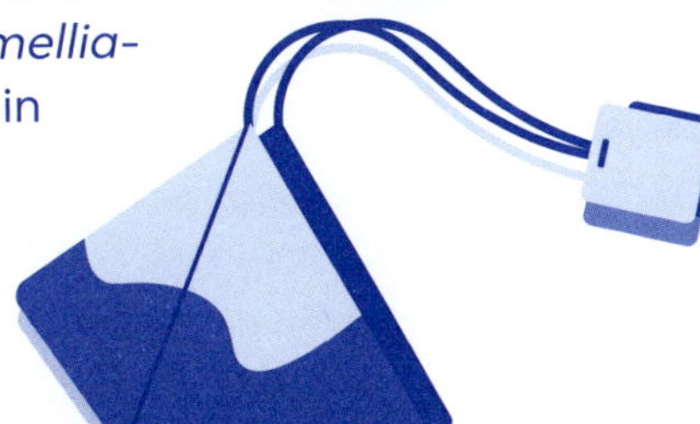

AILMENTS AND THEIR REMEDIES

Here is how our cupboard heroes, from apple cider vinegar to teas, can help various common ailments and some more serious conditions.

Acne

This can occur due to overproduction of the skin's oily sebum, caused by too much sensitivity of sebaceous glands to testosterone during puberty or after. Excess sebum may block skin pores. Another factor is a reduction in the skin's normal acidity. Other provoking factors are changes in sebum, and unusually sticky hair follicle cells. *Propionibacterium acnes* skin bacteria play a role in the inflammation of acne spots, as does imbalance or loss of microbial diversity of the skin's normal bacteria. An overactive immune system may contribute. The premenstrual fall in oestrogen, as well as humidity, polycystic ovary syndrome, stress and certain drugs (for example, the progestogen-only pill) can also be to blame.

APPLE CIDER VINEGAR

Some people report this helps. This could be because it increases skin acidity, emulsifies skin oil, and reduces inflammation. Also, *Propionibacterium acnes* can contribute to acne and apple cider vinegar has antimicrobial properties.

+ ACTION: Mix 1 part of apple cider vinegar with 4 parts of water. Apply with cotton wool, rinse off after 10 minutes and repeat 3 times a day.

LEMONS

Lemon juice may help as it kills acne bacteria, increases skin acidity, emulsifies skin oil and reduces inflammation.

+ ACTION: Apply lemon juice with a cotton pad 2 or 3 times a day.

HONEY

Honey does not kill those bacteria that are the major cause of acne. However, its high sugar content draws pus from spots, its anti-

inflammatories soothe skin, and it promotes wound healing.
+ ACTIONS: Three times a day, apply manuka honey with a UMF of 10 or more; or apply manuka-honey cream.

GARLIC

Skin needs sulphur to remain healthy, yet many people are sulphur-deficient. Garlic's sulphur compounds might help. They may also kill acne bacteria. Also, garlic's antioxidants reduce inflammation. Some people believe consuming or applying garlic helps acne, though there is no good evidence for this.
+ ACTIONS: First, do a patch test (p.82) to check garlic is safe for your skin. If so, rub spots with the cut surface of a garlic clove twice a day. Or bathe them with garlic water (p.81) twice a day. Include garlic in your daily diet or take a garlic powder supplement. You need both both water- and oil-soluble sulphur compounds (pp.78–9).

SPICES

Antibacterial, anti-inflammatory, astringent and and oestrogen-balancing spices may help. Also, try sesame seeds.
+ ACTIONS: Include these spices in your diet. Bathe affected skin twice a day with tea made from one or more of these spices.

TEAS

Antibacterial, anti-inflammatory and astringent teas may help. In particular, *Vitex agnus castus* may be useful for acne that flares before a menstrual period.
+ ACTIONS: Include these teas in your diet. Bathe affected skin twice a day with one of them.

Ageing-related health concerns

Conditions more likely in later life include Alzheimer's disease, artery disease, arthritis, cancer, depression, type 2 diabetes, heart disease, osteoporosis and strokes.

One reason is that some older people choose a less healthy diet, without enough vegetables, fruit, wholegrains, nuts, seeds and other sources of polyphenols and fibre. One consequence is an unhealthy

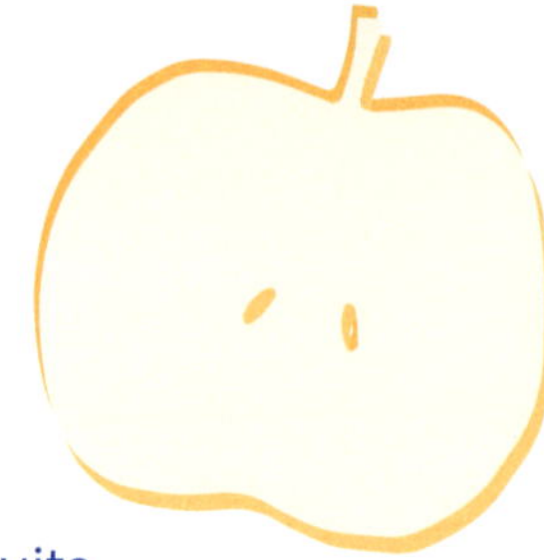

gut microbiome – with an imbalance of gut micro-organisms that encourages a variety of gut and general-health problems. Older people may also prioritise easy-to-eat food, such as white bread, biscuits and sugar, which also encourages an unhealthy gut microbiome. And the ageing process may reduce their absorption of nourishment from food.

See also *Premature ageing.*

APPLE CIDER VINEGAR

Particularly long-lived peoples include certain groups in Russia (the Georgians), Pakistan (the Hunzas), Ecuador, China and Peru. One link is that they tend to live at high altitudes: here, melting glacier water is rich in alkaline minerals such as calcium, which help the body maintain a healthy acid–alkali balance without drawing calcium from bones. Apple cider vinegar has an alkalinizing effect in the body, so helps conserve stored calcium.

Another possible factor encouraging their longevity is the consumption of fermented vegetables, fruit, milk, cereal grains, meat or fish. We don't know whether any benefit is caused by fermentation reducing the carbohydrate in these foods, by any remaining fermentation bacteria, or by the presence of fermentation acids (such as lactic or acetic). Apple cider vinegar is fermented apple juice, so may have the same effects.

Folk medicine has long held that apple cider vinegar helps protect against age-related disease. Certainly, consuming it before a meal discourages high blood sugar afterwards (see *Diabetes*). Also, one in two over-60s in Westernized cultures have an age-related reduction in stomach acid, which might reduce their absorption of many nutrients (including protein, carbohydrates, fats, vitamins A, B, C and E, and the minerals calcium, iron, magnesium, zinc, copper, chromium, selenium, manganese, vanadium, molybdenum and cobalt). Apple cider vinegar might help with this.

US researchers say mineral and vitamin deficiencies can accelerate age-related decay of mitochondria (tiny energy-producing "factories" in cells). Among the most important deficiencies are those of biotin, iron, magnesium, manganese, pantothenic acid and zinc.[4]

+ ACTIONS: Hedge your bets by adding 1 or 2 teaspoons of apple cider vinegar to your food, or taking it in a glass of water, once or twice a day.

LEMONS

A recent UK survey noted that one in ten over-65s were short of iron and vitamins B and C; lemons provide all three. Studies suggest that antioxidants such as vitamin C discourage premature ageing of skin. Lemons' antioxidants might help counter premature ageing elsewhere too – for example, in blood vessels, bones, cartilage, joints and muscle tendons. And in Westernized cultures, lemons' acids, as part of a healthy diet, could help the one in two over-60s with an age-related reduction in stomach acid.

Alkaline minerals such as calcium help the body maintain a healthy pH (acid–alkali balance) without drawing calcium from our bones. Lemon juice can have a similar effect.

Lemon acids help the body maintain a healthy acid–alkali balance. And the acids in lemon juice consumed before a meal are likely to discourage high blood sugar afterwards, both in healthy people and in those with diabetes.

Lemons' antioxidants may reduce inflammation associated with heart disease, arthritis and Alzheimer's disease. And consuming lemons may discourage certain cancers, and strokes.

Lemon juice is rich in vitamin C and a large US study found that, on average, men who consumed most vitamin C from the fruit and vegetables in their diet lived six years longer than those who consumed least, while women lived one year longer.[5]

Mice given a daily supplement of lemon polyphenols lived longer than other mice. Note that polyphenols are both antioxidant and anti-inflammatory.[6]

Finally, lemons' pectin encourages elimination of toxic heavy metals, such as aluminium and lead, from the gut (and is

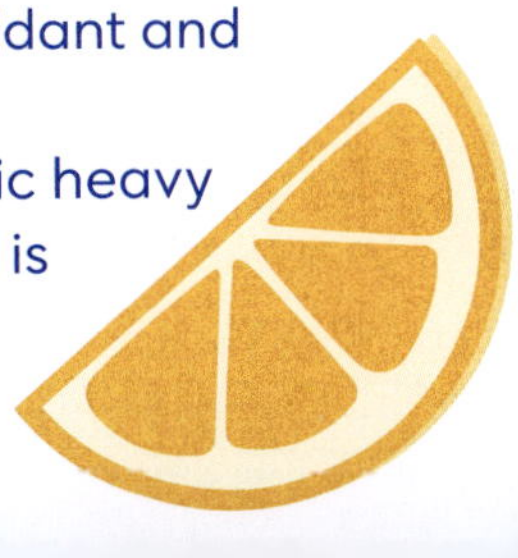

prescribed for this in Russia). Such metals encourage premature degeneration and ageing of brain and other cells. Lemons are rich in pectin.

+ ACTION: Consume the zest and juice of a lemon each day.

OLIVE OIL

Consuming this may be an important way of helping to delay the signs of premature ageing, thanks to its healthy fats and possible blood sugar-lowering properties. Consider these studies:

Researchers who followed 12,161 people in Spain for 10.7 years associated consuming 1½ tablespoons of virgin olive oil a day with a one-third lower risk of death from all causes, and half the risk of death from cardiovascular causes. These effects were not associated with other olive oils.[7]

US researchers examined nearly 30 years of information on 90,000 US health professionals in the Nurses' Health Study and Health Professionals Follow-up Study. They report that consuming more than 1½ teaspoons of olive oil a day reduced the risk of dying early from any cause by 19 per cent compared with consuming less.[8]

+ ACTION: Aim to consume at least 1½ tablespoons of extra-virgin olive oil a day.

HONEY

A survey in the 1980s of some of the world's oldest peoples found that three in four ate raw, unfiltered honey each day. If honey can indeed help maximize lifespan, one possible reason is that its antioxidants help prevent heart attacks, strokes and cancer.

Another is that honey can boost glutathione – a powerful antioxidant and detoxifier that slows ageing. To produce this from the amino acid homocysteine, our body requires vitamins B6 and B2 and zinc. These are quite often lacking, but honey can help fill the gap. Also, raw honey may help because it's an alkali-producing food (p.62).

+ ACTION: Take 1 teaspoon of raw honey 3 times a day.

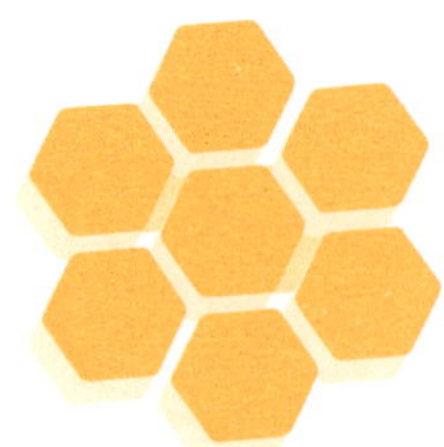

TEAS

Anti-inflammatory and antioxidant teas may help protect skin from damage and slow ageing.

A study of 5,998 Britons aged 37–73 and 7,931 Chinese aged 30–79 looked at the effects of daily consumption of green and black *Camellia-sinensis* teas on age markers including blood cholesterol, blood pressure and body-fat percentage. Drinking tea helped prevent crows' feet and slow the ageing process; 3 cups a day were associated with the most obvious benefits. Tea's polyphenols contributed to its anti-ageing benefits. These influence the gut microbiome, which in turn influences age-related changes in metabolism, immunity and cognitive function. There was negligible differences in ageing between black- and green-tea drinkers.[9]

+ ACTION: Include *Camellia-sinensis* teas in your diet.

Age-related cognitive decline

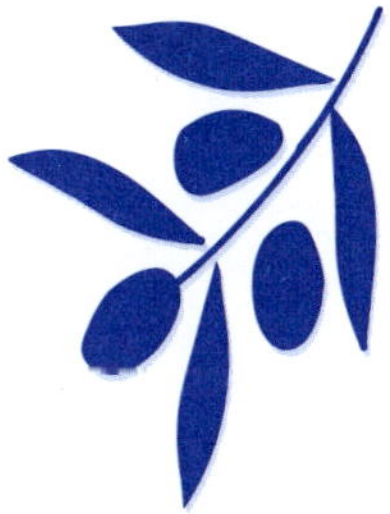

A healthy diet (p.58), regular exercise, keeping the brain active, social interaction and having a purpose in life help keep the brain in good condition.

OLIVE OIL

Olive oil's polyphenols are anti-inflammatory antioxidants that discourage memory loss and other cognitive decline. Its monounsaturated fatty acids help too, by keeping brain cell membranes healthy.

One study found that daily consumption of extra-virgin olive oil improved cognitive function in people with mild cognitive impairment.[10]

In a study of elderly people in southern Italy, age-related cognitive decline was least likely in those who consumed most monounsaturated fat. The amount of olive oil consumed was inversely proportional to memory loss.[11]

+ ACTION: Consume at least 2 tablespoons of extra-virgin olive oil each day.

GARLIC

Garlic's antioxidants discourage memory loss and other brainpower decline by helping prevent the oxidation of fatty acids, hormones and certain other substances in the brain. Garlic may also discourage artery disease, detoxify certain potentially damaging nerve-cell toxins, and encourage excretion of aluminium, lead and other heavy metals that can damage the brain.

A study reports that giving garlic extract to mice prone to early ageing increased their memory and learning ability. It also discouraged degeneration in the brain's frontal lobes. Nerve cells grew better too, suggesting enhanced memory.[12]

+ ACTION: Include garlic in your daily diet or take a garlic supplement. You need both water- and oil-soluble sulphur compounds (pp.78–9).

SPICES

Anti-inflammatory and antioxidant spices may help.

+ ACTION: Include these spices in your diet.

Age spots

The most common of these are freckles ("liver spots") caused by normal ageing, plus photo-ageing (accelerated ageing from sun exposure).

APPLE CIDER VINEGAR

Some people report that applying this – particularly if mixed with onion juice – lightens age spots.

+ ACTION: Finely chop an onion, wrap it in muslin and squeeze out the juice. Mix 2 teaspoons of cider vinegar with 1 teaspoon of onion juice, apply the mixture to the freckles twice a day and leave it on for 5 minutes. They may begin to lighten within 6 weeks.

LEMONS

Some people say lemon juice lightens age spots.

+ ACTIONS: Apply lemon juice each day, and the spots may begin to lighten within 6 weeks. Include the zest and juice of a lemon in your daily diet, as their antioxidants may delay age freckles and other signs of skin ageing.

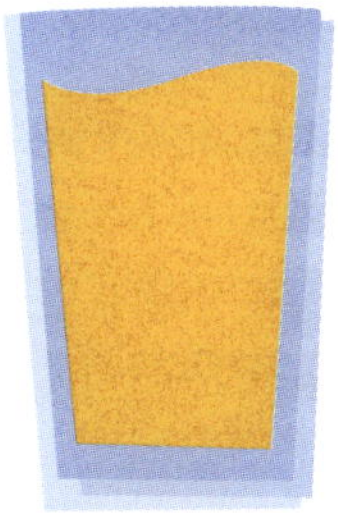

Alcohol intoxication

Alcohol can be enjoyable and relaxing but too much can be uncomfortable, even dangerous.

OLIVE OIL

Some people believe that consuming 1 tablespoon of olive oil before drinking alcohol discourages a hangover.

+ ACTION: Try swallowing 1 tablespoon of olive oil – either with food or on its own – before drinking alcohol.

SPICES AND TEAS

Anti-inflammatory, antioxidant and cholinergic spices and teas may help. In particular, try ginger, turmeric, or chamomile or mint tea.

+ ACTION: Include these spices and teas in your diet.

Alzheimer's disease

This causes seven in ten cases of dementia and is associated with several problems in the brain:

- Inflammation associated with clumps of amyloid protein between cells that control memory, and with tangled fibres of tau protein within brain cells.
- Low levels of the neurotransmitter (nerve message carrier) acetylcholine, which aids memory. Indeed, the level may be only 90 per cent of normal! This is now thought to result from the loss of acetylcholine-producing brain cells.
- Astonishingly, 81 per cent of people with Alzheimer's disease have type 2 diabetes! Their brain cells become more resistant to the sugar-regulating hormone insulin than do the brain cells of others with type 2 diabetes. This encourages poor brain-cell function. Some experts dub this subset of type 2 diabetes, "type 3 diabetes".

Alzheimer's disease is encouraged by a serious head injury. It can run in families and is associated with ageing. The underlying cause may be a combination of cardiovascular and metabolic diseases. Research suggests that inflammation and damage due to oxidation of the brain's two most abundant polyunsaturated fatty acids (docosahexaenoic and arachidonic acids) are partly to blame. Also, affected people have high levels of the amino acid homocysteine. A lack of B vitamins raises its levels, but people with Alzheimer's are particularly likely to eat a diet lacking in these vitamins.

Recent research found similarly changed patterns of gene expression in the brain in people with Alzheimer's and in those with "alcohol-use disorder", supporting the idea that alcohol could make Alzheimer's progress faster.[13]

The most reliable medical drugs for people with mild to moderate Alzheimer's disease are acetylcholinesterase inhibitors, such as donepezil. These work by preventing the enzyme acetylcholinesterase from breaking down acetylcholine, so raising the level of acetylcholine.

APPLE CIDER VINEGAR

Several studies suggest a small daily dose of aspirin or other non-steroidal anti-inflammatory drug discourages Alzheimer's disease. There isn't enough evidence for doctors to recommend such drugs long-term. But apple cider vinegar made from unpeeled apples is a good source of salicylates, which have aspirin-like qualities.

A study of mice indicated that cider vinegar may help protect against Alzheimer's.[14]

+ ACTION: Include apple cider vinegar in your daily diet, as this might help prevent Alzheimer's.

LEMONS

Lemons may help, as their polyphenols are anti-inflammatory. They also contain helpful B vitamins. Lemon peel is rich in flavonoid polyphenols such as hesperidin, nobiletin and quercetin that can slow or reverse memory impairment. Consider the following studies:

- A study lasting several years in Japan, involving more than 13,000 middle-aged or elderly people, found that consuming lemons or other citrus fruit daily can reduce the risk of Alzheimer's by almost 23 per cent compared with consuming them less than twice a week.[15]

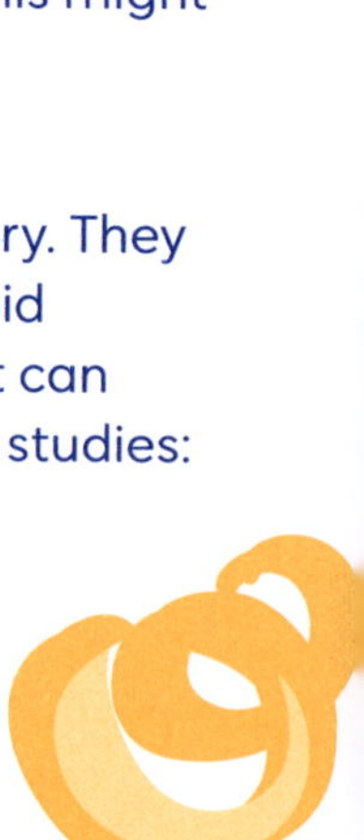

- Note that lemons' anti-inflammatory polyphenols can penetrate the blood–brain barrier.[16]
- Laboratory tests in the US and Korea found that quercetin helps protect against oxidation of rat brain cells.[17]

+ ACTION: Aim to include grated lemon peel and lemon juice in your daily diet.

OLIVE OIL

Extra-virgin olive oil's anti-inflammatory antioxidants counter the oxidation and inflammation of brain fats that accompanies Alzheimer's. Also, the oil's monounsaturated fats help to keep brain-cell membranes healthy. And:

- Researchers say the polyphenol oleocanthal can bind to amyloid protein and reduce its damaging effects. Oleocanthal is plentiful in olive oil.[18]
- An overview of studies, including one of over 1.5 million people found that strict adherence to the Mediterranean diet cuts the risk of Alzheimer's by 13 per cent, presumably partly because of its healthy balance of fats and its high content of anti-inflammatory polyphenols.[19]

+ ACTION: Have at least 2 tablespoons of extra-virgin olive oil each day.

HONEY

Honey discourages oxidation, can lower inflammatory prostaglandins and homocysteine, and contains small amounts of acetylcholine.

High blood sugar can encourage Alzheimer's by damaging ("glycating") brain-cell proteins. Honey triggers lower blood sugar spikes than does sugar.

In a five-year study, 2,290 "cognitively intact" people and 603 with mild cognitive impairment, all aged 65 and older, ate one tablespoon a day of Middle East honey or a placebo (dummy medication). Only 95 of the honey group developed dementia, compared with 394 of the others.[20]

+ ACTION: Eat 1 teaspoon of raw, antioxidant-rich honey 3 times a day, including 1 teaspoon within the hour before bedtime.

GARLIC

Possible culprits behind Alzheimer's include inflammation, as this encourages oxidation of brain fats, and high levels of the amino acid homocysteine. A lack of B vitamins raises homocysteine, and people with Alzheimer's are particularly likely to go short of this vitamin. Garlic's anti-inflammatory antioxidants and B vitamins may help.

In one study, Alzheimer's-prone mice were fed aged garlic extract, which helped prevent early memory loss.[21]

Bioactives in garlic boost the amounts of the neurotransmitter acetylcholine by inhibiting the enzyme acetylcholinesterase that breaks down acetylcholine. This can benefit memory and cognitive ability. Note that the Alzheimer's drug donezepil is an acetylcholinesterase inhibitor.

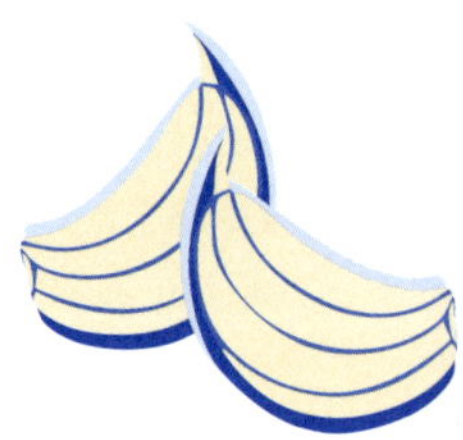

+ ACTION: Include garlic in your diet or take a garlic supplement. You need both water- and oil-soluble sulphur compounds (pp.78–9).

SPICES

Anti-inflammatory, antioxidant and cholinergic spices (p.89) may help. Both fennel seeds and saffron boost the activity of the brain's acetylcholine. Early research has found that cayenne pepper, cinnamon and turmeric contain compounds that reduce amyloid. Animal research suggsts that an alkaloid called piperine in black pepper helps protect against nerve-cell degeneration and cognitive impairment. And turmeric can help boost memory.

+ ACTION: Include these spices in your diet.

TEAS

A Polish review reports that *Camellia-sinensis* tea can help Alzheimer's disease. Analysis of *Camellia-sinensis* tea revealed acetylcholinesterase-inhibitor action. So it joins several other teas in having "cholinergic" action.[22]

Other researchers have correlated tea's strong anti-acetylcholinesterase activity with its high content of polyphenols. Epigallocatechin, epicatechin and rutin are among those that help protect cognitive function. One study found green tea more effective than black, thanks to it having more epigallocatechin gallate.

Studies confirm that regular tea-drinking can improve speech quality and fluency and help prevent cognitive function deteriorating.[23] Tea's caffeine can help symptoms too, thanks to its stimulatory effects on the brain.

Cholinergic, anti-inflammatory and antioxidant teas may be useful. Notably, laboratory research suggests that basil[24] can reduce amyloid, butterfly pea's flavonoids[25] can improve memory and prevent memory loss; mint[26] can improve cognitive ability; and lemon balm[27] can reduce the agitation often associated with Alzheimer's.

+ ACTION: Include these teas in your diet.

Anaemia

The most common type of anaemia is caused by iron deficiency and/or poor absorption of iron into the body.

APPLE CIDER VINEGAR

Iron-deficiency anaemia can be associated with having the low stomach acid that affects one in two over-60s. A lack of stomach acid can reduce iron absorption from food. Vitamin B12-deficiency anaemia is another possible result. Iron-deficiency anaemia can also result from stress, prolonged use of antacid or acid-suppressant medication, and not having a healthy diet (p.58).

+ ACTIONS: If you are anaemic, try improving your nutrient absorption by drinking a glass of water containing 2 teaspoons of cider vinegar in water before each meal, or by adding cider vinegar to a salad dressing or a soup.

LEMONS

In someone who lacks stomach acid, a lemon's acidity could aid digestion by raising stomach acidity. In addition, gut bacteria break down a lemon's pectin, releasing short-chain fatty acids which boost iron absorption by raising acidity.

+ ACTION: Drink a glass of water containing 2 teaspoons of lemon juice before each meal.

HONEY

Honey contains iron (vital for the production of haemoglobin – the red pigment that carries oxygen in the blood), copper (aids iron absorption) and manganese (helps build haemoglobin). The amounts are small, but nevertheless may help. Consider this study:

- When 10 volunteers in Dubai took a daily 1.2g of honey per 1kg (2.2lb) bodyweight for 2 weeks, blood tests revealed a 20 per cent increase in iron, a 33 per cent increase in copper, and slight increases in haemoglobin and red cells.[28]

+ ACTION: Eat 1 teaspoon of honey 3 times a day. Ideally, choose dark honey as it's richer in iron.

TEAS

If you have iron-deficiency anaemia, dandelion and nettle teas offer iron, and dong quai tea can boost blood cell production.
+ ACTION: Include these teas in your diet.

Ankle swelling

The many causes include too much salty food; obesity; pregnancy; arthritis; varicose veins; sitting or standing in the same position too long; certain medications (for example, certain blood pressure medicines and antidepressants, and steroids); deep vein thrombosis (a blood clot) in the leg; heart, kidney or liver failure; injury; and surgery.

LEMONS

These contain rutin, a flavonoid that strengthens vein walls, so may reduce ankle swelling caused by fluid seeping from varicose veins. Lemons may also help ease any fluid retention associated with heart or kidney disease as they have diuretic action – meaning they increase urine production.
+ ACTION: Include the zest and juice of a lemon in your daily diet.

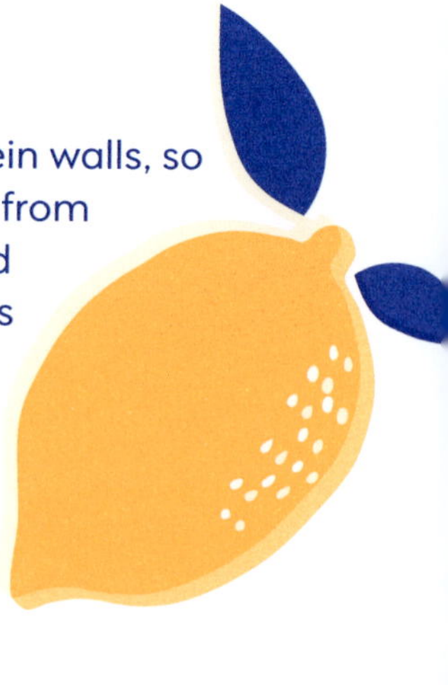

Anxiety

Continued anxiety, if not carefully managed, encourages long-term health problems, partly via its effects on the hypothalamus and the pituitary gland in the brain.

These can include addictive behaviours, arthritis, depression, digestive problems, fibromyalgia, headaches, high blood pressure, irregular heartbeat, infection, infertility, insomnia, irritable bowel syndrome, heart attacks, poor memory, aching muscles, peptic ulcers, polycystic ovary syndrome, premature ageing, psoriasis, sleep problems, social withdrawal, strokes, teeth grinding and weight gain or loss.

Not having a healthy diet (p.58) encourages an unhealthy gut microbiome, which may disturb our levels of calming neuro-transmitters (nerve message carriers) such as GABA (gamma-aminobutyric acid) and serotonin.

Also, dehydration can encourage anxiety. An increase in the "stress hormone" adrenaline tenses muscles, so boosting energy production in muscle cells and releasing acidic lactate. And severe, continued stress encourages mild acidosis (p.62) that in turn can encourage anxiety.

Importantly, a UK-biobank study of more than 144,000 people showed that those with anxiety and depression had increased inflammatory markers (C-reactive protein and interleukin 6).[29]

LEMONS

These might help as our need for vitamins B and C, calcium, magnesium, potassium and zinc rises during stress, and lemons are rich in these. Also, lemons can help the body maintain its normal acid–alkali balance and help counter the adverse effects of inflammation. Added to this, the scent of lemon oil is said to alleviate stress.

+ ACTIONS: Consume the zest and juice of 1–2 lemons a day. Consider using a few drops of calming lemon essential oil in an aromatherapy diffuser or massage blend.

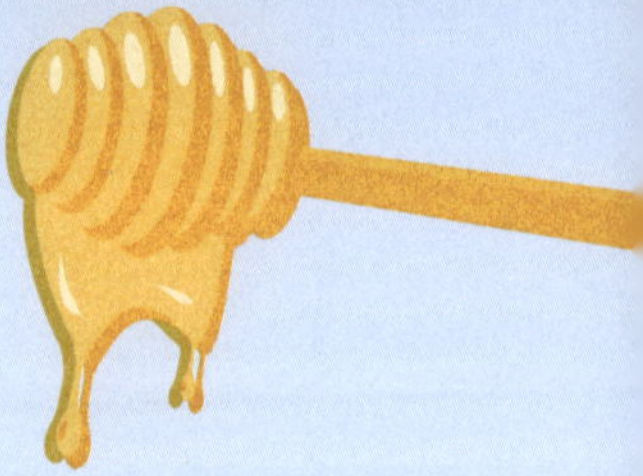

HONEY

This can help anxiety in several ways:

- Pleasure from its fragrance and flavour can boost the production of serotonin, a calming and "lifting" neurotransmitter.
- It contains tryptophan, which is needed for serotonin production.
- It's a high-carbohydrate, low-protein food, so helps tryptophan enter the brain.
- It's particularly good at boosting liver glycogen. A good store of this protects the brain's energy supply, preventing the need for adrenaline to increase blood sugar in response to stress – and in so doing increase anxiety.
- It's an alkali-producing food.

Consider these studies:

- A Malaysian analysis of 34 studies found honey had anti-stress effects.[30]
- In a study at Waikato University, New Zealand, 45 rats received a sugar-free diet or a diet containing sugar or honey. After 1 year, those in the honey group were less anxious.[31]

+ ACTION: Eat 1 teaspoon of raw honey 3 times a day, with the last one in the hour before bedtime.

SPICES

Studies suggest anti-adrenaline (p.87) and calming spices (p.89) help.
+ ACTION: Include these spices in your diet.

TEAS

Antispasmodic and tranquillizing teas may help (p.98) – in particular, passionflower tea. Research suggests this may be as good at relieving anxiety as the anti-anxiety drug oxazepam, but faster! Lavender tea can make GABA (gamma-aminobutyric acid) – a relaxing neurotransmitter – more efficient. Even inhaling the fragrance of a cup of lavender tea can reduce anxiety.
+ ACTIONS: Include these teas in your diet. Also, inhale the fragrance of the steam from any of these hot teas, especially lavender.

Artery disease

This causes poor circulation, encouraging thin dry skin, cold feet, leg pain on walking, impotence and dementia. It can also cause heart attacks, strokes and an aneurysm (p.132).

Not having a healthy diet (p.58) is a major risk factor, as it encourages high blood pressure and a tendency to inflammation. It also encourages obesity and unhealthy blood fats (high LDL cholesterol – which if oxidized is "bad"; and low HDL cholesterol – the "good" sort). The result is atherosclerosis (p.131), which narrows and stiffens arteries. High blood sugar from an unhealthy diet stiffens artery walls further by damaging ("glycating") their collagen. Other risk factors include smoking and inactivity.

Also, high blood levels of the amino acid homocysteine encourage inflammation, impairing artery-lining-cell function and encouraging blood clots. Possible causes include a lack of foods containing plant oestrogens (which help relax arteries), and low vitamin B6, B12 and folic acid. An underactive thyroid and certain medications can also be to blame.

Researchers in China who investigated 14,323 people to ascertain the association between dietary choline intake and cardiovascular disease (CVD) found that a higher dietary intake of the neurotransmitter choline was associated with a lower risk of CVD – especially of strokes. This suggests that besides eating choline-rich foods (such as eggs, other animal-source foods, almonds, broccoli, chickpeas, soybeans, kidney beans), cholinergic spices and teas may help.[32]

APPLE CIDER VINEGAR

A meta-analysis of nine studies, involving 686 people, found that taking apple cider vinegar improved total cholesterol, especially for people with diabetes. The authors suggest 15ml (1 tablespoon) a day is the ideal amount. But more research is needed.[33]

HONEY

Honey triggers lower blood sugar spikes than does table sugar. Consider the following studies:

- A laboratory study shows that honey discourages blood clotting, possibly thanks to its hydrogen peroxide, antioxidants or sugars.[34]
- In a study of 55 volunteers at Mashhad University of Medical Science, Iran, the 38 who included 70g of honey in their daily diet for 4 weeks had lower fasting levels in their blood of LDL cholesterol, triglycerides and C-reactive protein (a marker of inflammation) than those who had 70g of sucrose (table sugar).[35]
- Researchers at Qassim University, Saudi Arabia, found that giving honey to rats helped normalize high homocysteine.[36]
- A study in Dubai compared the effects of consuming 75g (2.6oz) of honey each day for 15 days in healthy people and those with high blood fats. Honey reduced blood cholesterol and a blood-marker of inflammation called C-reactive protein – but only in those with high blood fats.[37]

Also, honey's flavonoids and other antioxidants help protect collagen. This helps keep arteries pliable and strengthens capillary walls, encouraging good blood flow.

Chronic metabolic stress (p.152) can encourage artery disease by triggering pre-diabetes and high blood fats. Raw honey may help as it's an alkali-producing food (p.62).

+ ACTION: Eat 1 teaspoon of raw honey 3 times a day, including 1 teaspoon within the hour before bedtime. Antioxidant-rich honey (pp.74–6) might be especially useful.

GARLIC

Garlic is a traditional remedy for this ailment. Consider these reviews:

- A research review at John Moore University, Liverpool, suggests that the more garlic that's eaten, the less likely is artery disease to progress. This is extraordinary![38]
- A meta-analysis of 14 studies concluded that garlic can lower total cholesterol and LDL cholesterol (the sort that when oxidized is bad for us).[39]

Scientists believe garlic may have protective effects because various water- and oil-soluble sulphur compounds are anti-inflammatory; boost hydrogen sulphide; and inhibit ACE (see below) – which reduces blood pressure by expanding arteries. They also say that garlic's:

- Allicin derivatives produce nitric oxide, which reduces blood pressure by relaxing smooth muscle in artery walls; they also help counter atheroma
- Gamma-glutamyl cysteines act like ACE- (angiotensin-converting enzyme) inhibitor drugs, used for high blood pressure, heart failure and strokes
- Antioxidants discourage oxidation of LDL cholesterol, and inflammation
- Manganese aids certain antioxidant enzymes and boosts HDL cholesterol (the good sort)
- S-allyl cysteine acts like a statin (a drug that combats high cholesterol); and its vitamin B6 lowers the amino acid homocysteine (which can damage artery walls)

Bioactives in garlic boost the neurotransmitter acetylcholine by inhibiting the enzyme, acetylcholinesterase, that breaks it down. Good acetylcholine levels may help prevent or treat artery disease.

Garlic has antioxidant and blood pressure-reducing effects. It may also have modest anti-clotting and blood cholesterol- and blood triglyceride-reducing effects, and help ageing arteries stay stretchy. For example:

- An Indian study reports that garlic given to mice on a fatty diet reduced blood cholesterol. Garlic also acted like statins by blocking the enzyme (hydroxyl-methyl-glutaryl Co-A reductase) necessary for cholesterol production in the liver.[40]
- An Iranian study found that garlic extract strongly inhibited angiotensin-converting enzyme (ACE) production. ACE-inhibition lowers blood pressure by reducing angiotensin II and bradykinin. It also reduces extra-cellular fluid by diminishing secretion of the hormone aldosterone. All this would reduce high blood pressure.[41]

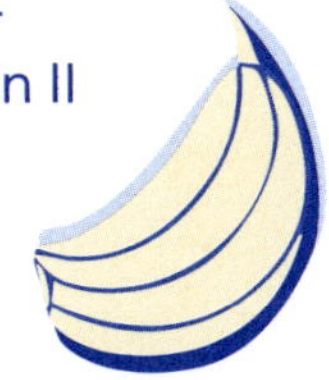

Giving garlic extract to volunteers with atherosclerosis for 6 months reduced oxidation in their blood. Garlic boiled for 20 minutes had the same effect as raw garlic.[42]

SPICES

Anti-inflammatory, antioxidant, anticoagulant, blood sugar-lowering and cholinergic spices may help. In particular, use cinnamon, mastic, cocoa (a high intake of which is associated with a halving of deaths from heart attacks and strokes) and sesame seeds.

Certain natural health practitioners even claim that drinking cayenne tea, or putting cayenne extract ("tincture") under the tongue or capsaicin cream on the skin can help prevent too much damage from a heart attack or a stroke. But there is no scientific proof.

+ ACTION: Include these spices in your diet.

TEAS

Anti-inflammatory, antioxidant, anticoagulant, blood sugar-lowering and cholinergic teas may help.

+ ACTION: Include these teas in your diet.

Arthritis

Inflammation links most of the many sorts of arthritis, so it's wise to eat a healthy diet as this is inflammatory (p.58). There is a lower likelihood of arthritis in Mediterranean countries, where the traditional diet contains little red meat.

Rheumatoid arthritis is less common in vegetarians and vegans. They are less likely than meat-eaters to have an acid-forming diet. It is also less common in people who eat more cruciferous vegetables (such as broccoli and cabbage) and fruit.

Rheumatoid arthritis is linked with the intake of wheat, sugar, salt and coffee – all of which are acid-producing. People with it are also more likely to have antibodies to milk, cereal, eggs, fish and pork, suggesting their body views these as threats; it's possible that such a diet might encourage rheumatoid symptoms as part of an immune response triggered by a food sensitivity. All this suggests an acid-producing diet encourages rheumatoid arthritis.

Osteoarthritis was once considered to result from "wear and tear" on joints. Now it's also known to involve inflammation – both generalized throughout the body and within affected joints.

Osteoarthritis can be linked with mild acidosis (p.62). If the kidneys excrete acidic salts fast enough, such salts can crystallize in joint fluid and trigger inflammation. The form of arthritis called gout can also be triggered by mild metabolic acidosis.

In one study, daily meat consumption was associated with double the risk compared with eating it less often. It also suggested a higher risk with more protein in general.[43]

APPLE CIDER VINEGAR

Although some people claim this helps their arthritis, others disagree. While it's certainly possible that people might react in different ways, the jury remains out.

+ ACTION: See if including cider vinegar in your diet helps. A folk remedy for arthritis in hands or feet is to soak them 3 times a day in a solution of 1 cup of cider vinegar and 3 cups of hot water.

LEMONS

Lemons' antioxidants help reduce inflammation.

Some people believe they should avoid lemons as they are acidic. But we metabolize lemon acids into potassium carbonate, which helps prevent excess acidity in the body. Indeed, consuming lemons helps prevent mild acidosis (p.62).

Consuming vinegar before a meal discourages high blood sugar after. Experts say lemon acids are likely to behave in the same way.

A study of more than 20,000 volunteers who kept diet diaries and were arthritis-free when the study began, indicates that vitamin C-rich foods such as lemons can help protect against inflammatory polyarthritis. This arthritis was more than three times as likely in those who consumed the least vitamin C-rich foods as in those who ate the most.[44]

A US study found that rheumatoid arthritis was less likely in women who ate more fruit and cruciferous vegetables (rocket, pak choi, broccoli, brussels sprouts, cabbage, cauliflower, collards, kale, radishes and watercress).[45]

The anti-inflammatory antioxidant hesperidin in lemons may reduce joint inflammation.[46]

+ ACTIONS: Include the zest and juice of a lemon in your daily diet. Massage the skin over your joints with 1 drop each of lemon and pine oils in 2 teaspoons of olive oil.

OLIVE OIL

This can help fight inflammation (p.224). A study of 365 people with rheumatoid arthritis found that consuming olive oil had a favourable effect, especially for those whose symptoms were more severe than average.[47]

+ ACTION: Consume 2 tablespoons of extra-virgin olive oil each day. If your symptoms are bad, try consuming 4 tablespoons a day.

HONEY

Honey contains anti-inflammatory compounds. Honey before bedtime can discourage inflammation (p.224). Honey's flavonoids and other antioxidants help protect collagen in joints, and honey lowers a raised level of the amino acid homocysteine, which is linked with a raised risk of rheumatoid arthritis. Raw honey may be particularly helpful as it's an alkali-producing food (p.62).

+ ACTIONS: Eat 1 teaspoon of raw honey 3 times a day, including 1 teaspoon within the hour before bedtime. Try massaging honey into the skin over a painful joint.

GARLIC

Early evidence suggests garlic's anti-inflammatory antioxidants benefit arthritic joints.

A UK study of more than 1,000 women found that osteoarthritis of the hip was less likely in those whose diet was high in garlic and other alliums. Also, in a laboratory experiment, diallyl disulphide reduced levels of cartilage-damaging enzymes.[48]

A study in Iran of 80 women with osteoarthritis in one or both knees and who were also obese found that eating garlic every day reduced their knee pain.[49]

+ ACTION: Include garlic in your daily diet or take a garlic supplement. You need both water- and oil-soluble sulphur compounds (pp.78–9).

SPICES

Anti-inflammatory, antioxidant, blood vessel-relaxing and pain-relieving spices may help. In particular, use chilli and cayenne. For osteoarthritis, try turmeric; for rheumatoid arthritis, ginger and nigella. Celery seeds inhibit certain inflammatory enzymes (COX-1 and COX-2) that encourage arthritis. Galangal makes cartilage stronger and healthier, and capsaicin cream is the preferred treatment for severe knee osteoarthritis.

+ ACTION: Include these spices in your diet. Apply a skin cream, massage oil, compress or poultice containing one of these spices over the affected joint, or apply capsaicin cream, available from a pharmacy or via the internet.

TEAS

Anti-inflammatory, antioxidant, antispasmodic and pain-relieving teas may help. In particular, note that rosehip tea may reduce pain and boost joint mobility in people with osteoarthritis. Also, nettle tea can reduce the need for medication for osteoarthritis.

+ ACTIONS: Include these teas in your diet. Apply a compress or poultice containing one of these teas to the affected joint.

Asthma

Inflammation and oversensitivity of the lungs' airways cause wheezing, difficulty in breathing (particularly breathing out), coughing and a tight chest. Triggers include cold air, exercise, certain foods, hormone changes, laughter, infection, various inhaled chemicals, a sudden fall in air pressure, thunderstorms, exposure to allergens and rapid breathing.

An unhealthy diet (p.58) can encourage asthma in asthma-prone people by causing mild acidosis (p.62) and inflammation. Such a diet is high in acid-forming foods (for example, red meat and ultra-processed foods) and low in alkali-forming ones (for example, vegetables and fruit). It can also make airway-widening asthma medication less effective early in an asthma attack.

All this is particularly likely in people whose weight is unhealthily high. One study, for example, showed that in overweight or obese children, a diet high in acid-forming foods was associated with a 95 per cent increase in the risk of asthma. One possible reason is that it causes slight inflammation throughout the body. This, in turn, could encourage asthma by inflaming the lining of the airways and making them over-react to asthma triggers.

The fluid in the lining of normal lung airways is slightly alkaline. But in people with mild asthma the fluid is slightly acidic. This slight acidity can cause a cough and make the airways narrower than they should be. It can also make the muscle fibres in the lining of the airways over-sensitive to such things as cold air and inhaled and irritating chemicals.

The following remedies are safe to try alongside any asthma medication prescribed for you.

LEMONS

These contain anti-inflammatory antioxidants. One of these, the polyphenol quercetin, acts as an antihistamine.

+ ACTIONS: If you suspect low stomach acid (for example, because you get indigestion that can't be relieved by antacids), try taking 2 teaspoons of lemon juice 3 times a day in the attempt to help prevent asthma. Or drink lemon juice early in an attack. For an adult, put 1 tablespoon of it in a glass of water and sip it over half an hour. Wait for 30 minutes, then repeat. For a child, use less, depending on their size.

OLIVE OIL

Researchers have linked olive oil consumption with lower rates of asthma, possibly thanks to its monounsaturated fats, oleocanthal and other anti-inflammatories. Also, olive oil's quercetin acts as an antihistamine. Oleocanthal and quercetin are both flavonoid polyphenols.

Italian researchers studied the association between asthma and dietary fats in 871 people aged 20–84. Of these, 145 currently had asthma, 77 had had it, 305 had rhinitis (nasal inflammation, causing, for example, nasal congestion) and 344 acted as "controls". High olive oil intake was associated with a lower risk of asthma.[50]

A study in Crete of nearly 700 children aged 7–18 shows that good adherence to the Mediterranean diet helped prevent asthma.[51]

+ ACTION: To help prevent asthma, consume 2 tablespoons of extra-virgin olive oil each day.

GARLIC

Garlic is a traditional remedy for asthma, and early evidence suggests its anti-inflammatory antioxidants (such as quercetin) may help. It may help in other ways too:

In one study, allicin-containing garlic extract relaxed smooth muscle in rats' windpipes. Aspirin and indomethacin, which inhibit the production of certain prostaglandins (hormone-like substances), reduced this relaxation. The conclusion was that garlic extract relaxed smooth muscle by stimulating the release of these prostaglandins.[52]

Iranian researchers report that giving aged garlic extract to mice with allergic airway inflammation decreased this inflammation. It also decreased eosinophil white cells and immunoglobulin-1 antibodies, which are markers of allergy.[53]

+ ACTION: Include garlic in your daily diet or take a garlic supplement. You need water- and oil-soluble sulphur compounds (pp.78–9).

HONEY

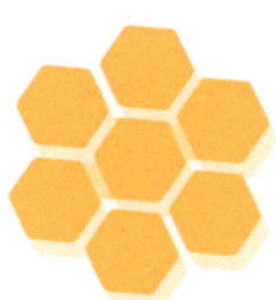

Its natural antihistamines might help.

+ ACTION: Include honey in your diet.

SPICES

Antihistamine, anti-inflammatory, antioxidant, astringent and antispasmodic spices may help prevent asthma. In particular, try cassia, cloves and nigella. Note that ajowan and aniseed can widen airways in the same way as the asthma drug theophylline.

+ ACTION: Include these spices in your diet.

TEAS

Anti-allergic, antihistamine, anti-inflammatory, antioxidant and antispasmodic teas may help.

+ ACTIONS: Include these teas in your diet. Also inhale steam from one of them once or twice a day.

Atherosclerosis

This is a major feature of artery disease and encourages high blood pressure, heart disease including heart attacks, poor circulation (p.261), poor memory and strokes.

It begins when high blood pressure, cigarette-smoke toxins, high blood fats, high blood sugar or mild acidosis (p.62), or any combination of these, damages the lining of artery walls throughout the body. This lets LDL cholesterol seep from blood into the artery lining. "Free radicals" (highly reactive oxygen particles in the blood, encouraged by not having a healthy diet (p.58) and by infection and smoking), can oxidize this LDL cholesterol, producing oxidized LDL cholesterol (the bad sort). White blood cells engulf this, swelling to become "foam cells" that inflame the lining of arteries. Calcium infiltrates the inflamed lining, and smooth muscle cells in the artery walls make collagen to help cover the damage. The resulting fatty, chalky, inflamed patches are called "atheroma" or plaque. This builds up, stiffening arteries and making them less elastic, so encouraging high blood pressure.

Particularly large, fatty or inflamed patches of atheroma are unstable. At worst, such a plaque can rupture, resulting in bleeding or encouraging a blood clot that can fully or partially block the artery. Or a bit of unstable plaque could break off and be swept away in the blood. An errant clot or bit of plaque reaching an artery in the heart can trigger a heart attack. One reaching a brain artery can partially block the artery, causing a "mini" thrombotic stroke (transient ischaemic attack or TIA), or block it fully, causing a thrombotic stroke. Bleeding in the brain from an atherosclerotic artery causes a haemorrhagic stroke. Atherosclerosis can also make an artery wall bulge. This bulge is called an aneurysm. Its rupture can cause life-threatening bleeding; and bleeding from an aneurysm in the brain can also trigger a haemorrhagic stroke.

GARLIC

This can discourage abnormal blood clotting by:

- Making tiny particles in blood called platelets less sticky, so less likely to encourage a clot
- Boosting production of nitric oxide, which helps prevent platelets sticking to artery walls and encouraging clots. Nitric oxide also dilates blood vessels, reducing blood pressure and the risk of a clot getting stuck

- Reducing inflammation and, perhaps, blood sugar (which is important because sugary blood clots more easily) and fibrinogen (a clotting factor)

Garlic may discourage permanent damage from a heart attack. Crushing it before cooking it for a short time helps conserve its anti-clotting ability.

+ ACTION: Include garlic in your diet or take a garlic supplement. You need water- and oil-soluble sulphur compounds (pp.78–9).

Athlete's foot

This fungal infection makes skin between toes sore and soggy and is often picked up in changing rooms or around swimming pools.

APPLE CIDER VINEGAR

Anecdotal reports suggest apple cider vinegar might help.

+ ACTION: Each day bathe feet for 5–10 minutes in warm water containing 4 tablespoons of cider vinegar and 10 drops of tea tree oil.

LEMONS

Anecdotal reports suggest lemon juice might help relieve athete's foot.

+ ACTION: Soak a cotton pad in lemon juice and apply to the affected area. Or bathe feet in a bowl of water containing 2 tablespoons of lemon juice.

GARLIC

Several studies report that garlic, or the compound found in garlic called ajoene, is a useful antifungal agent. For example:

A study of 50 people with athlete's foot in New Jersey compared 1 week's twice-daily application of a 1 per cent ajoene solution with the same-frequency application of the antifungal medication terbinafine. Ajoene had a 100 per cent cure rate; terbinafine 94 per cent.[54]

+ ACTIONS: Do a patch test (p.82) to check garlic is safe for your skin. Apply garlic oil macerate or garlic oil (p.80) twice a day. Or bathe the area with garlic water (p.81). Include garlic in your diet or take a garlic supplement. Choose an oil-soluble sulphur compound, in particular, ajoene (p.79).

Autoimmune diseases

In these, the immune system mistakenly attacks healthy parts of the body as if they were diseased. Examples include type 1 diabetes, multiple sclerosis, autoimmune thyroid disease (Graves' disease), pernicious anemia, rheumatoid arthritis, reactive arthritis, coeliac disease (sensitivity of the bowel to the protein gluten in many grains) and inflammatory bowel disease (Crohn's disease and ulcerative colitis).

APPLE CIDER VINEGAR

This has antioxidant and anti-inflammatory properties.

+ ACTION: Consume 1–2 tablespoons of cider vinegar each day for a few weeks to see if this reduces your symptoms.

OLIVE OIL

Italian researchers who studied 365 people with rheumatoid arthritis reported that higher consumption of olive oil had a favourable effect on symptoms and on the level of the inflammation marker C-reactive protein in blood.[55]

+ ACTION: Include olive oil in your diet.

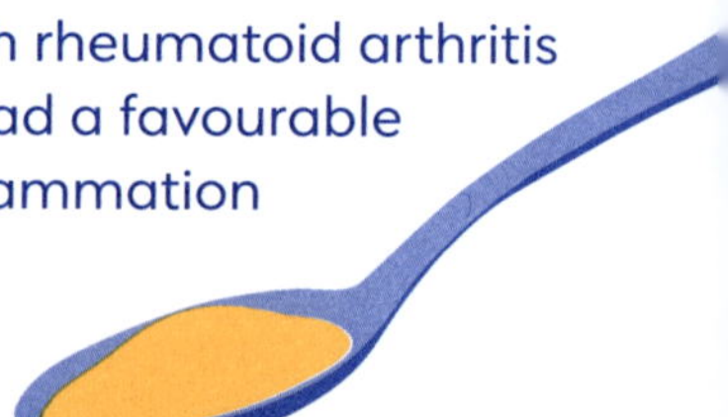

TEAS

Camellia-sinensis tea's catechins may reduce the raised levels of autoantibodies associated with diseases such as lupus.

+ ACTION: Include this tea in your diet.

Bad breath

Residues of meat or refined carbohydrate on or between teeth can cause bad breath. Their breakdown by mouth bacteria releases unpleasant-smelling compounds.

The body cells of people who eat a high-protein, low-carbohydrate diet, or have uncontrolled diabetes, produce energy from fats instead of sugar. This leads to a build-up of acidic ketones in blood. These taint breath with the scent of pear drops or nail-polish remover.

Good oral hygiene is essential, with twice-daily tooth-brushing, plus the use of dental floss or an inter-dental brush, to clean between teeth. Regular dental checks are also a good policy.

SODIUM BICARBONATE

A study at Duke University found that 63 per cent of people on a high-protein, low-carbohydrate diet reported bad breath.[56]

+ ACTIONS: Rinse your mouth with ½ a teaspoon of sodium bicarbonate in a glass of water. Eat a healthy diet (p.58).

CAUTION: Seek urgent medical help if your breath smells of ketones and you have diabetes, or suspect you have.

SPICES

Antibacterial spices such as allspice, cardamom, cinnamon or cloves may help.

+ ACTIONS: Chew a cardamom pod or a clove to clean teeth and reduce or disguise bad smells. Rinse your mouth with cinnamon or clove tea.

TEAS

Antibacterial tea may help, in particular barley or roasted-barley tea.

+ ACTION: Use these teas as a mouthwash.

Bedwetting

Many young children wet the bed. It's upsetting for a child to wake up with soggy bedsheets and pyjamas so it's a good idea to try to treat it.

HONEY

This is reputed to help prevent childhood bedwetting.
+ ACTION: Try giving 1 teaspoon of honey to your child within the hour before bedtime. (Make sure they rinse their mouth with water afterwards.)

Bronchitis and pneumonia

Bronchitis is inflammation of the lining of the lungs' main airways. It results from infection or allergy. Pneumonia is an infection of the lining of the lungs' tiny air-sacs.

LEMONS

Anti-inflammatory antioxidants seem to be protective, and quercetin (a flavonoid polyphenol) may play a key role. Pectin may help too.

Researchers have found that the high consumption of fibre and fruit is associated with less coughing. They believe flavonoids are partly responsible.[57]
+ ACTION: Include the zest and juice of a lemon in your daily diet.

GARLIC

People who eat garlic breathe out its volatile sulphur compounds. These have anti-infective, anti-inflammatory, detoxifying and immunity-stimulating properties. They can break down "biofilms" – thin sheets of bacteria in living tissue. They can also relax smooth muscle in airway walls – thus expanding airways and increasing airflow. Garlic syrup is an expectorant (encourages the coughing-up of phlegm). Garlic is a traditional remedy for pneumonia and studies suggest it can help viral pneumonia. It isn't yet certain if garlic is useful for bronchitis, but it's worth a try.
+ ACTIONS: Take 1–3 teaspoons of garlic syrup (p.81) 3 times a day to help cough up phlegm. Or include garlic in your diet or take a garlic supplement. Note that you need oil-soluble sulphur compounds (p.79).

Another option is to crush several garlic cloves, put them in a bowl, wait 30 minutes, then inhale the vapour from the garlic; repeat several times a day. Any stinging in the nose should quickly abate; if not, or if it's excessive, inhale from further away. Alternatively, do a patch test (p.82) and if there's no reaction, rub garlic oil over your chest.

Burns

Burns heal better when kept clean and covered. See also *Sunburn*.

CAUTION: Consult a doctor immediately if a burn is large, deep, on the face, or caused by chemicals or electricity.

SODIUM BICARBONATE

+ ACTION: For a small burn, apply a paste of sodium bicarbonate and cold water to help prevent blistering and scarring. The coldness takes heat from burnt skin. Also, sodium bicarbonate dissolves endothermically (removes heat from its surroundings as it dissolves).

OLIVE OIL

Applying olive oil to a small area of burnt skin can reduce pain. It also aids healing by keeping air from damaged skin and supplying antioxidants.

+ ACTION: Gently apply olive oil and repeat every hour or so.

HONEY

Medical-grade honey is an effective treatment for superficial burns as it has antibacterial and anti-Inflammatory properties. It also discourages blistering and infection, making a burn feel less sore and helping it heal faster.

Researchers in India used honey or the antibiotic silver-sulphadiazine on burnt skin in 100 people. After 1 week, 91 per cent of honey-treated burns were infection-free, compared with only 7 per cent of the others. And the honey-treated burns healed in 15 days, compared with 17 days for the others.[58]

+ ACTION: Choose a manuka honey with a UTM ("Unique Manuka Factor") of 10 or more for its particular anti-inflammatory and antibacterial properties. Gently apply a little honey to the burn, cover with a sterile, non-adherent dressing and secure the dressing in place with medical tape or a bandage.

Cancer

Cancers result from a mutation in a cell's DNA that allows the cell to keep multiplying instead of dying at its allotted time due to the natural process called apoptosis ("cell suicide"). Although malignant (cancerous) cells repeatedly arise in everyday life, most are destroyed by the immune system, but a few continue to multiply.

Lifestyle factors such as smoking, obesity, not having a healthy diet (p.58), inactivity, excess exposure to sunlight, sunbed use and excessive alcohol encourage cancers to develop.

- Obesity is associated with an increased risk of bowel, gallbladder, kidney and prostate cancers. Researchers speculate that mild acidosis (p.62) encourages obesity. So this might prove to be a factor behind both obesity and cancer.
- A high-protein intake can encourage bowel and prostate cancer; having plenty of vegetables discourages bowel, breast and stomach cancers.
- A lack of dietary antioxidants encourages certain cancers. Antioxidants normally mop up the free radicals (highly reactive, and inflammatory, oxygen ions) continually produced in the body. Chronic inflammation can damage cells' DNA (genetic material), encouraging cancer.
- Stomach cancer can be associated with *Helicobacter pylori* infection of the stomach lining (see *Peptic ulcer*).
- In two in three women with breast cancer, oestrogens fuel its growth by activating oestrogen receptors on cells. Overall, about one in eight breast cancers is "oestrogen-receptor positive" (ER+).

A study that analyzed data from 29 studies found that postmenopausal women with breast cancer had a 15 per cent higher average concentration of the oestrogen estradiol in their blood than did women without breast cancer.[59]

Oncologists commonly prescribe aromatase-inhibitor drugs to lower oestrogen in women with ER+ breast cancer. These can lower oestrogen by up to 95 per cent. They work by preventing the enzyme aromatase from converting androgens (hormones such as testosterone) to oestrogen in body fat. Low oestrogen encourages apoptosis of oestrogen-sensitive cancer cells.

It's possible, though unproven, that including more foods containing compounds with aromatase-inhibitor activity in the diet might discourage oestrogen-sensitive cancer by lowering the body's oestrogen. For example, certain flavonoids have some aromatase-inhibitor action, including:[60]

- Apigenin (in artichoke, chamomile, oregano, parsley)
- Chrysin (in honey, passionflower)
- Eriodictyol (in lemons)
- Hesperetin (in lemons, mint)
- Luteolin (in bell pepper, broccoli, carrots, celery, chamomile, chili, clover, dandelion, lemons, lettuce, olive oil, onion leaves, oranges, oregano, parsley, peppermint, rosemary, spinach, thyme)
- Naringenin (in beans, bergamot, cocoa, lemons, tart cherries, tomatoes, oranges, oregano)
- Pinocembrin (in ginger, honey, oregano, liquorice)
- Quercetin (in cloves, dill, fennel, lemons, oregano, parsley, sage, *Camellia-sinensis* tea, olive oil)

Other dietary aromatase-inhibitors include curcumin (a polyphenol) in turmeric and green tea.

CAUTION: If your oncologist has prescribed an aromatase-inhibitor, or tamoxifen (which prevents oestrogen reaching cancer cells), discuss whether increasing your intake of plant oestrogens is wise, as there is a suggestion that they might interfere with the stronger oestrogen-lowering action of aromatase-inhibitor medications and of tamoxifen (which helps prevent oestrogen getting to cancer cells).

Early and very limited research suggests that mild acidosis (p.62) might encourage cancer. First, laboratory studies show that cancer cells sometimes stop multiplying when their environment becomes more alkaline. Second, cancer cells can make their immediate environment more acid, which could make certain anti-cancer drugs less effective. Third, mild acidosis could theoretically encourage cancer formation via its effects on the hormone cortisol, as well as on insulin-like growth factor and on signalling by fat-cell cytokines. And fourth, studies suggest that mild acidosis encourages diabetes. This is important as diabetes itself encourages certain cancers (of the liver and pancreas, for example).

LEMONS

Lemons – especially their peel – contain many cancer-preventing and cancer-fighting compounds, including carotenoids, coumarins, flavonoids, glucaric-acid salts, limonene, limonoids and pectin. Potentially helpful lemon flavonoids include:

- Hesperidin, luteolin and quercetin, which have some aromatase-inhibitor qualities, so might help prevent oestrogen-sensitive breast cancers
- Nobiletin, which might help prevent breast and colon cancers and certain leukemias by inducing apoptosis of cancer cells, and make cancer cells less resistant to chemotherapy
- Naringenin and quercetin, which inhibit liver enzymes that convert the tobacco-related substance nicotine-derived nitrosamine ketone into a potent inducer of lung cancer
- Tangeretin, which might hamper cancer growth by disturbing the signalling between tumour cells

Research suggests that lemons' limonene helps prevent breast and colon cancers; their coumarins discourage cancer growth, and their limonoids help fight cancers of the mouth, stomach, colon, skin, lung and breast.

Lemons' glucaric-acid salts can discourage bowel cancer by promoting the production in the gut of butyric acid, which encourages apoptosis of malignant cells.

Lemon pectins' prebiotic properties help colon cells produce mucus, which helps stop carcinogens (compounds that encourage cancer) sticking to the gut lining. Pectin also reduces the progression of advanced prostate cancer and discourages the recurrence of mouth and throat cancers.

Interestingly, a US study linked a citrus-rich diet with a reduction in stomach cancer in men.[61]

+ ACTION: Include the zest and juice of a lemon in your daily diet.

SODIUM BICARBONATE

Researchers report that in mice with cancer, sodium bicarbonate by mouth decreased acidity around and within the cancer cells, reduced cancer growth, discouraged lymph node involvement and inhibited metastases (secondary cancers).[62]

+ ACTION: If you have cancer, it's certainly wise to eat a healthy – and therefore an "alkaline" – diet.

CAUTION: Sodium bicarbonate is not a proven treatment, so check with your oncologist (cancer doctor) before taking this or, indeed, using any other home remedies.

OLIVE OIL

Extra-virgin olive oil discourages inflammation. Several studies suggest that olive oil could help prevent certain cancers. A review and meta-analysis of 45 studies associated the highest olive oil consumption with a 31 per cent lower likelihood of any cancer.[63]

Research suggests that certain constituents of extra-virgin olive oil help prevent or treat certain cancers as they reduce oxidation damage to DNA or influence hormones, immunity, cell membrane composition or gene expression. The oil's antioxidants and anti-inflammatories may slow cancer development, encourage cancer cells to self-destruct, and boost enzymes that block the activation of carcinogens and boost their removal from the body. In particular:

- Virgin olive oil's polyphenols help prevent bowel cancer.
- Olive oil's lignans have anti-cancer effects in the breasts, lung, skin and colon. Some, indeed, are structurally similar to the breast cancer drug tamoxifen.
- Polyphenols from pinoresinol-rich extra-virgin olive oil have potent cancer-preventive properties. Note that the amount of pinoresinol

in this oil varies with the olive growing site, the agricultural techniques used, and the olives' maturity at harvest.

- Extra-virgin olive oil's polyphenols (especially secoiridoids and lignans) seem powerfully active against HER2-positive breast cancer cells. Such cells test positive for a protein called human epidermal growth factor receptor 2 (HER2), which promotes cancer cell growth. They tend to be more aggressive than other breast cancer cells.
- Oleic acid (olive oil's main fatty acid) reduces the effect of a particular oncogene (a mutated gene that encourages uncontrolled cell growth and division) associated with rapid breast cancer growth.
- Squalene (a terpenoid), beta-sitosterol (a plant sterol similar to cholesterol) and tyrosol (a polyphenol in beer, grapes, olive oil, olives, cider vinegar, wine) either inhibit the oxidation and production of inflammatory compounds from omega-6 fats (which we mainly get from red meat, corn oil and sunflower oil), or render them harmless.

Note that consuming olive oil is associated with a lower cancer risk, while eating a lot of meat is linked with a higher risk.

- Follow-up of 110,799 people in the UK Biobank cohort associated higher adherence to the Mediterranean diet with lower cancer mortality.[64]
- A review by Greek researchers concluded that the risk of gastro-intestinal cancer was 23 per cent lower for those who consumed the most olive oil.[65]
- Making olive oil the main dietary fat seems to halve the risk of developing bowel cancer.[66]
- Olive oil promotes the replacement of bowel-lining cells, so discouraging cancer.[67]

+ ACTION: Include olive oil in your diet.

HONEY

Laboratory and animal studies suggest honey has moderate anti-cancer effects and pronounced effects in stopping cancer from spreading. The constituents likely to be responsible include certain flavonoids and other polyphenols.

Honey's oligosaccharides aid the growth and activity of probiotic gut bacteria, which may help prevent colon cancer.

Raw honey may be particularly helpful because it's an alkali-producing food (p.62). Studies suggest honey:

- Discourages oxidation and inflammation
- Enhances immunity
- Reduces high homocysteine
- Kills bacteria and viruses
- Deactivates certain enzymes
- Detoxifies cancer-causing agents
- Reduces cancer cell formation
- Reduces cancer cell proliferation
- Discourages the new blood vessel growth that enables cancer growth
- Encourages apoptosis of cancer cells

Honey can be beneficial during cancer treatment, as it:

- Aids wound healing in people on chemotherapy or radiotherapy
- Reduces mouth soreness from head or neck radiotherapy
- Destroys *Helicobacter pylori* bacteria (which encourage stomach cancer)
- Helps prevent infection and odour in cancer involving skin and reduces fever plus a low white cell count, which are serious potential side effects of chemotherapy
- Potentiates the anti-cancer drugs 5-fluorouracil and cyclophosphamide
- Prevents the enzyme aromatase enabling oestrogen production from male hormones (androgens)
- Discourages adverse effects from certain cancer drugs
- Discourages multi-drug resistance

In addition, consider these research findings about a tree honey and thyme honey:

A Malaysian study reported that tualang honey (made from the nectar from the flowers of the very tall, south-east Asian rainforest, tualang tree) induced apoptosis of mouth and bone cancer cells.[68]

Research at Greek and Finnish universities suggested that thyme honey reduces oestrogenic activity in the body, so could deter oestrogen-dependent breast, prostate and womb cancers.[69]

+ ACTION: Consider consuming 1 teaspoon of raw honey 3 times a day, including one in the hour before bedtime.

GARLIC

Preliminary studies suggest garlic discourages several cancers, including mouth, gullet, stomach and bowel cancers.

Laboratory studies show that garlic might help prevent or treat cancer because it:

- Detoxifies certain cancer-causing agents, blocking their formation or halting their activation
- Discourages oxidation and chronic inflammation
- Enhances DNA repair
- Enhances immunity
- Helps prevent cancer cells becoming invasive
- Influences certain hormones
- Kills bacteria and viruses
- Promotes cancer cell apoptosis
- Reduces cancer cell multiplication
- Reduces cancer cells' promotion of the growth of the new blood vessels they need as they multiply

However, studies in people paint a much less rosy picture – as in this review (though the number of studies good enough to be selected was relatively small, as were the numbers of people studied):

A review of 19 trials found no credible evidence for a relation between garlic intake and a reduced risk of breast, lung, stomach or womb cancer. Also, only very limited evidence supported a relation between garlic intake and a reduced risk of colon, gullet, kidney, larynx, mouth, ovary or prostate cancer.[70]

+ ACTION: Including garlic in your daily diet or taking a garlic supplement is worth considering.

SPICES

Early evidence indicates that the anti-inflammatory action of antioxidant and salicylate-containing spices might aid the prevention and/or treatment of certain cancers.

CAUTION: Such constituents are present in spices mostly in very small quantities, and any benefits remain largely unproven. They are not a replacement for medical care.

Early research suggests these cancers may respond positively to the bioactive constituents in certain spices:

- Bladder: cumin, ginger, horseradish, mustard, saffron, turmeric
- Bone: sesame seeds, turmeric
- Bowel: caraway, cardamom, cinnamon, cocoa, coriander, cumin, horseradish, kokum, mustard, nigella, pepper, saffron, tamarind, turmeric, wasabi
- Brain: chilli, turmeric
- Breast: asafoetida, caraway, celery seeds, chilli, fenugreek, galangal, ginger, horseradish, juniper, nigella, pepper, poppyseeds, saffron, sesame seeds, turmeric, wasabi
- Cervix: cumin, fenugreek, nigella, saffron, turmeric
- Gullet: chilli, mustard, nigella, turmeric
- Kidney: ginger, sesame seeds
- Leukaemia: chilli, galangal, kokum, nigella, nutmeg, saffron, sesame seeds, turmeric, wasabi
- Liver: asafoetida, caraway, celery seeds, chilli, cumin, fenugreek, kokum, lemongrass, saffron, turmeric
- Lung: asafoetida, caraway, chilli, galangal, ginger, horseradish, mustard, nigella, pepper, saffron, sesame seeds, turmeric, wasabi
- Malignant melanoma: cinnamon
- Mouth: asafoetida, kokum, turmeric

- Multiple myeloma: galangal, nigella
- Neuroblastoma (the commonest cancer in babies): galangal
- Ovary: ginger, mustard, nigella
- Pancreas: chilli, fenugreek, ginger, horseradish, nigella, saffron, turmeric, wasabi
- Prostate: aniseed, caraway, chilli, cloves, coriander, cumin, dill seeds, fennel, fenugreek, ginger, green tea, horseradish, juniper, liquorice, mustard, nigella, turmeric, wasabi
- Skin: asafoetdia, cinnamon, galangal, ginger, lemongrass, nigella, sesame seeds, turmeric, wasabi
- Stomach: caraway, cumin, horseradish, turmeric, wasabi
- Womb: turmeric

+ ACTION: Include these spices in your diet.

TEAS

Early research suggests that certain constituents of teas may aid the prevention and/or treatment of certain cancers via their effects on particular enzymes, cell-signalling pathways and genes. This is because they modify cancer cell multiplication, or the formation of new blood vessels to support cancer growth, or cancer cell apoptosis. Discouraging apoptosis is considered the most common beneficial effect.

They include: alkylamides (in echinacea); antibacterial substances (p.97); antioxidants (p.98); beta-caryophyllene (in dong quai, echinacea, lavender, lemon balm, rosemary and *Vitex agnus castus*); beta-elemene (in ginseng); carnosol (in rosemary); chlorophyll (in nettle and peppermint); ellagic acid (in rosehip); farnesol (in linden); epicatechin and epigallocatechin gallate (in *Camellia-sinensis* tea); ginsenosides (in ginseng); limonene (in dong quai, peppermint, rosemary and verbena); flavonoids such as quercetin (in calendula, chamomile, elderflower, lemon balm, linden, nettle, passionflower), perillyl alcohol (in lavender, rooibos, rosehip, rosemary, tea and valerian); quinones (in chickweed, nettle, rosemary and verbena); various phenolic compounds; salicylates); selenium (in barley); trigonelline (in barley and corn); and valepotriates (in valerian and verbena).

Certain teas contain small amounts of other potentially beneficial ingredients:

- Aromatase inhibitors
- Beta-sitosterol – an antioxidant plant sterol similar to cholesterol (in chickweed, corn, dandelion, dong quai, elderflower, nettle and red clover) that inhibits the growth of oestrogen-receptor-positive and -negative breast cancer cells. (When combined with the medication tamoxifen, the inhibition of oestrogen-receptor-positive cells is greater.)
- Plant oestrogens (p.60) – in herb teas are weaker than an individual's own oestrogens, so may help prevent "oestrogen-receptor-positive" (therefore oestrogen-sensitive) cancer encouraged by high levels of a person's own oestrogen. However, they could reduce the beneficial effect of oestrogen-lowering medication for an existing oestrogen-sensitive cancer
- Ursolic acid (in elderflower, lavender, lemon balm, peppermint, rosemary, thyme and verbena) enhances chemotherapy for multiple myeloma

Early research suggests these cancers may respond positively to the bioactive constituents in certain teas:

- Bladder: *Camellia-sinensis* tea
- Bowel: barley, calendula, *Camellia-sinensis* tea, chamomile, corn, elderflower, lavender, lemon balm, linden, nettle, passionflower, peppermint, rooibos, rosehip, rosemary, valerian
- Brain: dong quai, lavender, green tea
- Breast: calendula, chamomile, cornsilk, dandelion leaf, dong quai, elderflower, ginseng, tea, lavender, lemon balm, linden, nettle, passion-flower, red clover, rooibos, rosehip, rosemary, green tea, valerian
- Cervix: barley, calendula, corn, green tea
- Fibrosarcoma: calendula
- Head and neck: calendula
- Leukaemia: barley, calendula, corn, dandelion root, echinacea, green tea, nettle, rosemary, *Vitex agnus castus*

- Liver: barley, calendula, corn, green tea, nettle, peppermint, rosemary
- Lung: calendula, ginseng
- Lymphoma (non-Hodgkin's): green tea
- Melanoma: calendula, dandelion root, green tea, nettle, peppermint, rosemary
- Multiple myeloma: elderflower, lavender, lemon balm, peppermint, rosemary, thyme, verbena
- Mouth: *Camellia-sinensis* tea
- Oesophagus (gullet): green tea
- Ovary: *Camellia-sinensis* tea
- Pancreas: calendula, lavender, green tea
- Prostate: barley, calendula, chamomile, dandelion, elderflower, green tea, ginseng, lavender, lemon balm, linden, nettle, passionflower, rooibos, rosehip, rosemary, valerian, *Vitex agnus castus*
- Stomach: calendula, *Camellia-sinensis* tea, ginseng, rosemary
- Uterus (womb): green tea

Please note that such constituents are present in teas mostly in very small quantities, and any benefits remain largely unproven; they are not a replacement for medical care.

One study found that daily consumption of lemon and ginger tea made cancers in mice shrink. This anti-cancer effect was caused by cancer-cell apoptosis and by inhibition of the formation of new blood vessels needed to supply cancer cells.[71]

Researchers at the University of Arizona noted that regular consumption of black *Camellia-sinensis* tea containing lemon zest was associated with a skin-cancer-risk reduction of more than 70 per cent. Regular consumption of black tea alone was associated with a reduction of 40 per cent.[72]

+ ACTION: Consider drinking an appropriate tea in case it helps prevent or treat cancer.

CAUTION: Consult your doctor before taking any tea as a possible treatment, as certain teas encourage unwanted weight loss while others might make particular anti-cancer medications less effective.

Cataracts

A cataract is a cloudy area in the eye's lens. It can make what you see blurry, hazy or less colourful. Many people aged over 65 have or have had a cararact, as have more than half of all Americans aged 80 or older. A healthy diet (p.58) and protecting the eyes against bright sunlight can help prevent cataracts.

APPLE CIDER VINEGAR

This is an unproven folk remedy for helping prevent cataracts worsening.

+ ACTION: If you would like to try apple cider vinegar, add it to recipes or take 2 teaspoons in a glass of water 3 times a day for 6 months.

SODIUM BICARBONATE

Cataracts can result from ageing or stress encouraging a build-up of insoluble calcium salts of phosphoric or uric acid in the eyes' lenses. Taking sodium bicarbonate might help dissolve these salts.

+ ACTION: Consider taking sodium bicarbonate by mouth (p.69).

Chapped lips

Dry, cracked lips can result from cold or dry weather, sun exposure, frequently licking your lips, or dehydration.

LEMONS

Lemon juice's antioxidant polyphenols and vitamin C can be soothing.

+ ACTION: Stir a few drops of lemon juice into half a teaspoonful of petroleum jelly ("Vaseline") or glycerine and smooth over your lips.

OLIVE OIL

This can soften dry skin on chapped lips.

+ ACTION: Smoothe a little olive oil into your lips several times a day.

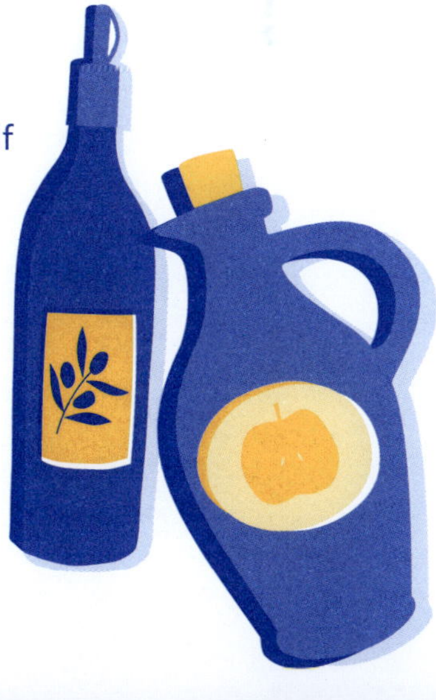

Chronic degenerative diseases

These include artery disease, diabetes and rheumatoid arthritis. A healthy diet (p.58) may help prevent and treat them.

OLIVE OIL

A high fat intake based on animal fats, corn and sunflower oil, and hydrogenated fats, is a risk factor for chronic degenerative diseases. In contrast, a high fat intake in which olive oil is the main fat – as with the Mediterranean diet – is associated with lower rates. This may be partly because the body uses olive oil's monounsaturated fats to produce substances that are relatively anti-inflammatory compared with the products of other fats.

Also, olive oil contains anti-inflammatory agents which could aid prevention or treatment. These include oleocanthal (a polyphenol) and squalene (an antioxidant terpenoid).

+ ACTION: Take 2 tablespoons of extra-virgin olive oil each day in food or on their own.

Chronic metabolic stress and metabolic syndrome

Chronic metabolic stress involves ongoing disruption to the body's normal metabolic processes. The usual causes are a poor diet, lack of exercise, smoking and stress. Mild acidosis (p.62) is a type of chronic metabolic stress. Chronic metabolic stress is also called insulin-resistance syndrome and is a harbinger of metabolic syndrome. A quarter of the world's population is thought to have metabolic syndrome.

The diagnosis of matabolic syndrome turns on having three or more of these conditions:

- Excess fat around the waist: in women this means a waist of 35in (88cm) or more, in men, 40in (102cm) or more
- High blood pressure
- Low HDL cholesterol (good cholesterol)
- High triglyceride blood fats
- High fasting blood sugar

Having metabolic syndrome encourages diabetes, heart disease and strokes. It is more likely with increasing age and can be associated with polycystic ovary syndrome (p.260). Most affected people are sedentary, obese and insulin-resistant, though it's unclear whether obesity and insulin resistance are direct causes, or consequences of a more general problem. Researchers suspect inflammation and oxidation play a part. Certainly, affected people are more likely to have high C-reactive protein in their blood, indicating inflammation.

Risk factors include a lack of exercise and not eating a healthy diet (p.58). Interestingly, people with fibromyalgia (p.188) are four times as likely as others to develop metabolic syndrome.

Treatment involves lifestyle modification through weight loss, a healthy diet and increased exercise, along with the medical treatment recommended by your doctor.

APPLE CIDER VINEGAR

Lebanese researchers found that consuming cider vinegar lowered weight, body mass index, waist/hip circumferences and body fat, and improved blood sugar, triglyceride blood fats, and cholesterol levels in overweight adults and obese adolescents. They say cider vinegar is known to slow stomach emptying, increase the feeling of fullness after eating, so decreasing hunger.[73]

Also, studies of rats on a high-calorie diet conclude that regular consumption of apple cider vinegar discourages inflammation, high blood sugar, unhealthy blood fats and obesity.

+ ACTION: Include it in your diet.

LEMONS

Lemons' antioxidants and acids may help prevent pre-diabetes, high blood pressure, obesity and unhealthy levels of cholesterol and triglycerides.

+ ACTION: Consume the zest and juice of a lemon each day.

OLIVE OIL

Extra-virgin olive oil seems to discourage atheroma in arteries, so improving the overall health status of people with metabolic syndrome.

- A large Italian review concluded that the Mediterranean diet is a cornerstone in treating metabolic syndrome and lowering cardiovascular risk. Extra-virgin olive oil is an essential component, partly because it is high in polyphenols and monounsaturated fatty acids that could optimize blood sugar control and lipid metabolism, reduce damage to the linings of arteries, lower blood pressure and provide anti-inflammatory activity.[74]
- A study of 20 people with metabolic syndrome found changes in genes whose activity is regulated by olive oil polyphenols. Virgin olive oil suppressed 98 genes, many of them linked to obesity, high blood fats, diabetes and heart disease, and several concerned with pro-inflammatory processes. The researchers suggest olive oil can "switch off" certain genes that control immune cells, so these are less likely to induce inflammation.[75]
- A study of 808 people at high risk of cardiovascular disease found the Mediterranean diet discouraged metabolic syndrome. Those with the highest adherence were only half as likely to have low HDL cholesterol and high triglycerides as those with lowest adherence.[76]

+ ACTION: Consume at least 2 tablespoons of extra-virgin olive oil each day.

HONEY

Eating honey (which has a moderate glycaemic index) instead of table sugar (which has a high glycaemic index) could theoretically help prevent and treat metabolic syndrome by preventing "spikes" of high blood sugar and insulin and discouraging chronic metabolic stress (p.152).

A Malaysian review concludes that honey has potent healing actions against metabolic syndrome. This is mainly because of its polyphenols' antioxidant and anti-inflammatory properties, which help prevent obesity and high blood fats. They help widen blood vessels by increasing nitric-oxide production. And they decrease a group of proteins ("nuclear factor-kappa B") that help regulate the body's response to inflammation.[77]

+ ACTION: Consume low glycaemic-index honey instead of table sugar, including 1 teaspoon within the hour before bedtime.

GARLIC

Recent research suggests garlic discourages metabolic syndrome:

- In an Indian study, rats ate a diet of 65 per cent fruit sugar (a diabetes-inducing diet), or a diet of 65 per cent fruit sugar and raw garlic, or a control diet of 65 per cent cornflour. After 8 weeks, the first two groups had raised blood sugar, insulin, triglycerides, uric-acid and insulin resistance. But the gains were lower in the group that also consumed garlic. The conclusion was that garlic improves insulin sensitivity and metabolic syndrome in rats on a diabetes-inducing diet.[78]

+ ACTION: Include garlic in your daily diet or take a garlic supplement. You need water- and oil-soluble sulphur compounds (pp.78–9).

Cold sores

These lip sores are caused by reactivation of a *Herpes simplex* virus infection by triggers such as stress, menstrual periods, infection, skin damage, sunshine and fatigue.

APPLE CIDER VINEGAR

This is an old home remedy for cold sores. It can help by removing dead skin cells and discouraging an overlying bacterial infection. However, it can't cure them.

+ ACTION: If you suspect a sore is imminent, dilute 1 tsp of apple cider vinegar with 1 tsp of water and dab the mixture on to the affected lip with a paper tissue or clean cotton pad 3 times a day. You can also apply neat cider vinegar to an actual sore, though it might sting a bit!

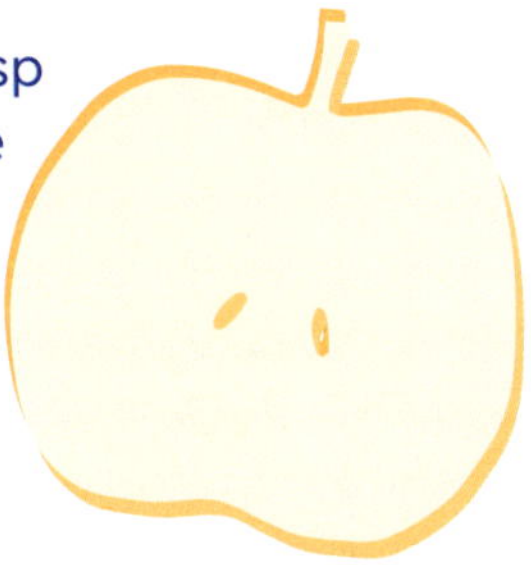

LEMONS

The limonene in a lemon's juice and particularly in its oil has antiviral properties. Lemon oil can also help, by excluding air from a sore.

+ ACTION: Apply lemon juice to a cold sore several times a day, using a clean cotton pad each time. Or add 1 drop of lemon oil to 1 teaspoon of sweet almond oil and apply this to the cold sore.

HONEY

Applying honey to cold sores excludes air, so reducing pain, and providing antiviral and anti-inflammatory agents. Honey can also help relieve the symptoms of shingles and genital herpes.

Researchers in Dubai compared honey with acyclovir cream for 8 volunteers with cold sores and 8 with genital herpes. Honey was up to 43 per cent better at reducing pain from cold sores and helping them heal. A similar benefit was found with genital herpes.[79]

+ ACTIONS: Apply raw honey 3 times a day. Or apply manuka honey cream.

GARLIC

In the laboratory – at least, *Herpes simplex virus* type 1, which causes cold sores – is sensitive to allicin and its derivatives, particularly the oil-soluble compound ajoene.

+ ACTIONS: If a patch test (p.82) shows that garlic won't cause irritation, smear a little petroleum jelly ("Vaseline") on the skin around the sore, then press on to it a sliver of garlic cut from a garlic clove. Leave it there for as long as it will stay. Repeat twice a day.

You could instead apply the oil from garlic oil macerate or a garlic perle to the sore, several times a day (p.80). These methods exclude air from the sore, which is helpful. Another option is to bathe the infected area with garlic water (p.81). A final option is to apply allicin cream. Any stinging and smell should be short-lived.

It's also a good idea to include garlic in your diet or take a garlic supplement. You need oil-soluble sulphur compounds (p.79).

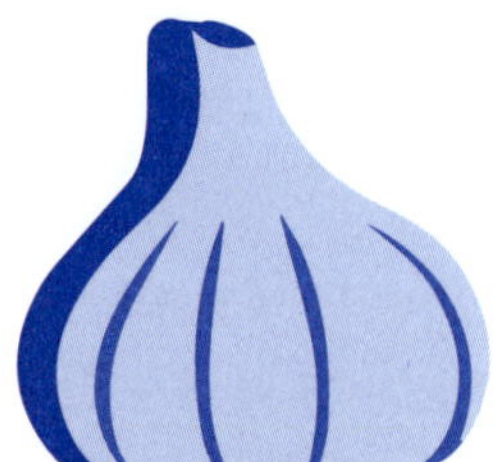

TEAS

Antiviral teas can help with cold sores.

+ ACTIONS: Drink one of these teas. Also apply them frequently as a wash.

Colds, flu, laryngitis, sore throat, sinusitis

These upper respiratory infections are among the most common ailments we encounter.

APPLE CIDER VINEGAR

Apple cider vinegar has antibacterial and anti-inflammatory properties, and its acidity can kill bacteria in the throat. However, it can erode tooth enamel, so should be used with care.

+ ACTION: Possible ways of using it are to:

- Mix a teaspoon of apple cider vinegar in warm water. Gargle for 20–30 seconds, 2–3 times a day
- Drink a cup of warm water mixed with a tablespoon of cider vinegar and a teaspoon of honey twice a day
- Add it to food (such as a soup or stew) just before eating it
- Heat cider vinegar until it steams, then pour it into a bowl. Lean over the bowl, put a towel over your head and the bowl and inhale the steam for 5 minutes. Do this twice a day

LEMONS

Lemons' flavonoids have antibacterial, anti-inflammatory and antiviral properties.

The water in home-made lemonade helps replace the fluid lost in sneezes, catarrh and – if you are feverish – sweat. Water makes catarrh moister and easier to shift, and helps prevent dehydration, which can cause headaches.

The decongestant vapour from lemon oil can shrink the swollen mucous membrane lining the air passages and Eustachian tubes. This eases breathing and discourages deafness.

Another benefit of lemons is that bowel bacteria ferment their pectin. This releases butyric acid and other short-chain fatty acids with prebiotic qualities – meaning they nourish "good" probiotic bowel bacteria such as lactobacilli and bifidobacteria. These, in turn, benefit our immunity in general, including our immunity to infection.

A German study of 479 volunteers found that taking tablets containing lactobacilli and bifidobacteria reduced the severity of colds, shortened their length by two days and increased the number of immune cells.[80]

+ ACTIONS: Drink 3–6 glasses of lemonade each day. Add two or three cloves or a small pinch of dried cinnamon to each glass to ease a fever. Gargle with 1 teaspoon of lemon juice in a glass of warm water twice a day. If you have temporarily gone a bit deaf because of congestion, put a few drops of lemon oil on a paper tissue and inhale its vapour.

HONEY

Its soothing, anti-inflammatory and antimicrobial properties may help these ailments, as may its oligosaccharides, which aid the growth and activity of probiotic gut bacteria.

+ ACTION: Consume 1–2 teaspoons of raw honey 3 times a day, or chew some honeycomb (meaning some of the honeybees' honey-store construction, not the confectionery item called honeycomb) for 15 minutes every few hours. Try gargling with 1 teaspoon of honey in ½ a glass of warm water.

GARLIC

This is a traditional remedy for these ailments. Any success may be because of its antimicrobial, anti-inflammatory and immunity-enhancing compounds. For example, laboratory studies show that the symptoms of infection with parainfluenza virus type 3 and human rhinovirus type 2 may be eased by taking garlic.

This study suggests garlic helps to prevent and treat colds: 146 volunteers took either an allicin-containing garlic supplement or a placebo for 12 weeks in winter. Those taking garlic had only 24 colds while those on the placebo had 65. Also, their colds didn't last as long and their chances of re-infection were reduced.[81]

+ ACTIONS: Take garlic in honey, as garlic is powerfully antiseptic, while honey is soothing and healing. To do this, crush 10 garlic cloves, then leave to stand for 10–90 minutes before stirring the garlic into a 450g (1lb) jar of clear honey. Take 1 teaspoon every 2 hours. Alternatively:

- Take a teaspoon of garlic syrup (p.81) every 2 hours.
- Crush several garlic cloves, then wait for 30 minutes before inhaling the fumes from up to 20cm (8in) away. Repeat several times a day. Any initial stinging in the nose should quickly abate; if not, or if the stinging is excessive, inhale from further away or take garlic in another form.
- Take a garlic supplement. You need one containing garlic's oil-soluble sulphur compounds (p.79).
- Take a pure allicin supplement.
- Have a warm garlic bath (p.81).
- For a sore throat, gargle with garlic water (p.81).

SPICES

Astringent, antibacterial, anti-inflammatory, antiviral and decongestant spices may help. In particular, try ginger. For a feverish cold, consider diaphoretic (cooling) spices. For flu, consider asafoetida, which kills certain flu viruses more effectively than the flu drug amantadine. If lymph nodes are enlarged, consider fenugreek.
+ ACTIONS: Include these spices in your diet. For example, drink cinnamon and clove tea mixed with the juice of ½ a lemon, 2 teaspoons of honey and a tot of whisky. Or gargle with cayenne or clove tea if you have a sore throat. Soak your feet in a basin containing 2 teaspoons of mustard in hot water for general relief from symptoms.

TEAS

Astringent, antibacterial, anti-inflammatory, antiviral and decongestant teas may help. If feverish, consider drinking diaphoretic (cooling) teas.
+ ACTIONS: Include these teas in your diet. Also inhale the steam from these teas several times a day.

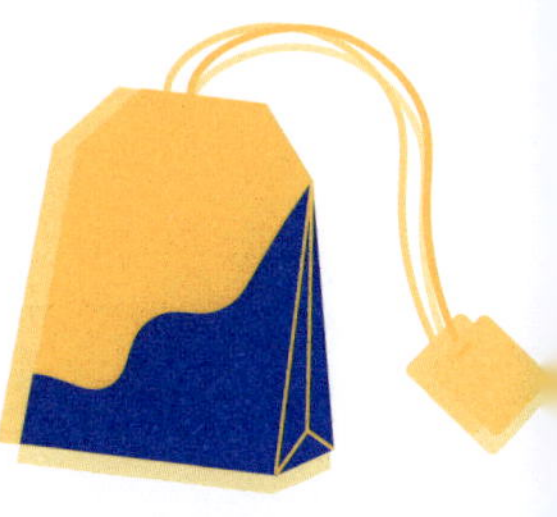

Conjunctivitis

Conjunctivitis is inflammation and, perhaps, infection, of the layer of cells covering the surface of the eyes. It is also known as "pink eye" due to the effect it has on the eye's appearance.

TEAS

Antibacterial, anti-inflammatory, antiviral and immunity-boosting teas may help.
+ ACTIONS: Include these teas in your diet; also try bathing your affected eye with one of these teas in an eyebath. To do this, remove glasses or contact lenses, if worn, then half fill the eyebath with your chosen tea. Leaning forward, position the eyebath around your eye socket. Keeping your eye open, tilt your head up until the eye wash flows over your eye, then rock your head from side to side for half a minute. Repeat 2 or 3 times a day but consult a doctor if the conjunctivitis does not rapidly improve, or worsens.

Constipation

The most likely causes are not eating a healthy diet (p.58), dehydration, stress and anxiety, lack of exercise, irritable bowel syndrome and depression. Antacids containing aluminium can also be to blame. Disruptions to a person's normal daily routine can disturb a normal "bowel habit", as can not using the lavatory when you feel the urge. Note that repeated constipation can be a sign of bowel cancer or intestinal obstruction. And abdominal surgery and certain medications (for example, anticonvulsants, antacids, anticholinergics, antispasmodics, chemotherapy drugs, calcium channel blockers, diuretics and narcotic pain relievers) can be the trigger.

LEMONS

These are mildly laxative, partly because they are rich in pectin. This dissolves to form a gel in the bowel that makes stools softer and easier to pass. Lemons' cellulose also attracts water, making stools bulkier, softer and easier to pass, and reducing their transit time through the bowel
+ ACTION: Include the zest and juice of a lemon in your daily diet.

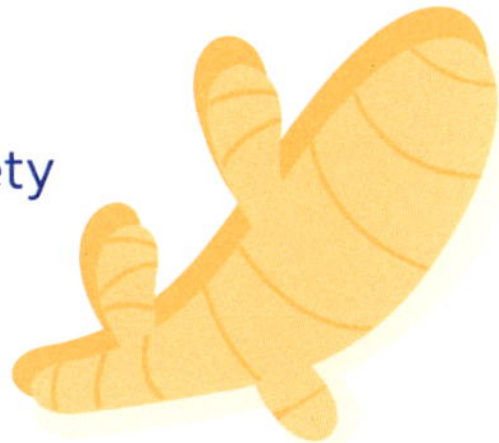

SPICES AND TEAS

Try spices and teas with these properties: anti-anxiety (if you are stressed), cholinergic and laxative, as well as those containing serotonin (p.61).

+ ACTION: Include these in your diet.

Convulsions

Also known as fits or seizures, these result from bursts of abnormal electrical activity in the brain causing momentary loss of awareness, or longer episodes together with uncontrolled jerking of the limbs. Having epilepsy means having repeated convulsions. Convulsions occur in 20–30 per cent of people with epilepsy despite their medication.

Researchers believe the mild acidosis (p.62) associated with most modern Western diets encourages chronic epilepsy by over-exciting brain cells.[82] Convulsions can also result from a slow-onset immune reaction caused by a food sensitivity encouraged by mild acidosis.

+ ACTION: Eat a healthy diet (p.58).

Corns and calluses

These uncomfortable hard areas on the feet are usually caused by ill-fitting footwear.

APPLE CIDER VINEGAR

Soaking feet in a cider vinegar solution is reputed to soften corns and calluses and hasten their demise.

+ ACTION: Add a cup of apple cider vinegar to a large bowl of warm water and soak your feet for 10 minutes a day. Afterwards, rub softened skin from the surface of the corn or callus.

LEMONS

Soaking the hard skin regularly in lemon juice and water, or lemon essential oil, should soften and hasten its replacement with healthy skin.

+ ACTION: Add the juice of 2 lemons to a bowl of warm water and soak your feet for 10 minutes a day. Then rub softened skin from the surface of the corn of callus.

Alternatively, add 1 drop of lemon oil to 2 teaspoons of sweet almond or other carrier oil, rub the mixture into the hard skin and cover with clingfilm (plastic wrap) for 20 minutes. Repeat daily for a week.

Coughs

Common causes include acid reflux from stomach to throat; hay fever; throat and chest infections; dust, mould and pollens in the air; and smoking or breathing in second-hand smoke. Certain medications (for example, ACE-inhibitor drugs for high blood pressure) can also be to blame.

APPLE CIDER VINEGAR AND HONEY

Both have been used for millennia to fight infections. The ancient Greek physician Hippocrates (460–370 BC), for example, prescribed oxymel – a mixture of apple cider vinegar, honey and herbs – for coughs. Its name is derived from the Greek “oxys”, meaning sour, and “meli”, meaning honey.

+ ACTIONS: Include cider vinegar and honey in your daily diet. To do this, you can make your own oxymel by mixing: 2 tablespoons of organic cider vinegar, 6 tablespoons of raw honey, 2 tablespoons of dried herbs or 4 tablespoons of chopped fresh herbs – choose from infection-fighting and anti-inflammatory herbs (p.98).

Take 1–2 tablespoons of oxymel 2 or 3 times a day.

LEMONS

A five-year study of 63,257 people in Singapore suggested a diet high in fruit fibre discourages coughs.[83]

+ ACTIONS: Include the peel and juice of a lemon in your daily diet. You could also try one of the following to soothe a cough:

- Drink home-made lemonade (p.xx).
- Put 2 tablespoons of cracked linseeds and half a lemon, sliced, into 570ml (1 pint) of water, simmer for 20 minutes, then strain, sweeten with honey and drink.
- Put 2 drops each of lemon essential oil, eucalyptus oil and tea-tree

oil into a bowl of just-boiled water; then put a towel over your head and inhale the vapour.

HONEY

Honey's soothing, anti-inflammatory and antimicrobial properties may help, as may its oligosaccharides, which aid the growth and activity of probiotic gut bacteria. Also, honey is safe, whereas certain cough medications can have adverse effects.

In a study at Penn State College of Medicine, 105 children aged 2–18 with an upper respiratory infection and night-time cough had buckwheat honey, honey-flavoured dextromethorphan or no treatment 30 minutes before bedtime. Honey had the best results.[84]

+ ACTIONS: Consume 1–2 teaspoons of raw honey 3 times a day; every few hours, chew some honeycomb for 15 minutes or gargle with a solution made by mixing 1 teaspoon of honey into half a glass of warm water.

SPICES

For a dry cough, anti-inflammatory, antioxidant and antiviral spices can help. In particular, use ajowan, aniseed and ginger. For a productive cough, use antibacterial, anti-inflammatory, antioxidant, astringent, decongestant and expectorant spices – in particular, aniseed and mustard.

+ ACTIONS: Include appropriate spices in your diet. For a cough caused by bronchitis or pneumonia, apply a mustard-seed poultice to your chest.

TEAS

For a dry cough, anti-inflammatory, antioxidant, antiviral and demulcent teas can help. For a productive cough, try antibacterial, anti-inflammatory, antioxidant, astringent, decongestant and expectorant ones.

+ ACTIONS: Include these teas in your diet. Also, inhale the steam from one of these teas several times a day. Do this by leaning over a bowl of the steaming tea, covering your head and the bowl with a towel, and inhaling the steam for several minutes.

Cramp, including period pain

This sudden severe clenching of muscle can be excruciatingly painful. The various sorts include cramp from too much exercise, period pains (from intense contractions of the muscular uterus), and night cramp. Keeping warm can help prevent certain cramps. Not eating a healthy diet (p.58) encourages mild acidosis (p.62) that can reduce the kidneys' normal re-absorption of magnesium from urine into blood. The body's resulting low magnesium encourages cramp.

Period pain results from the cells that line the uterus breaking down before a menstrual period, releasing prostaglandins that constrict local blood vessels, cause local inflammation and trigger uterine contractions. The higher the prostaglandin levels, the worse the pain. Non-steroidal anti-inflammatory drugs (NSAIDs) such as aspirin – which contains salicylates – block the effects of prostaglandins. Other causes of period pains include a narrow cervix, endometriosis, uterine fibroids, ovarian cysts, pelvic inflammatory disease, uterine infection and an intra-uterine contraceptive device.

APPLE CIDER VINEGAR

This is a folk remedy for cramp. One possible reason is that its acidity in the stomach improves calcium and magnesium absorption in those of us (for example nearly one in three of those aged over 60) who produce sub-optimal levels of stomach acid. Another is that cider vinegar – like aspirin – contains salicylates.

+ ACTIONS: Include apple cider vinegar in recipes or take 2 teaspoons in a glass of water 3 times a day. Soak a face cloth in a mixture of 2 tablespoons of vinegar in a cup of warm water, put it over the painful area and cover with a thick towel.

SODIUM BICARBONATE

This can ease mild acidosis and help restore a low magnesium level.

+ ACTION: If you get repeated cramp, consider taking sodium bicarbonate (p.69).

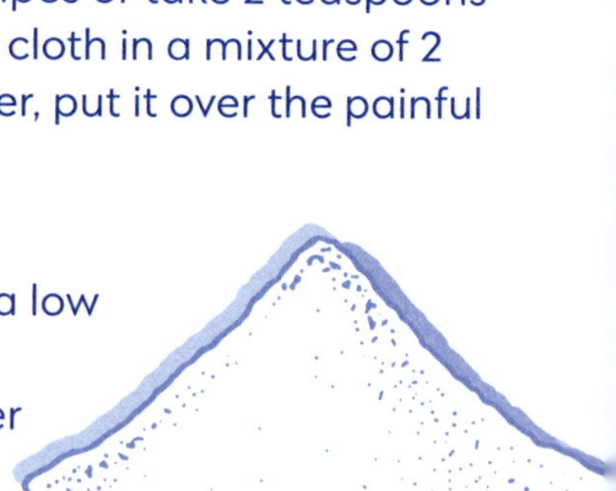

HONEY

Honey's reputed usefulness for preventing cramp may stem from its easily digested sugars and its minerals, as well as its anti-inflammatory effects.

+ **ACTION:** Take 1 to 3 teaspoons of honey before going to bed.

SPICES

Anti-inflammatory, antispasmodic and pain-relieving spices may help. For period pain, try celery seeds, fennel seeds and saffron.

+ **ACTION:** Include these in your diet.

TEAS

Anti-inflammatory, muscle-relaxing and pain-relieving teas may help.

+ **ACTION:** Include these in your diet.

Cuts and grazes

Treatment aims to prevent infection and encourage healing. So clean a wound well and apply a sterile dressing, changing it as necessary.

HONEY

People have anointed cuts and grazes with honey since ancient times. After cleaning the wound well, apply a manuka-honey dressing (p.74). Manuka honey has antibacterial, anti-inflammatory properties. It also encourages damaged skin to regenerate.

Applying honey to a wound:

- Provides a barrier against infection
- Attracts water, helping to flush out dirt, draw out pus, prevent waterlogging of tissue, activate hydrogen-peroxide release, enable moist wound healing and discourage thick scarring (keloid)
- Contains antimicrobials
- Reduces odour within 24 hours by killing infecting bacteria
- Contains anti-inflammatories that reduce swelling. This reduces pressure on tiny blood vessels, increasing their blood flow and so increasing the cells' oxygen and nutrient supply
- Stimulates skin-cell multiplication and gives new cells energy to migrate across the wound

- Prevents blood and wound secretions adhering to dressings, so these can be changed without damage and pain
- Digests dead cells

Yemeni researchers treated 50 women with a wound infection after a Caesarean section or a hysterectomy with raw honey or an antiseptic twice daily. The honey-treated women were infection-free sooner (6 days on average, compared with 15 for the antiseptic group). They also needed antibiotics for less time (7 days instead of 15) and had faster wound healing (11 days instead of 22). The average scar was only 3mm long instead of 7mm. None of the 26 in the honey group needed re-stitching, compared with 4 of the 24 in the other group. Their average hospital stay was 9 days instead of 20.[85]
+ ACTION: Apply a home-made honey dressing. Any honey helps, but certain honeys are preferable. For infected skin, or to help prevent infection, choose manuka honey with a UMF (p.74) of 10–20 or higher, as this is particularly rich in antibacterial power; for inflamed skin, choose this honey or any other antioxidant-rich honey. To apply a honey dressing:

- Put honey on one side of a sterile cotton dressing (this need not be non-adherent, as honey will help prevent the dressing sticking).
- Apply honey-side down.
- Secure with tape.
- A larger wound should have a secondary dressing – ideally, an occlusive one (meaning its wound-side surface is made of plastic film, hydrogel or hydrocolloid to prevent it absorbing honey).
- Change the dressing at least once a day.
- You could also use a commercially produced honey dressing.

TEAS
Antibacterial, anti-inflammatory, antiviral and wound-healing teas may help.
+ ACTION: Include these in your diet. Bathe affected skin with one of them or apply a tea-soaked compress.

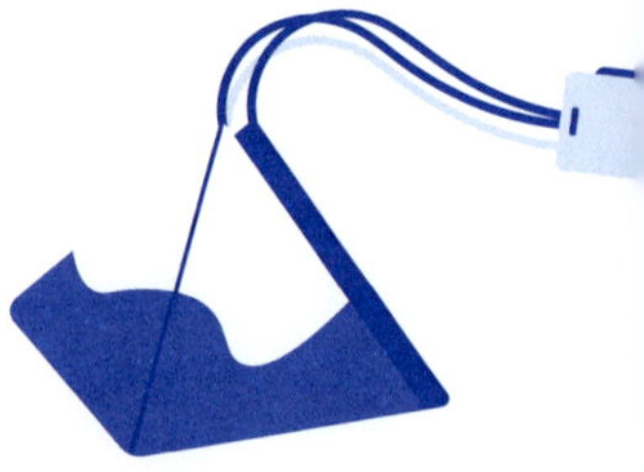

GARLIC

This is a useful treatment for bacterial, viral and fungal skin infections. During World War I, the British Government paid a shilling a pound for garlic to prevent wound infections!

+ ACTION: First, do a patch test (p.82) to check garlic won't irritate your skin. Apply garlic oil macerate or garlic oil twice a day (p.80). Alternatively, bathe the infected area with garlic water (p.81). Include garlic in your daily diet or take a garlic supplement. You need oil-soluble sulphur compounds (p.79).

Cystitis

This inflammation of the bladder lining usually results from infection, causes painful, frequent urination and is more common in women. Interstitial cystitis ("bladder pain syndrome") is a chronic inflammatory condition causing discomfort in the bladder and pelvic region. Someone with mild acidosis (p.62) – for example, from not eating a healthy diet (p.58) – makes urine that is more acidic. This can inflame the bladder, encouraging infection and inflammation. Urine's normal pH (acid–alkali balance) varies from 4.5 to 9, the ideal perhaps being 5.8 to 6.8. The lower its pH, the more acidic the urine. Dehydration (p.64) concentrates urine and makes it more likely to irritate the bladder lining.

SODIUM BICARBONATE

This can help prevent mild acidosis, and help neutralize excess acid in urine. It also kills bacteria and makes certain antibiotics more effective.

+ ACTION: Consider taking sodium bicarbonate (p.69) as it is as effective as the potassium-citrate cystitis remedies available from pharmacies. See a doctor if this is your first attack, or you are no better within 2–3 days. Men and children who develop cystitis should always see a doctor.

OLIVE OIL

Its anti-inflammatory quercetin might be soothing.

+ ACTION: Consume 1 tablespoon of olive oil twice a day.

HONEY

If honey helps, as reputed, this is probably thanks to its anti-inflammatories and antimicrobials. Raw honey may be particularly useful as it's an alkalinizing food.

+ ACTION: Consume 1 teaspoon of raw honey 3 times a day.

GARLIC

Any of its anti-inflammatory and antimicrobial agents that make it to the bladder may help counter a urine infection. Also, it is possible, though unproven, that garlic's smooth muscle-relaxing properties might help cystitis-like symptoms caused by unusually tense smooth muscle in the bladder wall.

+ ACTION: Include garlic in your daily diet or take a garlic supplement. You need both water- and oil-soluble sulphur compounds (pp.78–9).

SPICES

Antibacterial and anti-inflammatory spices may help. Celery seeds, horseradish and juniper could also be useful as they are urinary antiseptics.

+ ACTION: Include these in your diet.

TEAS

Antibacterial and anti-inflammatory teas may help.

+ ACTION: Include these teas in your diet.

Dandruff

This is often associated with an infection of the scalp with the fungus *Malassezia furfur.*

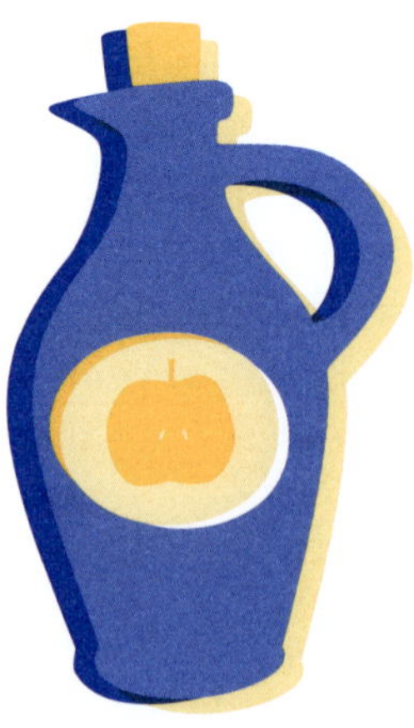

APPLE CIDER VINEGAR

This is a popular home remedy.

+ ACTIONS: Mix 1 cup of apple cider vinegar with 1 of warm water, apply this solution to the scalp, cover with a towel and wait an hour before rinsing and shampooing. Alternatively, massage neat cider vinegar into the scalp, cover with a towel and leave on for an hour. Repeat once or twice a week.

LEMONS

Lemon juice or oil may help with dandruff.

+ ACTIONS: Apply 1 cup of lemon juice to the scalp, cover with a towel for 1 hour, then rinse and shampoo. Repeat once or twice a week. Alternatively, if your scalp is dry, warm 2 teaspoons of coconut oil and mix with 1 drop each of lemon and chamomile essential oils. Massage your scalp with the mixture for 5 minutes, then cover with a hot towel for 20 minutes. Shampoo to remove.

OLIVE OIL

Sometimes dermatitis coexists with dandruff (see *Seborrhoeic dermatitis*). Extra-virgin olive oil's antifungal properties may help.

+ ACTIONS: Consume at least 2 tablespoons of extra-virgin olive oil each day. To treat dandruff, apply extra-virgin olive oil to your scalp. Put a shower cap or plastic carrier bag over your hair and cover with a towel wrapped turban-style. Relax for 1 hour, then shampoo your hair. Repeat twice a week. To prevent dandruff, use a home-made shampoo containing olive oil.

GARLIC

Garlic's antifungal activity means it might be effective in treating dandruff.

+ ACTIONS: First, do a patch test (p.82) to check garlic doesn't irritate your skin. Apply garlic water (p.81) to your scalp, cover with a towel for 1 hour, then rinse off the bits of garlic before shampooing. Repeat once or twice a week. Or mix 2 crushed cloves of garlic with 1 tablespoon of coconut oil. Use the mixture to massage your scalp for 5 minutes, then cover with a hot towel for 20 minutes before shampooing. Try the same process with garlic oil, or use a garlic shampoo and conditioner (available on the internet). Include garlic in your daily diet or take a garlic supplement. You need both water- and oil-soluble sulphur compounds (pp.78–9).

TEAS

Antifungal teas (p.97) may help.

+ ACTION: After washing your hair, apply a hair rinse of an antifungal tea mixed with 1 tablespoon of cider vinegar.

Dementia

This condition gradually destroys memory and understanding; it also causes behavioural changes such as agitation, unease, dissatisaction and apathy.

Of the two most common sorts of dementia, one is Alzheimer's disease (see *Alzheimer's disease*), the other is vascular dementia (see *Artery disease*). Mild cognitive impairment – meaning poor understanding – can be an early warning sign of dementia so is an excellent reason to improve general health.

Depression

This is all too common a condition, and difficult to treat, but consider the following natural remedies.

Depression is sometimes reported as a side effect of not eating a healthy diet (p.58), which in turn is associated with mild acidosis (p.62). It can also result from a slow-onset immune reaction caused by a food sensitivity enabled by this acidosis.

+ ACTION: Eat a healthy diet.

LEMON

The scent of lemon oil can affect mood positively, possibly via the brain's limbic system.

Backing for the suggestion that inhaling lemon-oil vapour can ease a depressed mood comes from researchers at Ohio State University.[86]

+ ACTION: Put a few drops of lemon essential oil into a diffuser or on a paper tissue and inhale the vapour every so often.

OLIVE OIL

Diet is one of several lifestyle factors that can either trigger or treat depression.

A Spanish study of 10,094 healthy people found that those who followed the Mediterranean diet most closely had a more than 30 per cent reduction in their risk of depression compared with those who adhered to it least well.[87]

+ ACTION: Consume at least 2 tablespoons of extra-virgin olive oil each day.

GARLIC

One study shows that garlic extract has antidepressant activity. This was thought to be probably because its action resembled that of compounds called MAOI inhibitors which break down the neurotransmitter (nerve message carrier) monoamine oxidase, and because it affected the brain's levels of other neurotrasnmitters called adrenaline, dopamine, serotonin and GABA. These actions increase the levels of these neurotrasnmitters in the brain by preventing their breakdown. Garlic's antidepressant-like action was comparable to that of the antidepressant drugs imipramine and fluoxetine.[88]

+ ACTION: Include garlic in your diet.

SPICES

Early research suggests that depression might be improved by cardamom, liquorice, pepper, saffron and turmeric.

Note too that aniseed, black pepper, cinnamon, cloves, coriander, cumin, ginger, nutmeg and vanilla are traditionally reputed to be uplifting.

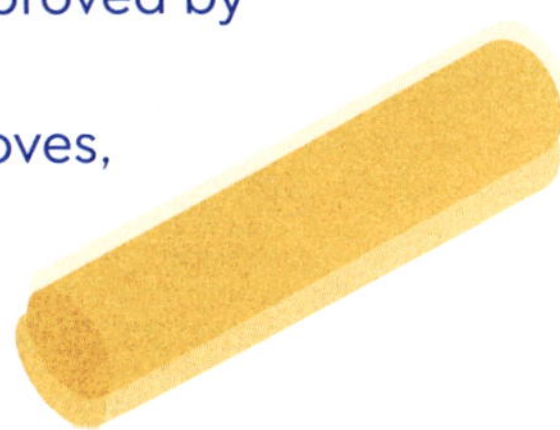

+ ACTION: Include these spices in your diet.

TEAS

Antidepressant teas may help, as may those containing monoamine-oxidase inhibitors (p.101) and serotonin (p.102).

+ ACTION: Include these teas in your diet. Also try inhaling the scent from lavender, lemon balm or rosehip tea every 2 hours or so.

Diabetes – type 2

Of those with diabetes, only 8 per cent have type 1 – the type requiring insulin injections. The other 92 per cent have type 2.

Type 2 diabetes is associated with eating an unhealthy diet (p.58), being overweight or obese, not exercising enough, and, perhaps, having mild acidosis (p.62), which researchers believe encourages cells to become resistant to insulin. Normally, this hormone enables blood sugar to enter cells. But if cells are insulin-resistant, blood sugar rises. The pancreas then produces extra insulin to prevent high blood sugar, but may fail to produce enough.

Blood sugar is constantly raised with diabetes. Having pre-diabetes means having high fasting blood sugar, and repeated spikes of high blood sugar interspersed with slightly higher than normal blood sugar. Pre-diabetes affects one in three adults in the UK and US, one in six in Australia. Up to seven in ten people with pre-diabetes develop diabetes at some time. But with a healthy diet the blood sugar levels stand a good chance of reverting to normal.

The high blood sugar and insulin of type 2 diabetes can cause dry and/or darkened skin, faintness, fatigue, fluid retention, frequent urination (especially at night), hair loss on the lower legs, high blood pressure, itching in moist skin folds, mood swings, patches of raised brown skin on the neck or in the armpits or groins, slow wound healing, raised LDL (bad) cholesterol, low HDL (good) cholesterol, skin tags and thirst.

Longer-term problems from untreated pre-diabetes include brain, eye, kidney, heart and nerve disease. With continuing pre-diabetes, the body becomes less sensitive to insulin. This "insulin resistance" encourages chronic inflammation. More inflammation causes more insulin resistance and vice versa. The chronic inflammation caused by the high blood sugar of untreated diabetes is responsible for most of the ill health caused by diabetes.

APPLE CIDER VINEGAR

This may help reduce the high blood sugar of pre-diabetes and type 2 diabetes. Experts believe vinegar delays stomach emptying, inactivates gut enzymes that convert complex sugars to glucose, and reduces the liver's production and release of sugar from non-carbohydrate sources. Indeed, certain acidic foods have as powerful an effect on a meal's glycaemic index (blood sugar-raising ability). as the diabetes drug metformin. Frequent consumption of acidic foods is traditional in many countries and may help explain national variations in diabetes rates.

- A meta-analysis of six trials, involving 317 people with type 2 diabetes, reports that taking 1–2 tablespoons of vinegar a day

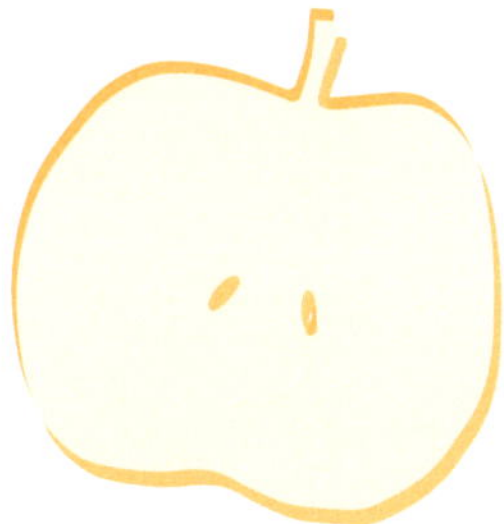

decreased fasting blood sugar and HbA1c (a marker of long-term blood sugar levels). Apple cider vinegar was more effective than other vinegars.[89]

- In a study at Arizona State University, 21 people with diabetes or pre-diabetes each drank water containing 2 tablespoons of apple cider vinegar before a carbohydrate breakfast. Vinegar increased insulin sensitivity by 34 per cent in those with insulin resistance and 19 per cent in those with diabetes. This meant they were better able to get sugar from blood into cells. Blood sugar was 25 per cent lower in those with diabetes, and nearly 50 per cent lower in those with pre-diabetes.[90]
- Japanese researchers report that acetic acid inactivates the gut enzymes that convert sugars to glucose. This would help prevent blood sugar rising too high or too quickly.[91]

All this suggests that vinegar can reduce a meal's glycaemic index. This could slow the progression of pre-diabetes to diabetes, and aid blood sugar control in people with diabetes.

Other studies suggest that acetic acid – as in vinegar – helps normalize the release of sugar from the liver, and the production of sugar in the liver from non-carbohydrate sources.

Some studies report that other acidic foods – such as lemon juice, yogurt, traditionally made slowly fermented bread, kenkey (fermented corn) and turmeric – also reduce post-meal blood sugar spikes. Certain foods are as powerful as the oral diabetes drug metformin! Frequent consumption of acidic foods is traditional in many countries and may help explain national differences in diabetes rates. Many such foods contain acetic acid, including Japanese sunomono (vinegar-treated vegetables), sumeshi (vinegared rice), potato salad, mustard, vinegared fish and chips, and vinegar-based dressings.

+ ACTIONS: It seems sensible for people with pre-diabetes or diabetes to add apple cider vinegar to their food, or drink 2 teaspoons of cider vinegar in a glass of water 3 times a day, with meals, or eat other fermented foods, or foods pickled in vinegar.

LEMONS

Acid-containing foods seem useful for those with type 2 diabetes. A lemon's acidity is similar to that of vinegar. Experts believe that lemon juice behaves in a similar way to cider vinegar in helping prevent high blood sugar. One study found that drinking 250ml (8½fl oz) of lemon juice lowered the blood sugar rise after eating 100g (3½oz) of bread by 30 per cent.

A lemon's fibre may help, too. "Good" bowel bacteria break down pectin, liberating short-chain fatty acids, which reduce the release of sugar from the liver. Short-chain fatty acids also inhibit C-reactive protein – a blood marker of inflammation and a predictor of diabetes.

+ ACTION: Include the zest and juice of a lemon in your daily diet.

OLIVE OIL

With diabetes, the pancreas makes little or no insulin, so there is too much sugar in the blood but insufficient in the cells. High blood sugar can damage arteries and veins; a lack of sugar in cells stops them functioning properly. The olive oil-rich Mediterranean diet helps prevent and treat type 2 diabetes.

- One study suggests the elenolic acid in mature olives and extra-virgin olive oil can lower blood sugar and promote weight loss in mice. The blood sugar-lowering effect was comparable with that of injections of the diabetes medication liraglutide, and better than that of the oral diabetes drug metformin. While olive oil has only a very low concentration of elenolic acid, there's reason to believe it may have similar, though smaller, effects in humans.[92]
- In an Italian study of overweight adults with type 2 diabetes, one group ate a diet low in total fat and saturated fat, the other a Mediterranean diet. All exercised and reduced their calorie intake. After four years, 56 per cent of those on the Mediterranean diet could control their blood sugar without medication, compared with 30 per cent of the low-fat group.[93]
- A Spanish study of 13,380 people found that a Mediterranean diet discourages type 2 diabetes.[94]

+ ACTION: Consume 2–3 tablespoons of extra-virgin olive oil a day.

HONEY

Most honeys raise blood sugar less than sugar does. More importantly, we tend to use less honey than we would sugar, producing an even smaller rise in blood sugar. In addition:

- Honey's antioxidants have a bigger than predicted effect and may, for example, reduce diabetes-related inflammation in blood vessels. In addition, honey is proven to reduce inflammatory prostaglandins.
- Honey's flavonoids aid cell communication. For example, eating honey with a starchy food such as bread slows the release of amylase (the enzyme that converts starch to sugar), making blood sugar lower than after starchy food alone.
- Honey's trace elements and other minerals may be useful. For example, chromium, magnesium, manganese and zinc are vital for healthy blood sugar control; vanadium decreases the need for insulin; and potassium improves insulin sensitivity.

In a study in Pakistan, 26 volunteers consumed 1g per kg bodyweight of honey, artificial honey-flavoured sugar syrup, or glucose. After 1 hour, blood sugar had increased by 20 per cent in the honey group, 47 per cent in the simulated-honey group, and 52 per cent in the glucose group.[95]

In a study in Iran, 55 overweight volunteers ate 70g of honey or sugar daily for 30 days. The honey group had lower fasting blood sugar.[96]

In people with pre-diabetes, blood sugar 60 and 90 minutes after eating honey was lower than after eating sugar.[97]

High levels of the amino acid homocysteine (which are usually linked with a dietary deficiency of vitamin B) are linked with diabetes. Honey can help reduce high homocysteine.

+ ACTIONS: Use honey (preferably raw) instead of sugar in your diet because it's alkali-producing. Consume a teaspoon of honey within the hour before going to bed.

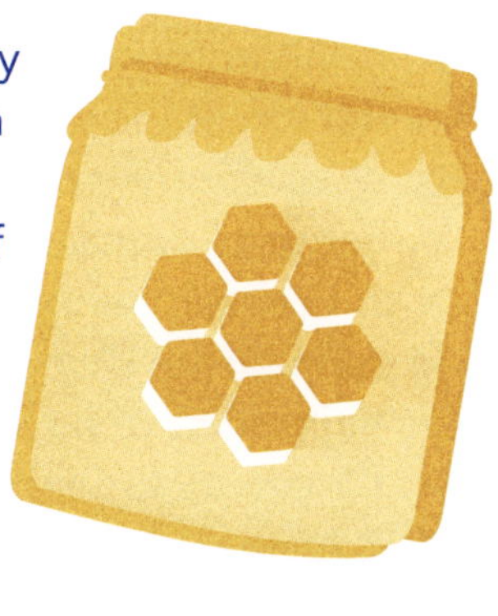

GARLIC

Many studies show that raw garlic reduces blood sugar in animals with type 2 diabetes. Researchers attribute this to garlic's allicin and allicin derivatives.

In an Indian study, rats were given a diet of 65 per cent fruit sugar (which induces type 2 diabetes); or 65 per cent fruit sugar and raw garlic; or a "control" diet of 65 per cent cornflour. After 8 weeks, the fruit-sugar group had higher blood sugar, insulin and insulin resistance than the controls, but the gains were lower in those who had consumed garlic.[98]

It isn't yet known whether garlic helps to prevent or treat diabetes in humans, but research suggests it might help to prevent diabetes-associated heart disease, which is responsible for most deaths in people with diabetes.

+ ACTION: Include garlic in your daily diet or take a garlic supplement. You need both oil- and water-soluble sulphur compounds (pp.78–9).

SPICES

Anti-inflammatory and blood sugar-lowering spices may help. Indeed, galangal lowers blood sugar as effectively as the diabetes drug gliclazide.

Sweeten food with the "sweet" spices – allspice, cardamom, cinnamon and cloves, because, unlike sugar, these don't raise blood sugar levels.

+ ACTION: Include these spices in your diet.

TEAS

Anti-inflammatory and blood sugar-lowering teas may help. If you prefer sweet teas, drink those that have a touch of natural sweetness (such as chamomile and peppermint) to avoid sweetening with sugar. Several studies report that *Camellia-sinensis* tea has beneficial effects in people with diabetes; this might be because of its high levels of flavonoid catechins.

+ ACTION: Include these teas in your daily diet.

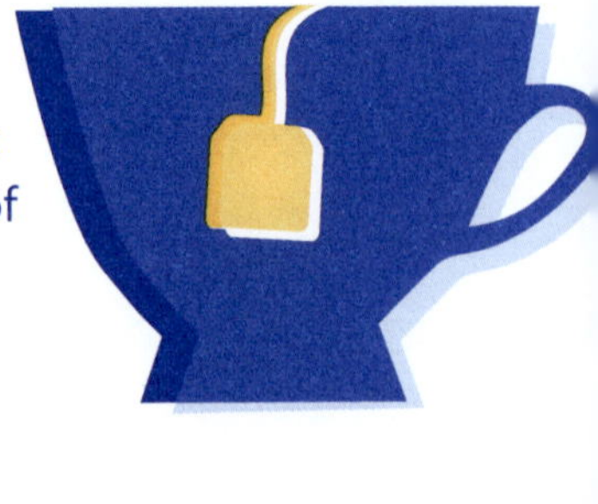

Diarrhoea

The many causes include certain artificial sweeteners (mannitol, sorbitol, xylitol), bowel infection, food allergy, magnesium-containing antacids, inflammatory bowel disease, and side effects from certain medications – for example, antibiotics; antidepressants; magnesium-containing antacids; metformin for diabetes; nonsteroidal anti-inflammatory drugs; and proton pump inhibitors (such as omeprazole, for heartburn and stomach ulcers). Digoxin (for atrial fibrillation/irregular heartbeat and heart failure) and lithium (for mood disorders) can cause diarrhoea as an early sign of toxicity.

Persistent severe diarrhoea originating in the small intestine can cause mild acidosis (p.62) owing to loss of bicarbonate (which is alkaline) in stools. The type of diarrhoea originating in the large intestine can cause metabolic alkalosis (too much alkali and not enough acid in the body) from the loss of chloride, which is acidic.

APPLE CIDER VINEGAR

This can help destroy diarrhoea-causing bacteria such as *Escherichia coli* (*E. coli*), so is useful for those people (including one in two of those aged over 60) who have low production of stomach acid that would otherwise attack bacteria.

+ ACTION: Try drinking 2 tablespoons of apple cider vinegar in a glass of water 3 times a day.

LEMONS

These might help in several ways. Their pectin dissolves in the gut to form a gel that helps bind the bowel contents into stools, which increases transit time. Also, "good" gut bacteria break down some of the pectin. This forms a coating for the gut lining, which soothes irritation. It also releases butyric acid and other short-chain fatty acids with prebiotic qualities, meaning they nourish good (probiotic) bowel bacteria such as lactobacilli and bifidobacteria. All this helps colon cells produce mucus, which helps prevent irritants sticking to and inflaming the gut lining.

Their cellulose attracts water in the bowel, making its contents more bulky and less runny.

Food acid, like stomach acid, helps kill diarrhoea-causing bacteria such as *Escherichia coli* (*E. coli*). Lemons are particularly useful for people (such as one in two over-60s) with poor stomach acid production. Indeed, certain West African villagers consume citric acid with a meal to protect themselves from cholera. The acidity of lemons (pH 2.1) is only a little less than that of stomach acid (pH 1–2).

One study found that hesperidin in lemons may reduce bowel inflammation.

+ ACTION: Include the zest and juice of a lemon in your daily diet.

SODIUM BICARBONATE

+ ACTIONS: Eat an alkali-producing diet. Consider taking oral rehydration salts (from a pharmacy) or sodium bicarbonate (p.69).

GARLIC

Garlic's allicin and certain allicin derivatives (such as diallyl disulphide) can kill bacteria such as *Escherichia coli* (*E. coli*) and salmonella, which can cause gastroenteritis. Garlic can also help to cure diarrhoea caused by gut infection with the protozoon *Cryptosporidium*.

In addition, garlic can help to relieve diarrhoea associated with antibiotics, or with irritable bowel syndrome, by restoring a normal balance of gut bacteria.

+ ACTION: Include garlic in your daily diet or take a garlic supplement. You need both water- and oil-soluble sulphur compounds (pp.78–9).

SPICES

Anti-inflammatory, antioxidant, antibacterial, antispasmodic, antiviral, astringent, demulcent and gut microbiome-enhancing spices may help. Cumin helps to disable the bacteria that cause food poisoning.

+ ACTIONS: Include these spices in your diet. For traveller's diarrhoea, chew 1 teaspoon of ajowan or cumin seeds and wash them down with water.

TEAS

Anti-inflammatory, antioxidant, antibacterial, antispasmodic, antiviral, astringent and demulcent teas may help.
+ ACTION: Include these teas in your diet.

Dizziness, light headedness and fainting

Common causes include:

- Low blood sugar from an unhealthy diet that causes blood sugar spikes followed by blood sugar dips 2–4 hours later
- Pre-diabetes
- Mild acidosis (p.62)
- Poor digestion from having low stomach acidity, plus being a "fast oxidizer" of sugar, so being hungry after a meal sooner than most people. This latter condition is said to affect many people, including one in two over-60s, and is more likely in people who are stressed
- Poor circulation

Other causes include:

- Repeated vomiting
- Certain diuretics ("water tablets")
- Chronic liver disease
- A problem with the balance organ in the inner ear, such as an infection causing vestibular neuronitis; this may also cause vertigo (the feeling that your surroundings are spinning around you)

APPLE CIDER VINEGAR AND LEMONS

Their acidity can improve protein digestion in people with low stomach acid, so enabling such people to produce energy from protein when they have used up their readily available sugar. In addition, lemons' acidity and fibre slow the absorption of sugar from the gut. This helps prevent blood sugar rising too high then dipping too low.
+ ACTIONS: Include cider vinegar and lemons in your main meals. Include the zest and juice of a lemon in your daily diet.

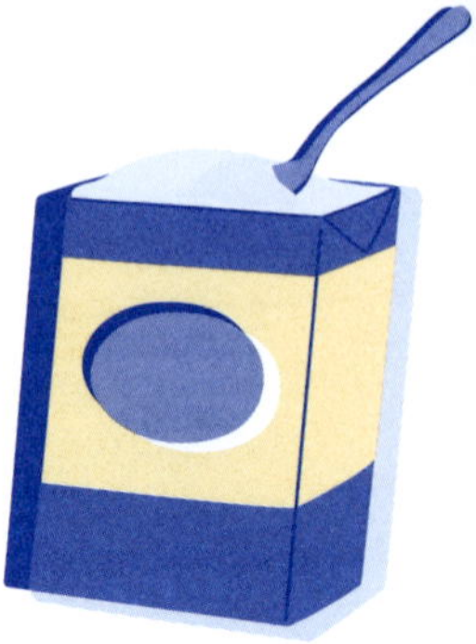

SODIUM BICARBONATE

+ ACTION: Eat a healthy, alkali-producing diet to help your body avoid chronic metabolic stress (p.152). Consider taking sodium bicarbonate (p.69).

Ear infection

If you have an infection in your middle ear, follow the general advice for infection (p.220). If you have an outer-ear infection, try using apple cider vinegar.

APPLE CIDER VINEGAR

This is a traditional treatment for infection in the outer ear.

+ ACTION: Add 2 teaspoons of cider vinegar to an eggcup of water and apply with a cotton bud 3 times a day.

Ear wax

If wax in the outer ears hardens and becomes stuck, it can reduce hearing and cause tinnitus (ringing in the ear).

OLIVE OIL

Room-temperature olive oil can soften hard ear wax, so helping it come out or aiding its removal.

+ ACTIONS: Put one or two drops of warmed olive oil into the ear canal twice a day for a week. Alternatively, soak a ball of cotton wool in warmed olive oil. Squeeze the oil into your ear then gently plug the ear with the cotton wool for an hour. Repeat daily for a week.

Eczema and dermatitis

Atopic eczema is a chronic inflammatory condition that makes skin itchy and irritated. It is most common in young children. Other sorts of dermatitis include contact dermatitis (for example from contact with cosmetics, dyes, nickel and soap); seborrheic dermatitis (which affects the scalp and is thought to be associated with the *Malassezia* yeasts that normally inhabit the skin); and stasis dermatitis in the legs (resulting from poor blood flow – see *Poor circulation*).

Researchers have found a lack of stomach acid in many adults with atopic eczema.

SODIUM BICARBONATE

This can have a soothing effect.

+ ACTION: Try having a daily alkaline bath (p.69).

OLIVE OIL

Applying olive oil may help dermatitis, thanks to its anti-inflammatories. Consuming it can help, too. This is because:

- It contains antioxidant – and therefore anti-inflammatory – compounds such as polyphenols and a terpenoid compound called squalene.
- Its particular balance of omega-3 and omega-6 fatty acids, plus its omega-9 fatty acids and its monounsaturated fats, mean it can help reduce inflammation.

+ ACTIONS: Consume at least 2 tablespoons of extra-virgin olive oil each day. Smoothing extra-virgin olive oil on your skin may help to ease irritation and prevent cracking. Also, aim to consume olive oil in place of saturated-fat containing foods, such as butter and red meat.

HONEY

Anecdotal evidence and early scientific research suggests that honey can help. If so, this could be because of its anti-inflammatory qualities.

+ ACTION: Apply medical-grade honey cream. Consume 1 teaspoon of raw honey 3 times a day.

SPICES

Antihistamine and anti-inflammatory spices may help, as may certain coumarin-containing ones (p.90). In particular, try cassia, cloves and nigella. For eczema over varicose veins, try including circulation-boosting spices in your daily diet.

+ ACTIONS: Include these in your diet. Apply fresh ginger juice to the affected areas. For eczema, try bathing affected skin with anti-inflammatory or antihistamine herb tea or spice tea twice a day.

TEAS

Anti-allergic, antihistamine, anti-inflammatory, antioxidant and astringent teas may help. Also for eczema over varicose veins, try circulation-boosting teas.

+ ACTIONS: Include these teas in your diet. In addition, use these teas, and emollient teas, in a bath or in a compress, poultice or wash for the affected skin.

Eye problems

These include blepharitis (inflamed eyelid margins), cataracts, conjunctivitis, corneal injury, keratitis (inflamed cornea), and macular degeneration (p.234). (See also *Conjunctivitis*; *Macular degeneration*.)

HONEY

Honey applied topically is traditionally reputed to help blepharitis, cataracts, conjunctivitis, keratitis and corneal injury. If it does, this is probably thanks to its antimicrobials and anti-inflammatories. Ideally, see a doctor before applying honey to your eye.

It's suggested that eating raw honey can help cataracts because it's an alkali-producing food (p.62). High blood sugar encourages eye diseases such as cataracts and age-related macular degeneration by damaging ("glycating") proteins in the eye. Honey triggers lower blood sugar spikes than does sugar.

+ ACTIONS: With an eye dropper or straw, put 1 honey eye drop into the outer corner of the affected eye 3 times a day. To make these drops, put ½ a teaspoon of honey and 1 tablespoon of warm water into a container and mix very well, until there are no lumps of honey. Make a fresh mixture each day. To combat infection, for example, with conjunctivitis or blepharitis, use manuka honey with a UMF of at least 10 (p.74). For other eye inflammation, use any antioxidant-rich honey (pp.74–6). It's suggested, but not proven, that eating honey (for example, 1 teaspoon 3 times a day) might help prevent or treat cataracts and age-related macular degeneration.

CAUTION: Consult a pharmacist or doctor before applying honey, or diluted honey, to your eye.

SPICES

Antioxidant and circulation-boosting spices may help cataracts and age-related macular degeneration; antibacterial and anti-inflammatory spices may ease conjunctivitis. Cumin, fennel seeds, fenugreek and ginger may be useful for cataracts.

+ ACTION: Include these in your diet.

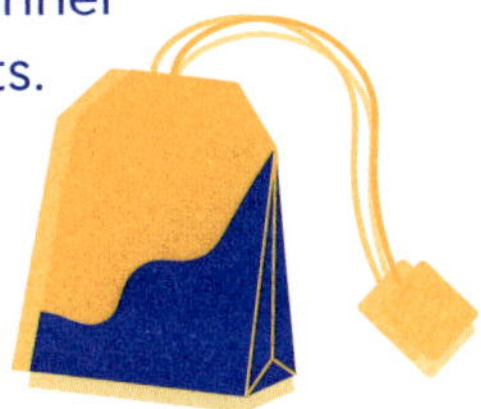

TEAS

Antioxidant and circulation-boosting teas may help cataracts and age-related macular degeneration. Antibacterial and anti-inflammatory teas may ease conjunctivitis.

+ ACTION: Include these in your diet.

Fatigue

The many reasons for fatigue include:

- Doing too much in general
- Doing too much exercise
- Chronic fatigue syndrome, also known as myalgic encephalomyelitis (ME)
- Not eating a healthy diet (p.58), as an unhealhy diet can cause blood sugar spikes followed maybe 2 hours later by fatigue-inducing low blood sugar "troughs". An unhealthy diet may also lack various vitamins (including vitamin B), minerals and polyphenols (p.20) which discourage fatigue by reducing oxidative stress and inflammation)
- Mild acidosis (p.62)
- A weight-loss diet, particularly if low in carbohydrate
- Too little stomach acid: this prevents proper absorption of nutrients such as protein. Low stomach acid is more likely with stress and with prolonged use of acid-suppressant medication. It affects one in two people aged over 60. Finally, fatigue is more likely with stress and can result from many illnesses
- A slow-onset immune reaction associated with a food sensitivity enabled by mild acidosis

Researchers in the UK have developed an ATP profile test to indicate how well mitochondria (our cells' "power plants") are working. Their study of 71 people with chronic fatigue syndrome and 53 healthy controls suggested that fatigue can result from mitochondrial dysfunction – meaning poor working of the energy-producing "factory" in each of the body's cells.[99]

US researchers say deficiencies of certain minerals and vitamins (including iron, magnesium, manganese, zinc and B vitamins) – all present in small amounts in lemons – accelerate age-related decay of mitochondria.[100]

APPLE CIDER VINEGAR

This might ease tiredness from a lack of sufficient stomach acid or a lot of exercise. Research at Nagoya University, Japan, found that including acetic acid – the main component of cider vinegar – in the diet of rats enhanced the replenishment of stored sugar (glycogen) in their liver and muscle. This suggests it might help prevent fatigue associated with endurance exercise.[101]

+ ACTION: Try taking 2 teaspoons of apple cider vinegar 3 times a day.

LEMONS

These may help because:

- They have small amounts of B vitamins.
- Their fibre slows sugar absorption from the stomach, so helping prevent blood sugar dips.
- Lemon acids could aid digestion in those with low stomach acid.
- Japanese researchers (see above) found that giving rats acetic acid (as in vinegar) helped replenish sugar stores in their liver and muscle, suggesting food acids in general may help prevent fatigue associated with low blood sugar.[102]

+ ACTION: Include the zest and juice of a lemon in your daily diet.

SODIUM BICARBONATE

A lack of energy can result from chronic low-grade metabolic stress (p.152).

+ ACTION: Eat a healthy diet to help counteract this. Consider taking sodium bicarbonate (p.69)

HONEY

Consuming honey before, during and after aerobic exercise reduces post-exertion fatigue as its carbohydrates, minerals and vitamins aid recovery. Studies suggest honey reduces cortisol during resistance exercise, which would also reduce fatigue.

In a study at the University of Memphis, 39 athletes ate protein, plus sugar, maltodextrin or honey, after weight lifting. Only honey maintained optimal blood sugar for 2 hours (which would aid muscle recovery, glycogen restoration and energy repletion). Blood tests indicated good muscle recovery.[103]

Raw honey may be particularly helpful as it's an alkali-producing food (p.62).

+ ACTION: Take 1 teaspoon of honey 3 times a day.

GARLIC

Garlic is a traditional remedy for fatigue. Early research suggests it promotes exercise endurance. It also promotes the production of hydrogen sulphide and nitric oxide: both relax arteries, which increases the blood flow to muscles. This enhances energy, post-exercise recovery and muscle growth.

A study in which rats did endurance exercise 5 times a week found that giving aged garlic extract 30 minutes beforehand facilitated aerobic sugar metabolism, reduced oxidation and, by widening arteries, promoted the muscles' oxygen supply.[104]

+ ACTION: Include garlic in your daily diet or take a garlic supplement. You need both water- and oil-soluble sulphur compounds (pp.78–9).

SPICES

Warming spices may be invigorating, thus combating fatigue. Fenugreek and pepper are traditional remedies.

+ ACTION: Include these in your diet.

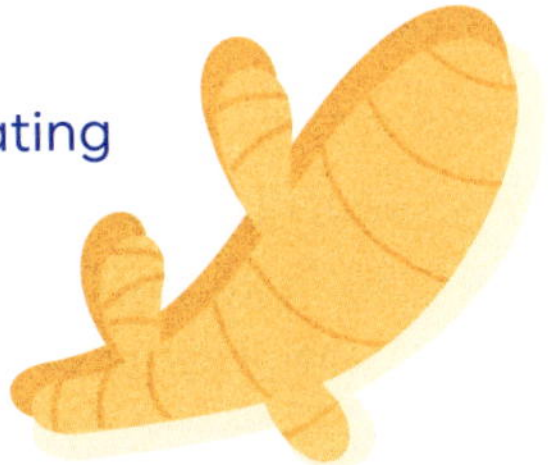

TEAS

Warming and tonic teas may be invigorating. Rosehip tea may help as well.

+ ACTIONS: Include these teas in your diet. Also try inhaling the scent of linden or rosemary teas as this can have an energizing effect.

Fatty liver

One cause of a fatty liver is too much alcohol.

A fatty liver bad enough to cause "non-alcoholic fatty liver disease" can result from the various factors that cause chronic metabolic stress (p.152), including diabetes, high blood fats, high blood pressure, high cholesterol, and overweight and obesity (especially if there is a lot of belly fat). Each of these can result in mild acidosis (p.62) – most often from an unhealthy diet – and this may be a linking factor. At worst, there may be serious liver damage, including a type called cirrhosis.

+ ACTIONS: Eat a healthy diet (p.58) and either drink no alcohol or substantially limit its intake.

APPLE CIDER VINEGAR

Early research suggests this may help, so include it in a healthy diet.

LEMONS

Including these in your diet is a valuable adjunct to a healthy diet.

Fertility problems

These are surprisingly common in both men and women. It's wise to eat a healthy diet (p.58), exercise regularly and use stress management strategies as necessary. Hormone tests in the second half of the menstrual cycle may reveal low progesterone, implying ovulation hasn't happened.

SPICES

Progesterone-balancing spices may be useful for a woman who is not ovulating.

+ ACTION: Consider including progesterone-balancing spices in your diet.

TEAS

Dong quai tea contains an antioxidant called ferulic acid that can improve sperm quality. Progesterone-balancing teas may be useful for a woman who is not ovulating.

+ ACTIONS: Men can try drinking dong quai tea each day. Women can consider drinking progesterone-balancing teas.

Fever

Infection is the most likely cause of a raised body temperature. Other common causes include sustained physical exertion, a hot environment and immunization.

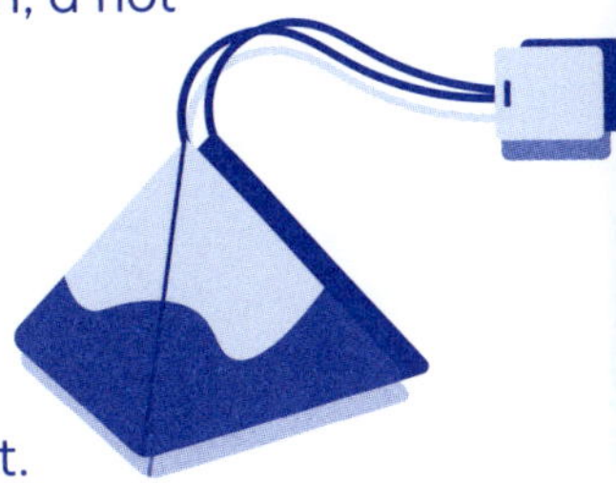

SPICES AND TEAS

Antibacterial and antiviral spices and teas can help a fever associated with infection. Diaphoretic spices are cooling (p.90).

+ ACTION: Include these, as appropriate, in your diet.

Fibroids

Too much oestrogen is one possible reason for these non-cancerous growths in the womb. This could activate genes that encourage womb muscle fibres to proliferate. Another possibility is being very overweight, partly because fat cells produce oestrogen, and partly because very overweight women tend to have high levels of blood sugar and growth hormone. A third possibility is pressure on and in the womb from congestion of blood and lymph in the pelvis.

Women with fibroids have a higher than normal risk of also having atherosclerosis and high blood pressure.

LEMONS

Normally, the liver gets rid of excess oestrogen in the blood by secreting it into the gut, from where it is excreted.

However, certain gut bacteria produce the enzyme beta-glucuronidase which enables the absorption of oestrogen from the gut into the blood. This in turn enables continuing high levels of oestrogen in the blood.

Lemons can help reduce high levels of oestrogen in the body. This is because their fibre reduces the numbers of gut bacteria that produce beta-glucuronidase. Also, lemons' B vitamins encourage the liver to break down surplus oestrogen.
+ ACTION: Include the zest and juice of a lemon in your daily diet.

SPICES
The phytoestrogens in certain spices may help.
+ ACTION: Consume oestrogen-balancing spices: for example, aniseed, caraway, cloves, coriander, cumin, dill seeds, fennel, fenugreek, ginger, juniper, liquorice, nigella, green-tea, sesame and turmeric.

TEAS
+ ACTION: Consume oestrogen-balancing teas: for example, chamomile, fennel, ginger, ginseng, green tea, nettle, red clover, rooibos, thyme, valerian and verbena.

Fibromyalgia

This involves having stiff, weak, knotted shoulder and back muscles and tender points on hips, knees, neck, spine, elbows or buttocks. Associated with this may be anxiety, depression, dizziness, fatigue, headaches, irritable bowel and bladder, numbness, over-sensitivity to noise, light and temperature, poor memory and concentration, poor sleep, Raynaud's phenomenon (white, blue, red or purple discolouration of fingers and toes induced by a sudden change in ambient temperature), and restless legs. Fibromyalgia is more common with increasing age. Some experts blame mild acidosis (p.62), caused by an unhealthy diet, suggesting this deposits acidic ions in muscles and connective tissue. Various studies support this idea, for example:

- A study in Turkey found that people with fibromyalgia had a four times greater risk than others of having metabolic syndrome.[105]
- A study at the University of Oslo in which most of the volunteers with fibromyalgia who ate a vegetarian diet for 3 weeks reported less pain and better wellbeing.[106]

- Research suggests that smokers are more likely to have fibromyalgia.[107]

NOTE: Discuss with your doctor whether any form of chronic metabolic stress (p.152) – for example, high blood fats and high blood pressure – could be encouraging your fibromyalgia. If so, take steps to treat it.

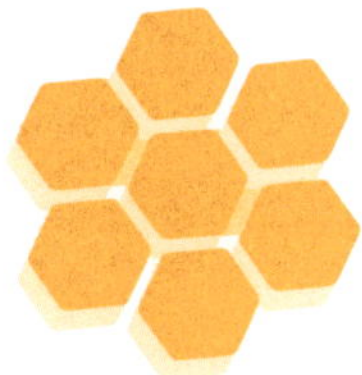

HONEY

Raw honey may help fibromyalgia.

+ ACTION: Eat 1 teaspoon of raw honey 3 times a day.

SPICES

A review of laboratory and animal studies reports that ginger and turmeric have the potential to help the symptoms of fibromyalgia.[108]

+ ACTION: Include ginger and turmeric in your diet.

TEAS

Anti-inflammatory, antispasmodic and diuretic teas may help.

+ ACTION: Include these teas in your diet. Also put them in your bathtub water.

Fluid retention

The many possible causes include being overweight or obese, having a sedentary lifestyle and not eating a healthy diet (p.58). Others include kidney or thyroid problems and heart failure.

GARLIC

Garlic is a traditional remedy for fluid retention in certain countries.

An Iranian study found that garlic extract strongly inhibited the formation of angiotensin-converting enzyme (ACE). ACE inhibition is known to reduce fluid retention by diminishing secretion of the hormones aldosterone and anti-diuretic hormone.[109]

A study in Chile found that garlic powder capsules increased urine production in dogs. The effects were dose-dependent, peaked within 40 minutes and fell to their initial levels within 2½ hours.[110]

+ ACTION: Include garlic in your daily diet or take a garlic supplement. You need both water- and oil-soluble sulphur compounds (pp.78–9).

SPICES

Circulation-boosting (warming) and diuretic spices can help.
+ ACTION: Include these in your diet.

TEAS

Circulation-boosting (warming) and diuretic teas may be useful. Note that unlike many diuretic drugs, dandelion tea replaces the potassium lost from the blood as more urine is produced.
+ ACTION: Include these teas in your diet.

Fractures

After having routine first aid and medical attention for a broken bone, it's a good idea to take advantage of the healing power of lemons.

LEMONS

Vitamin C aids collagen production, so may help the healing of fractured bones and sprained ligaments.
+ ACTION: Include the juice of a lemon in your daily diet.

Fungal infections

See also *Athlete's foot, Dandruff, Ringworm* and *Thrush*.

HONEY

Honey is reputed to help with fungal infections, and research offers some backing.

A laboratory study at Erciyes University, Turkey, tested the effects of various honeys on yeasts such as *Candida albicans, Trichosporon* and certain strains resistant to fluconazole. Honey inhibited their growth, the degree of inhibition depending on the type and concentration of honey and type of yeast. Rhododendron and multifloral honeys had more effect than eucalyptus and orange honeys.[111]
+ ACTION: Apply raw honey twice a day, covering with a dressing if necessary. Manuka honey with a UMF of at least 10–15 is reportedly effective.

Gallstones and gallbladder inflammation

These small, hard "stones" form in bile while it is stored in the gallbladder. Most contain cholesterol, others bile pigments or calcium salts. They are caused by excess cholesterol in bile and by poor emptying of the gallbladder, encouraged by the muscular wall of the gallbladder contracting only feebly. Each of these is more likely with constipation, diabetes or obesity. The risk of gallstones or an inflamed gallbladder (called cholecystitis) rises in people who lose weight rapidly, as this can cause mild acidosis (p.62). The risk also rises with obesity – and certain experts believe this type of acidosis encourages obesity.

Gallstones may also be linked with a lack of stomach acid, as this makes the gallbladder's contractions weaker, allowing the bile in it to stagnate. Note that a lack of stomach acid is more likely with ageing and stress and in people taking antacid or acid-suppressant medication. Encourage gallbladder contractions with frequent healthy meals including something sour (such as lemons and apple cider vinegar) or bitter (such as certain spices – p.88, or teas – p.98).

Bile itself can be over-acidic – for example, in people who eat an unhealthy diet. Such a diet can cause mild acidosis which, in turn, encourages an immune response to certain proteins, perhaps triggering food sensitivity. Indeed, people with gallstones have a raised risk of food sensitivity, the most likely culprits being eggs, pork, chicken, milk, onions and coffee. So mild acidosis might indirectly encourage gallstones. One suggested mechanism is that a food-sensitive immune response inflames the bile duct, making bile stagnate in the gallbladder and so encouraging stones. Studies suggest that dietary antioxidants (such as vitamin C and polyphenols) discourage gallstones.

+ ACTIONS: Include the juice of a lemon in your daily diet. Eat a healthy diet (p.58) and note whether any particular foods make your symptoms worse.

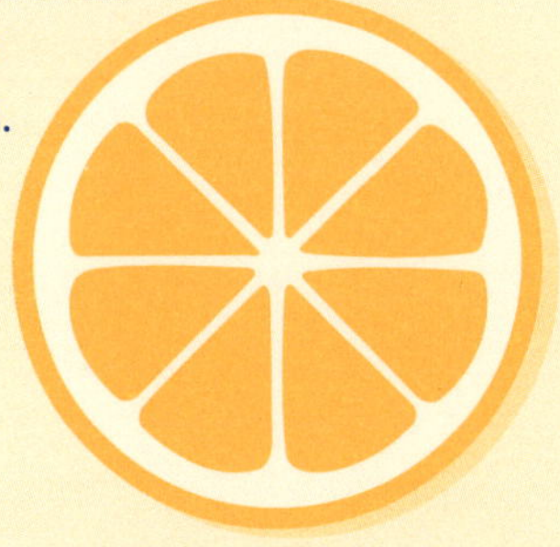

APPLE CIDER VINEGAR

This may help constipation, diabetes and obesity, all conditions that could encourage gallstones.

Consider taking apple cider vinegar in a glass of water or added to a starter before a meal to increase stomach acidity. Apple cider vinegar's pH (acidity measure) is 5, whereas stomach acid is more strongly acidic, with a pH of 1–2, but a little extra acid might be useful.

+ ACTION: Incorporate 1–2 tablespoons of apple cider vinegar into your daily diet.

LEMONS

These have many ways of helping:

- A lemon's pectin helps bind bile acids in the gut, which prevents them from being reabsorbed and used to make gallstones.
- Lemon acids encourage the gallbladder to contract and expel bile and small stones.
- Lemon juice before a meal can mimic stomach acid.
- Lemons as part of a healthy diet discourage any tendency of the body to become relatively more acidic.
- Lemons' acids may also discourage gallstones, and certain practitioners suggest, though their suggestions are unproven, that lemons' acids may encourage the production of stomach acid.
- Studies suggest antioxidants discourage gallstones; lemons are rich in antioxidants.
- Cholesterol dissolves in limonene (albeit in large amounts). Lemon peel contains some limonene.

+ ACTION: Include the zest and juice of 1 or 2 lemons in your daily diet to help prevent or treat gallstones.

SODIUM BICARBONATE

This might help, as people with gallstones have a raised risk of food sensitivity, and any mild acidosis (p.62) – which is common – might encourage this because it raises a person's risk of having an unhelpful immune response to certain proteins.

+ ACTION: Consider taking sodium bicarbonate (p.69).

OLIVE OIL

This oil discourages any tendency to unhealthy acidity in the body. Also, its slight acidity may encourage the normal gallbladder contractions that help prevent bile accumulating in the gallbladder and causing gallstones. Olive oil can help prevent the obesity, constipation and diabetes that can encourage gallstones to form. It is also relatively rich in antioxidants, which studies suggest may help prevent gallstones.

+ ACTIONS: Consume 2 tablespoons of extra-virgin olive oil each day. You can also try taking 1 tablespoon each of olive oil and lemon juice 1 hour before breakfast each day.

GARLIC

This has been claimed to increase bile flow. If so, it would discourage gallstones, which are more likely when bile in the gallbladder stagnates. What's more, garlic is rich in antioxidants, which, studies suggest, discourage gallstones. Garlic may also have a cholesterol-lowering effect in both blood and bile.

Researchers in India found that when mice on a gallstone-promoting diet were given raw or cooked garlic, the bile's cholesterol concentration was reduced and gallstones discouraged. Raw garlic was the most effective.[112]

+ ACTION: Include garlic in your daily diet or take a garlic supplement. You need both water- and oil-soluble sulphur compounds (pp.78–9).

SPICES

Antispasmodic and bitter spices can help, as can limonene-containing spices, because limonene helps dissolve gallstones.

+ ACTION: Include these in your diet.

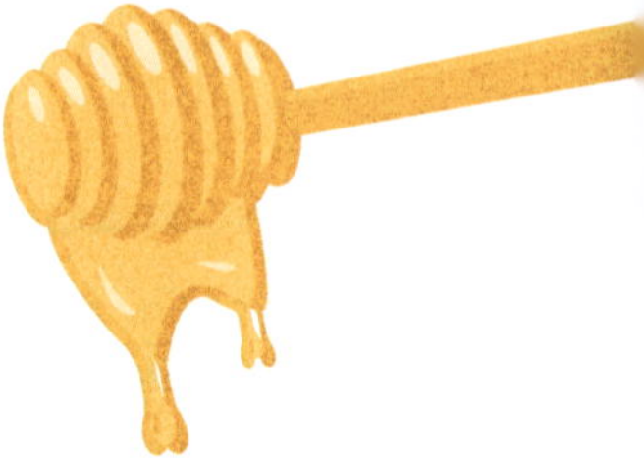

Gastroenteritis

This inflammation of the stomach and gut can result from infection and inflammation.

HONEY

Honey's antimicrobials and anti-inflammatories make honey useful for bacterial gastroenteritis. Its simple sugars make it easier to digest if gastroenteritis provokes a lack of the digestive enzymes that break down complex sugars. Its oligosaccharides aid the growth and activity of probiotic gut bacteria, which may also help.

Researchers at the University of Natal, South Africa, treated 36 children with bacterial gastroenteritis. Those given oral rehydration solution containing honey recovered in 58 hours on average; those given oral rehydration solution containing sugar recovered in 93 hours.[113]

+ ACTION: Consume 2 teaspoons of antimicrobial-rich honey 3 times a day. If unable to keep food down, drink at least 3 litres (5¼ pints) a day of a honey-containing oral rehydration solution made by mixing:

- 1 litre (35fl oz/5 cups) water (boiled if necessary)
- ¼ teaspoon salt
- ¼ teaspoon sodium bicarbonate
- 2 tablespoons runny honey

Gout

This can cause acute pain resulting from irritation by needle-like crystals of sodium urate in joints or under skin.

These crystals are associated with high uric acid in the body. One in five Americans has high uric acid. An unhealthy diet high in sugar – especially sucrose ("table sugar") – and alcohol encourages high uric acid. The kidneys normally excrete any excess, but with mild acidosis (p.62) they may not do this fast enough. High uric acid can also be associated with atrial fibrillation, diabetes, heart disease, gallstones, high blood pressure, kidney stones, metabolic disease, obesity and strokes. A healthy diet (p.58) is a good way of helping to prevent this condition.

LEMONS

Their vitamin C may aid the excretion of uric acid in urine, so reducing high uric acid in the body and discouraging gout.
+ **ACTION:** Consume the juice of half a lemon twice a day.

SODIUM BICARBONATE

Some people find this alleviates an attack. Presumably – though this is unproven – it encourages urate crystals in joints to dissolve. Gout attacks are more likely at night, as the body is relatively more acidic then. In an online poll of people with gout, 85 per cent said that taking sodium bicarbonate helped.
+ **ACTION:** See if taking sodium bicarbonate helps (p.69).

SPICES

Celery seeds and juniper may promote excretion of uric acid.
+ **ACTION:** Include these in your diet.

Hair loss

One reason for this is a poor blood supply to the hair follicles. Others include a diet lacking enough of those nutrients – such as catechins – that stimulate hair growth by encouraging hair follicle cells to multiply and discouraging their apoptotis ("cell suicide").

Flavonoids called catechins may help by prolonging the "anagen" stage of hair growth. This is when hair follicles are busy producing new hairs to replace ones that have fallen out. During this stage, hair follicle cells divide rapidly and hair grows at about half an inch a month. It can last for up to six years, and about 90 per cent of the hairs on the head are in this stage at any one time. Generalized thinning or even total loss of hair differs from the male-pattern hair loss that affects many men as they grow older. The good news is that several natural approaches may help. For example:

- Hesperidin, a flavonoid in lemons, might slow hair loss or stimulate hair growth.
- The flavonoid quercetin and the phytoestrogen genistein may help prevent the patchy balding called alopecia areata.

- Vitamin C improves blood vessel formation, so increasing the blood flow in the scalp.
- Garlic can boost the circulation in the scalp.
- Ginseng may increase hair growth and hair life, so enabling hair to grow longer.
- Italian researchers who reviewed several foods reputably useful for hair loss concluded that *Camellia-sinensis* tea, garlic and ginseng are particularly promising.[114]
- Butterfly pea tea contains a flavonoid called anthocyanin that increases the blood flow in the scalp. This enables hair follicles to do their job of growing hair well. Drinking the tea may darken hair, according to animal studies. And this tea is thought by some to be one of nature's most effective ingredients for promoting hair growth. One study found that an alcoholic extract of butterfly pea flowers was more effective than minoxidil at promoting hair growth![115]

LEMONS

Their hesperidin may help.

+ ACTION: Try consuming the juice of half a lemon each day.

OLIVE OIL

Some people find that consuming olive oil and/or applying it to the scalp helps with hair loss.

+ ACTIONS: Consume at least 2 tablespoons of extra-virgin olive oil each day. Also, apply extra-virgin olive oil to your scalp, Put a shower cap or plastic carrier bag over your hair and cover with a towel wrapped turban-style. Relax for 1 hour, then rinse, shampoo and rinse again. Repeat twice a week.

HONEY

One study reports that honey slows hair loss in people with seborrheic dermatitis and dandruff.[116]

+ ACTION: Once or twice a week, massage 2 tablespoons of warmed runny honey into the scalp. Wait 30 minutes, then shampoo.

SPICES

Fenugreek may help as its trigonelline increases the scalp's blood supply, enabling more nutrients and oxygen to nourish hair roots. Trigonelline resembles minoxidil, a drug that encourages hair growth.
+ ACTION: Include fenugreek in your diet.

TEAS

Camellia-sinensis and ginseng teas may help, as may butterfly pea tea.
+ ACTION: Include these teas in your diet.

Hangover

Although hangovers are avoidable, this unpleasant "morning after" temporary condition affects many and includes headache, dizziness, fatigue, irritability and anxiety.

HONEY

Honey's fructose speeds the breakdown of alcohol in the liver; it also aids recovery by providing sodium, potassium and vitamin B6.
+ ACTION: Consume 1 tablespoon of honey after drinking alcohol.

Hay fever

Also called "allergic rhinitis", its triggers can include, for example, exposure to certain pollens, house dust mites, animal dander (flakes of skin in animals' fur) and moulds.

APPLE CIDER VINEGAR

Apple cider vinegar is a traditional remedy for allergic rhinitis. Dr DC Jarvis, of Vermont, studied 24 people over two years in the 1950s and found their urine became highly alkaline before and early on in an allergic attack. On following his suggestion to drink cider vinegar, their urine rapidly returned to a normal acid pH and the attack became less severe. He attributed this to cider vinegar's organic acids and potassium.

I can find no confirmatory studies. However, it's possible that apple cider vinegar might help because it has anti-inflammatory effects and can

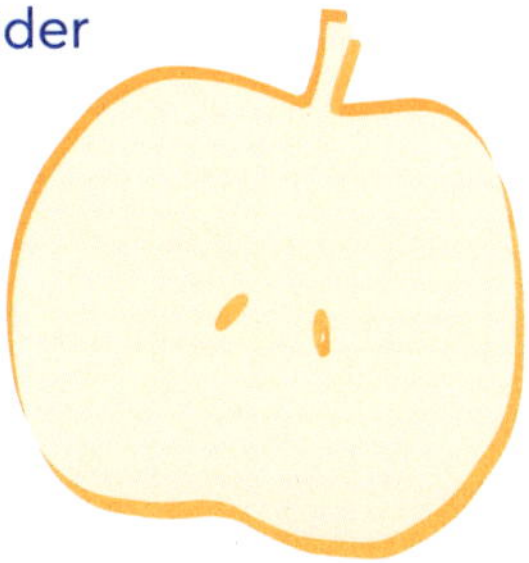

also thin the mucus made by the lining of the nose. It should do no harm to try apple cider vinegar early in an attack.

+ ACTIONS: Put 1 tablespoon of apple cider vinegar into a glass of water and sip the mixture over half an hour. Wait half an hour then repeat. Alternatively, add 1 tablespoon of apple cider vinegar to soup or other food.

LEMONS

Try consuming lemon juice as part of your daily diet, as well as during an attack, as its anti-inflammatories and antihistamines could help prevent or ease hay fever.

+ ACTIONS: Include the zest and juice of a lemon in your daily diet. During an attack, consume 2 tablespoons of lemon juice in a glass of water 3 times a day. If your throat is sore, gargle with 1 tablespoon of lemon juice in a cup of warm water.

OLIVE OIL

Consuming this may help to discourage the allergic inflammation of hay fever because some of its constituents are anti-inflammatory and because its quercetin acts as an antihistamine.

A study in Crete of nearly 700 children aged 7–18 suggests the Mediterranean diet (which includes olive oil) helps prevent hay fever. Conversely, a high consumption of margarine is associated with double the risk.[117]

+ ACTION: Consume at least 2 tablespoons of extra-virgin olive oil each day.

HONEY

Eating locally produced honey for several months before a person's particular "hay-fever season" reputedly helps. Honey made locally is best as it contains anti-inflammatory-rich pollens and a natural antihistamine as well as local wind-borne pollens.

In a Finnish study, 44 volunteers with birch-pollen allergy consumed honey with added birch pollen, or regular honey, daily from November, and 17 had no honey. In April and May, those taking either honey had fewer and milder symptoms. Those taking honey with added birch pollen used less medication than the regular-honey group and only half that of the non-honey group.[118]

Wind-spread pollens are much more likely to provoke hay fever as they are easily inhaled. Pollens collected by bees are larger and stickier, so don't hang in the air. However, nectar is sticky, so may attract wind-blown pollens. Also, bees mix pollen with anti-inflammatory-containing saliva and nectar, and some of this gets into the honey they store in their hives. Honey contains vitamin B5, a natural antihistamine.

However, the following study questions the efficacy of any honey, so the picture isn't clear:

Researchers at the University of Connecticut worked with 36 volunteers with hay fever. One group took 1 tablespoon a day of locally produced unfiltered, unpasteurized honey. The second took non-local filtered, pasteurized honey. The third took corn syrup flavoured with artificial honey. Symptoms were similar in each group.[119]

+ ACTION: Try having 1 to 2 teaspoons of locally produced raw multi-floral honey 3 times a day, starting 3 months before you expect hay fever.

GARLIC

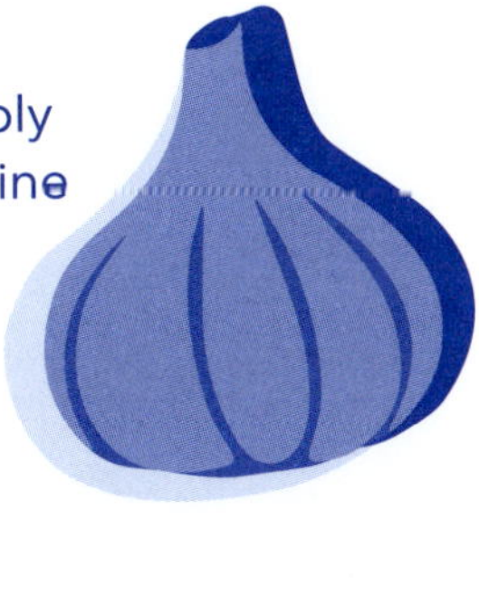

Garlic is a traditional remedy. Any success probably stems from its anti-inflammatory and antihistamine constituents.

+ ACTION: Eat more garlic or take a garlic supplement in the weeks before and during your usual hay-fever season. You need both water- and oil-soluble sulphur compounds (pp.78–9).

SPICES

Antihistamine, anti-inflammatory, antioxidant, astringent and antispasmodic spices may help. In particular, try cassia, cloves and nigella.

+ ACTIONS: Include these spices in your diet. Inhale the steam from spice tea once or twice a day.

Headache, including migraine

Headaches are a possible symptom of mild acidosis (p.62). It's also possible, though unproven, that such acidosis can cause headaches as a result of the body's buffer systems working extra hard to keep the blood's acid–alkali balance within its normal tightly controlled range.

Another cause of headaches is a slow-onset immune reaction associated with a food sensitivity enabled by this acidosis.

Interestingly, vinegar – which is acidic – is a folk remedy familiar from the nursery rhyme "Jack and Jill" in which Jack mends his hurting head with "vinegar and brown paper". It may be that headaches can result from the body's normal acid–alkali balance being at either extreme of its usual range.

APPLE CIDER VINEGAR

It's worth trying this to see if this vinegar's acidity help – as it did in the nursery rhyme!

+ ACTIONS: Sponge your forehead or head with apple cider vinegar, or apply a face cloth soaked in 570ml (1 pint) of water containing 2 tablespoons of cider vinegar. Inhale organic acid vapour by putting 1 tablespoon of apple cider vinegar into a vaporizer and staying nearby for, say, 15 minutes. Or drink 1 cup of hot water containing 3 teaspoons of cider vinegar 3 times a day.

LEMONS

Lemons' acidity may help with headaches.

+ ACTIONS: Sponge your head with lemon juice, or apply a facecloth soaked in 570ml (1 pint) of water containing 2 tablespoons of lemon juice. Inhale mildly acidic vapour by putting 1 tablespoon of lemon juice into a vaporizer and staying close by until it has evaporated. Alternatively, drink a cup of hot water containing 1 tablespoon of lemon juice three times a day.

SODIUM BICARBONATE

While a healthy – therefore alkali-producing – diet, plus regular exercise and effective stress management, can help prevent headaches associated with chronic mild acidosis, taking sodium bicarbonate may help relieve a heachache in the here and now.

TEAS

Pain-relieving teas may help: in particular, those containing salicylates. Also use anti-inflammatory and antispasmodic teas.
+ ACTION: Include these teas in your diet. Apply a compress made with one of them – hot or cold according to what you find works best.

Head lice

These little insects and their eggs – known as "nits" – are common in young schoolchildren, and often easily passed to their parents!

APPLE CIDER VINEGAR

This can loosen the glue that sticks nits to hairs.
+ ACTION: Mix a cupful with a cup of water. Apply to dry hair then leave for half an hour. Wet the hair with water and smooth in lots of silicone-based conditioner (such as Pantene). Comb the hair first with a wide-toothed comb, then a fine-toothed one to remove any lice. Now shampoo. Some nits may stay stuck to hairs, so do this wet-combing twice weekly for 2 weeks to catch newly hatched lice.

LEMONS

Lemon oil discourages lice from settling on scalps.
+ ACTION: Add 2 drops of lemon essential oil to your shampoo and another 2 drops to your conditioner or final rinse.

Heart disease

See also *Artery disease, Atherosclerosis, Heart attack.*

Heart disease can lead to angina ("heart pain") and a heart attack. These usually result from atheroma in the lining of the heart's coronary arteries becoming so thick that the heart muscle can't get enough blood.

Mild acidosis (p.62) encourages an irregular heartbeat (atrial fibrillation), chest pain on exercise (angina), heart attacks and heart failure.

Many studies also show that mild acidosis can:

- Reduce energy production from sugar in heart muscle cells. Energy production from fats and proteins takes longer than from sugar. So low energy is an early problem associated with heart disease
- Irritate coronary arteries, encouraging tiny tears that in turn encourage atherosclerosis
- Interfere with the passage of potassium, sodium and calcium through cell membranes. Also, rob the body of calcium, magnesium and potassium as these must be used to neutralize acids excreted in urine. All this weakens heart muscle, prevents its normal conduction of electrical messages, and makes sodium and calcium accumulate in the blood, encouraging high blood pressure and atheroma
- Increase LDL cholesterol (the potentially "bad" sort, especially if oxidized) and decrease HDL cholesterol (the "good" sort)
- Increase adrenaline, which speeds the heart and boosts its cells' need for oxygen
- Encourage insulin resistance: blood sugar can't enter cells as well, so its level in the blood rises, triggering greater insulin production. But high insulin has adverse effects, such as boosting LDL cholesterol
- Raise fibrinogen, encouraging blood clots, which can block a coronary artery

Mild acidosis reduces the passage of calcium into heart muscle cells, preventing the heart pumping efficiently and rhythmically. The greater the acidosis, the less well the heart pumps. A healthy (and therefore alkaline) diet, regular suitable exercise and effective stress management may help your heart by reducing mild acidosis.[120]

Blood is most acidic during sleep, which is when most fatal heart attacks occur. High blood pressure and atrial fibrillation are sometimes associated with high uric acid (see *Gout*). Heart palpitations can result from a slow-onset immune reaction associated with a food sensitivity enabled by mild acidosis.

APPLE CIDER VINEGAR

Researchers at Harvard University followed 76,283 women for 10 years. Those who consumed 1 to 2 tablespoons of oil and vinegar salad dressing most days had only half the average risk of heart disease. The oil contained alpha-linolenic acid, a polyunsaturated fat with heart-health benefits, and the dressing's apparent benefit was attributed to this. But the vinegar might have played a part.[121]

+ ACTION: Do your heart a favour by consuming apple cider vinegar each day.

LEMONS

These can reduce many risk factors, including obesity, high blood pressure, diabetes and high cholesterol, homocysteine (via lemons' folate) and C-reactive protein (via lemons' anti-inflammatories). Lemons' antioxidants can reduce the oxidation associated with smoking and stress; and their flavonoids can help lower blood pressure and improve blood vessel function.

A review at Boston University suggests flavonoids improve the behaviour of artery-lining cells and help prevent blood clots.[122]

In addition, studies suggest flavonoids (as in lemon peel) discourage heart disease: Finnish scientists who followed 5,133 people found the risk of heart disease deaths was lowest in those who ate most foods rich in flavonoids.[123]

"Good" micro-organisms in the bowel degrade pectin from lemons, freeing short-chain fatty acids such as butyric acid. These, in turn, reduce LDL cholesterol, increase HDL cholesterol (the potentially protective sort) and inhibit C-reactive protein.

Researchers at Florida University found that giving pigs pectin reduced their expected artery calcification.[124]

+ ACTION: Include the zest and juice of a lemon in your daily diet.

OLIVE OIL

Extra-virgin olive oil, the Mediterranean diet's main fat, discourages oxidation, inflammation, high blood pressure, unhealthy blood clotting, atherosclerosis, endothelial dysfunction (badly behaved artery-lining cells making arteries shrink) and an unhealthy blood fat profile (high LDL cholesterol and triglycerides and low HDL cholesterol). It also guards against heart disease risk factors such as obesity, high blood pressure and diabetes.

When olive oil is the main dietary fat, oleic acid is the main fatty acid in cholesterol. This is good because oleic acid is more resistant than other fatty acids to oxidation. If extra-virgin olive oil rather than refined olive oil is consumed, the oleic acid and other fats are further protected by polyphenols and other antioxidants. Many other constituents of extra-virgin olive oil are heart-protective too; they include the following anti-inflammatories:

- Antioxidants – discourage oxidation of LDL cholesterol. Squalene, beta-sitosterol and tyrosol also discourage the production of inflammatory compounds from omega-6 fats, or render them harmless
- Polyphenols – help prevent white blood cells from sticking to the artery lining: one of them, hydroxytyrosol acetate, directly inhibits clotting
- Monounsaturated fatty acids – once absorbed into blood, these are either surrounded by protein molecules and disguised as HDL or LDL cholesterol, or converted into other compounds. This happens much more quickly than the 6–12 hours it takes to clear saturated fatty acids from blood. Scientists believe this speed of clearing fatty acids from blood helps prevent atherosclerosis. Monounsaturated fats also help prevent blood becoming sticky after a fatty meal and forming dangerous clots

Indeed, the US Food and Drug Administration allows olive oil bottle labels to claim: "Limited and not conclusive evidence suggests that eating about 2 tablespoons of olive oil daily may reduce the risk of coronary heart disease due to the monounsaturated fat in olive oil." However, labels must also say: "To achieve this possible benefit, olive oil is to replace a similar amount of saturated fat and not increase the total number of calories you eat in a day."

Research suggests that if we don't overeat, and if we eat a healthy diet, then a well-balanced intake of different fats, without too much food high in saturated or trans fat, is what's best for the heart. What seems more important is what we should eat rather than what we should not.

- A huge meta-analysis of 30 studies, involving 2,710,351 people, linked a high olive oil intake with a reduced risk of cardiovascular disease (and cardiovascular mortality) and coronary heart disease. For each 10g a day increment of olive oil intake, cardiovascular-disease risk fell by 7 per cent and cardiovascular disease mortality by 8 per cent.[125]
- Evaluation of the effects in 50 people of consuming high- or low-polyphenol olive oil found the antioxidant and anti-inflammatory effects of high-polyphenol extra-virgin olive oil more pronounced in those at high risk of cardiometabolic disease (a group of conditions including diabetes, fatty liver disease, heart attacks and strokes). Its risk factors include obesity, smoking, lack of exercise, poor diet, high blood pressure, high fasting triglyceride blood fats, and low HDL cholesterol.[126]
- The PREDIMED study of 7,216 people aged 55–80 at high risk of cardiovascular disease, found that those who consumed the most extra-virgin olive oil had a 39 per cent reduction in risk. Each extra 10 g per day consumed reduced their risk of this disease by 10 per cent and of dying from it by 7 per cent.[127]
- A Spanish study of 13,609 people found that those with the highest adherence to the Mediterranean diet had a lower heart disease risk than those with the lowest adherence. In this study participants ate a breakfast of bread and either

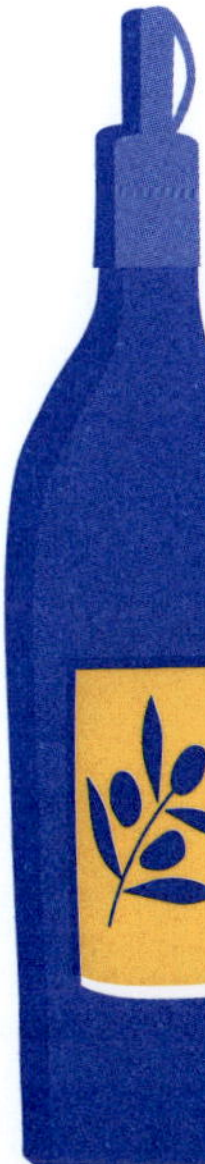

extra-virgin or refined olive oil. After a breakfast containing extra-virgin olive oil (which is relatively high in polyphenols), their arteries were more elastic. But after a breakfast containing olive oil (which is low in polyphenols) there was no change in their arteries' usual elasticity.[128]

+ **ACTION:** Take at least 2 tablespoons of extra-virgin olive oil a day.

SPICES

Anti-inflammatory, antioxidant, anticoagulant and blood sugar-lowering spices may help. In particular, use cinnamon, mastic, cocoa (a high intake of which is associated with a halving of deaths from heart attacks and strokes) and sesame seeds.

+ **ACTION:** Include these spices in your diet.

TEAS

Anti-inflammatory, antioxidant, anticoagulant, cholesterol-lowering and blood sugar-lowering teas may help.

+ **ACTION:** Include these teas in your diet.

Heavy periods

Possible triggers include fibroids, hormone imbalance, inelastic blood vessels (possibly due to a poor diet), inflammation from an intra-uterine contraceptive device, iron-deficiency anaemia, womb infection and stress.

APPLE CIDER VINEGAR

This is sometimes claimed to ease heavy periods.

+ **ACTIONS:** See if it helps to drink 2 teaspoons of apple cider vinegar in a glass of water 2 or 3 times a day, or add some to your food.

LEMONS

Lemon juice is a folk remedy. If it works, it's probably because of some combination of its minerals (such as calcium, iron, magnesium and zinc), vitamins (such as beta-carotene and vitamin C) and flavonoids (such as rutin).

+ **ACTION:** Include the zest and juice of 2 lemons in your daily diet.

SPICES AND TEAS

Oestrogen-balancing and astringent spices and teas might help.
+ ACTION: Include these in your diet.

Hiccups

Possible causes of this irksome phenomenon are an overfull stomach after eating too much; low stomach acid slowing protein digestion; or fatty, sugary food slowing stomach emptying and encouraging fermentation.

APPLE CIDER VINEGAR

Apple cider vinegar is a traditional remedy for hiccups.
+ ACTIONS: To prevent frequent attacks, try adding apple cider vinegar to your food, or drink 1 teaspoon in a glass of water before a meal. To stop hiccups, try very slowly sipping the same solution or swallowing 1 teaspoon of neat apple cider vinegar.

High blood pressure

Risk factors include obesity, partly because more weight means more work for the heart, and also because visceral fat encourages inflammation. Other risk factors include age, genetics, not eating a healthy diet (p.58), atherosclerosis, over-activity of renin (a kidney hormone), insulin resistance (pre-diabetes) and salt. In addition, high blood sugar can encourage high blood pressure by damaging ("glycating") collagen in artery walls and thus stiffening the arteries. Sometimes there is no obvious cause.

The charity Blood Pressure UK points out that salt is the single biggest cause of high blood pressure. It advises checking food labels and avoiding products that are high in salt, defined as 1.5g or more per 100g of food.

Note that while some people are "salt-sensitive", meaning that consuming salt raises their blood pressure, others are not salt-sensitive, so salt does not raise their blood presssure. Mild acidosis (p.62) may encourage high blood pressure. One possible reason is that it might make cells more resistant to insulin. The pancreas then produces extra insulin to prevent high blood sugar. This makes arteries over-sensitive to adrenaline, so encouraging high blood pressure.

A study of 15,385 women found that those whose diets had a higher potential acid load had higher blood pressure than those with a lower load. The probable culprit is an unhealthy diet, with a lack of vegetables, fruit and nuts and a surfeit of meat, sugar and refined-carbohydrate foods.[129]

Another study reported that consuming sodium bicarbonate and having a low-salt diet can lower blood pressure by reducing calcium excretion in urine.[130]

APPLE CIDER VINEGAR

There are several reasons why vinegar may help lower blood pressure.

- It increases nitric oxide (which relaxes blood vessels).
- It acts like ACE-inhibitor blood pressure medication (by inhibiting angiotensin-converting enzyme, so decreasing production of the blood vessel-constricting hormone angiotensin II).
- It adds flavour, which helps salt-sensitive people reduce their salt intake.
- It encourages weight loss.
- Adding it when cooking casseroles or stocks containing bones releases some of the bones' calcium: this could help the many people whose diet is low in calcium, as calcium helps maintain healthy blood pressure.

When researchers in Iran reviewed randomized controlled trials of vinegar's effect, they found it reduced both systolic blood pressure (a reading's upper figure) and diastolic (the lower figure) blood pressure. So it may be considered an adjunct to drug treatment for high blood pressure.[131]

Japanese researchers found that long-term dosing of rats with vinegar or acetic acid lowered blood pressure. They attributed this to vinegar's acetic acid. They believe this reduces renin activity, so decreasing angiotensin II. This, in turn, lowers blood pressure by decreasing blood volume and relaxing blood vessels.[132]

+ ACTION: Include apple cider vinegar in 2 or 3 meals a day, or take 1 teaspoon in a glass of water 3 times a day.

LEMONS

These can affect several high blood pressure risk factors, including age, insulin resistance (pre-diabetes), obesity, overactivity of the kidney hormone renin, salt sensitivity and atherosclerosis (see *Atherosclerosis*). Lemons aid weight loss, their potassium helps regulate body fluids, their magnesium relaxes arteries, their fibre encourages weight loss, their flavonoids promote artery health, and their acids discourage pre-diabetes. Interestingly, note that Russian folklore recommends lemon juice to help prevent atherosclerosis.

Studies suggest that hesperidin, a lemon flavonoid, reduces blood pressure in rats.[133]

Japanese researchers found that when rats with high blood pressure consumed lemon juice, their blood pressure tended to fall. They attributed this to the inhibition of angiotensin-converting enzyme (ACE) by flavonoids such as hesperidin and eriocitrin. (Note that doctors may prescribe ACE-inhibitor medications for high blood pressure.)[134]

+ ACTION: Include the zest and juice of a lemon in your daily diet.

OLIVE OIL

Including olive oil in your diet discourages obesity and atherosclerosis. Also, its polyphenols and magnesium may help. Note that adding it to your diet while on high blood pressure medication might lower your blood pressure enough to make your current dose of medication too high. So monitor your blood pressure and if necessary discuss with your doctor whether you can change the dose.

A review of studies done up to 2015 concluded that consuming at least 2 tablespoons of extra-virgin olive oil a day can lower blood pressure. The higher the oil's polyphenol content, the better.[135]

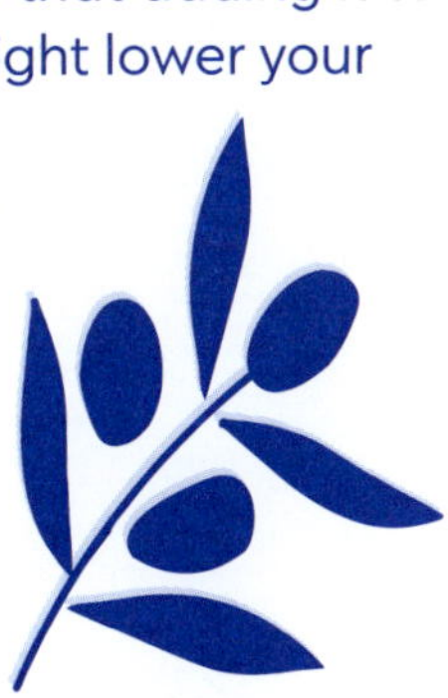

- A Greek study of more than 20,000 people eating the Mediterranean diet associated extra-virgin olive oil and vegetables with lower blood pressure; and cereals, meat and alcohol with higher blood pressure. Olive oil was the main factor in lowering blood pressure, probably thanks to its polyphenols rather than its monounsaturated fats.[136]
- A Spanish study reported that women with high blood pressure experienced a lowering of their readings when they added olive oil to their diet. In contrast, adding a type of sunflower oil rich in oleic acid had no effect. This suggests that components of olive oil other than its monounsaturated fat are responsible.[137]

+ ACTION: Consume at least 2 tablespoons of extra-virgin olive oil each day.

HONEY

Honey's antioxidants discourage artery disease; its acetylcholine dilates blood vessels; and its oligosaccharides may aid the growth and activity of probiotic gut bacteria. Honey also helps prevent stress hormone release (p.123). Honey triggers lower blood sugar spikes than sugar; while raw honey may be particularly useful as it's an alkali-producing food (p.62).

However, more research needs to be done to confirm whether honey can help prevent or lower high blood pressure.

+ ACTION: Take honey, in particular, raw honey, instead of sugar. Have a teaspoon of honey within the hour before bedtime.

GARLIC

Research suggests this traditional remedy reduces high blood pressure. Falls in blood pressure produced by taking garlic compare with those from common blood pressure medications (such as ACE inhibitors and beta-blockers). Some of the many studies undertaken use garlic cloves, others garlic supplements. For example:

- A review and meta-analysis of 12 trials involving 553 people with high blood pressure confirmed that garlic supplements lower systolic blood pressure (the upper of a reading's two numbers) by an average of 8.3mmHg and diastolic blood pressure (the lower of the two numbers) by 5.5 mmHg. Note that this equates to the results from taking standard anti-hypertensive medications! This reduction in blood pressure was associated with a 16–40 per cent reduction in the risk of suffering from cardiovascular events.[138]

- A meta-analysis of studies by Chinese researchers found that garlic can reduce high blood pressure.[139]
- In a study at the University of Adelaide, 50 volunteers with high blood pressure, despite taking medication, were put into two groups. One took aged garlic extract plus their medication for 12 weeks; the other just their medication. Those on garlic had an average fall in their systolic blood pressure of 10 mmHg.[140]

Garlic probably helps because it:

- Discourages atherosclerosis (see *Artery disease*; *Atheroscerosis*)
- Contains gamma-glutamyl cysteines – natural angiotensin-converting enzyme inhibitors (ACE inhibitors) that reduce blood pressure by expanding arteries
- Releases hydrogen sulphide (from polysulphides in chopped or crushed raw garlic), which expands arteries
- Promotes nitric oxide production, which expands arteries (this ability is retained by heat-treated and aged garlic products)
- Has prostaglandin-like effects that reduce blood pressure by relaxing artery wall muscle
- Contains substances that activate sodium-pump enzymes, which maintain low sodium levels in cells

One small study suggests vitamin C enhances garlic's blood pressure-lowering effect. Also, studies suggest this effect lasts for up to 24–48 hours.

+ ACTIONS: Include garlic in your daily diet or take a garlic supplement. You need both water- and oil-soluble sulphur compounds (pp.78–9). Eat plenty of vitamin C-containing foods.

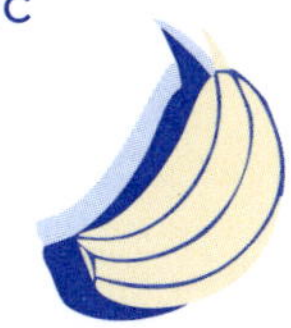

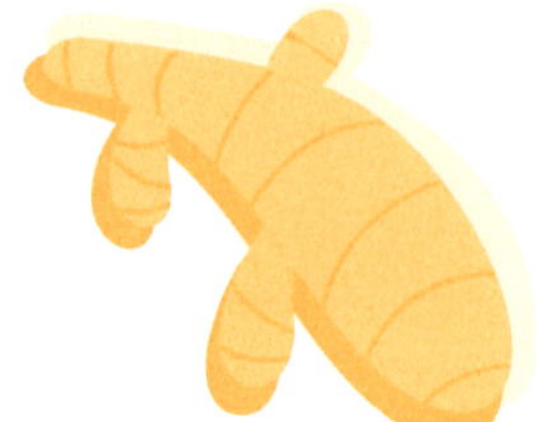

SPICES

Anti-adrenaline, anti-inflammatory, antioxidant, antispasmodic, blood pressure-lowering, calming, cholesterol-lowering and choline-containing spices (p.89) may help. In particular, use celery seeds, cinnamon, fennel seeds, ginger and mastic. Cardamom is also useful, because it acts like the blood pressure-reducing drugs called calcium channel blockers.

+ ACTION: Include these spices in your diet.

TEAS

Anticoagulant, anti-inflammatory, antioxidant, antispasmodic, blood pressure-lowering, blood sugar-lowering, choline-containing (p.98), cholesterol-lowering, diuretic and relaxing teas may help. In particular, try hibiscus tea.

Note that rooibos tea can act like an ACE-inhibitor blood pressure drug. Even just inhaling the fragrance of lavender tea can reduce high blood pressure. And 3 cups a day of black tea can reduce blood pressure by 2–3 points.

+ ACTION: Include these teas in your diet.

High cholesterol

Cholesterol is vital for the production of vitamin D, steroid hormones, neurotransmitters (nerve message carriers) and bile acids. But the presence in the bloodstream of too much LDL cholesterol (sometimes called the "bad'"sort) and not enough HDL cholesterol (sometimes called the "good" sort) encourages heart disease and strokes.

HDL-C is considered good because the higher its level, the lower the risk of cardiovascular disease. Note, though, that certain rural people in Japan not only have the world's lowest rate of heart disease but also have very low HDL-C. So other protective factors (perhaps a high oily fish intake and a low alcohol intake, together with exercise and low body weight) are clearly more important.

Note that high LDL-C is "bad" only if oxidized. This is because it is oxidized LDL-C that encourages inflammation and plaque formation in artery walls. Oxidation involves having an increased amount of "free radicals" (reactive oxygen ions). These encourage an imbalance between antioxidants and pro-oxidants in the body, resulting in oxidative stress.

Possible causes of oxidation of LDL-C include:

- An unhealthy diet, with low antioxidants (such as polyphenols; the mineral selenium; vitamins C and E and beta-carotene) and high saturated fat
- High blood sugar from pre-diabetes and untreated diabetes
- Smoking
- High blood pressure
- Lack of exercise
- Poorly managed stress
- Too much sunlight   d

In most people, the liver makes 80 per cent of the body's cholesterol from triglyceride blood fats and from a compound called apolipoprotein B. Dietary cholesterol is only a minor source for them. For others, though, dietary cholesterol is more important, and lowering their intake of cholesterol-rich foods has a bigger effect on their cholesterol levels. No test can currently identify this group.

A protective level of HDL-C in the blood is considered to be 60mg/dl (1.55mmol/l) or higher. The higher it is above this, the better your protection against heart disease.

In the US, India and many other countries, blood tests report blood-cholesterol levels in mg/dl; in Europe and Australia in mmol/l:

- To convert mmol/l to mg/dl, multiply by 18.
- To convert mg/dl to mmol/l, divide by 18.

When considering the results of blood tests looking at blood fats, doctors are more interested in the overall profile. This includes total cholesterol, HDL-C, LDL-C and triglycerides. Having high total cholesterol and LDL-C, plus low HDL-C, makes a person particularly susceptible to heart attacks and strokes. Having low HDL-C is better at predicting heart attacks than high LDL-C, and much better than high total cholesterol.

Doctors use particular ratios of various types of cholesterol to help assess a person's risk of heart disease and strokes – for example:

HEART DISEASE AND STROKE RISK

RISK	TOTAL:HDL RATIO IN MEN	TOTAL:HDL RATIO IN WOMEN
Very Low	Less than 3.4	Less than 3.3
Low	4.0	3.8
Average	5.0	4.5
Moderate	9.5	7.0
High	More than 23	More than 11

APPLE CIDER VINEGAR

It's possible that apple cider vinegar as part of a healthy diet might help reduce high cholesterol. A review of nine studies found that consuming apple cider vinegar decreased total cholesterol in blood (especially in those who had diabetes).[141]

A meta-analysis of six trials involving 317 people with diabetes taking 1–2 tablespoons of vinegar a day noted a remarkable reduction in total cholesterol and LDL-cholesterol.[142]

+ ACTION: Consume at least 1 tablespoon, preferably more, of apple cider vinegar each day.

LEMONS

Various constituents can influence the balance and levels of cholesterol. Lemons' vitamin C, phenolic compounds, pectin, limonin and acids encourage healthy cholesterol levels.

- A study found that citrus flavonoids reduce LDL cholesterol in hamsters, probably by reducing its production in the liver.[143]

- Lemons – especially their peel – are rich in a type of fibre called pectin. This thickens the bowel's contents, which reduces absorption of cholesterol from food and bile and helps eliminate it. Also, certain good gut bacteria degrade pectin, liberating short-chain fatty acids (such as butyric acid) which inhibit cholesterol absorption, suppress its production in the liver, reduce LDL cholesterol and boost HDL cholesterol. These short-chain fatty acids also inhibit inflammation in the body.
- Studies show that pectin plus vitamin C lowers cholesterol more than pectin alone, and pectin plus phenolic compounds lower cholesterol and triglycerides more than either alone.
- Researchers in Iran report that participants who ate 20g of garlic (about 4 cloves) and 1 tablespoon of lemon juice daily for 8 weeks had lower cholesterol.[144]
- The US Agricultural Research Service found that liver cells produce less of the protein apo B (needed to make LDL cholesterol) when exposed to limonin.[145]
- Research suggests a lemon's glucaric-acid salts reduce LDL cholesterol by up to 35 per cent.[146]

+ ACTION: Include the zest and juice of 1 or 2 lemons in your daily diet.

OLIVE OIL

Several constituents in olive oil, including fatty acids and polyphenols and other antioxidants, have beneficial effects on cholesterol production and metabolism. Also, its sitosterol reduces the intestinal absorption of dietary cholesterol. If you take statins for high cholesterol, note that taking olive oil may lower your cholesterol, so get your cholesterol level checked in case you can lower your dose of statins. Consider the results of these studies:

- A study of diets high in carbohydrate, protein or unsaturated fat (from olive oil, canola oil and olive oil spread – each rich in monounsaturated fat) found each reduced total cholesterol and LDL ("bad") cholesterol.[147]

- Consuming olive oil improved the fatty-acid profile of LDL cholesterol and reduced its oxidation.[148]
- Consuming extra-virgin olive oil (which is rich in clot-fighting polyphenols) discourages blood clots (such as those causing heart attacks and strokes) after a meal in people with high cholesterol.[149]
- Researchers report that the higher an olive oil's polyphenol content, the higher the resulting increase in HDL ("good") cholesterol. The ratio of total cholesterol to HDL cholesterol, and the degree of oxidation of LDL cholesterol, decreased with increasing polyphenol content.[150]
- When 21 volunteers with a high cholesterol level ate a breakfast containing virgin olive oil, their blood contained far fewer free radicals than normal after a meal. But when they ate breakfast containing olive oil with a lower polyphenol concentration, the beneficial effects were virtually absent.[151]

+ ACTION: Consume 2 tablespoons of extra-virgin olive oil each day.

HONEY

Honey raises HDL cholesterol. Honey's vitamin B3 can reduce LDL cholesterol, and its antioxidants help protect LDL cholesterol from oxidation. In one study, a group of 80 obese and 80 normal-weight volunteers took 80g of honey a day and a group of equal numbers of obese and normal-weight volunteers did not. After 4 weeks, the honey group had lower total cholesterol and higher HDL cholesterol. Obese honey-eaters also had lower LDL cholesterol.[152]

Scientists at the National Research Center Dokki in Egypt found honey highly effective at preventing oxidation of LDL cholesterol.[153]

+ ACTION: Eat 1 teaspoon of honey 3 times a day.

GARLIC

Many early studies suggested garlic might help to inhibit cholesterol production, increase cholesterol excretion and protect LDL cholesterol from oxidation. But since then, high-quality studies suggest it does not help significantly.

+ ACTION: Until we know more, include garlic in your daily diet.

SPICES

Cholesterol-lowering spices can reduce high total cholesterol (p.89). Also, chilli, cayenne and paprika discourage the formation of the oxidized LDL cholesterol that encourages heart attacks and strokes.

+ ACTION: Include these spices in your diet.

TEAS

Antioxidant and cholesterol-lowering teas should help (p.99), as should teas rich in beta-sitosterol (which may reduce fat absorption from the gut).

+ ACTION: Include these teas in your diet.

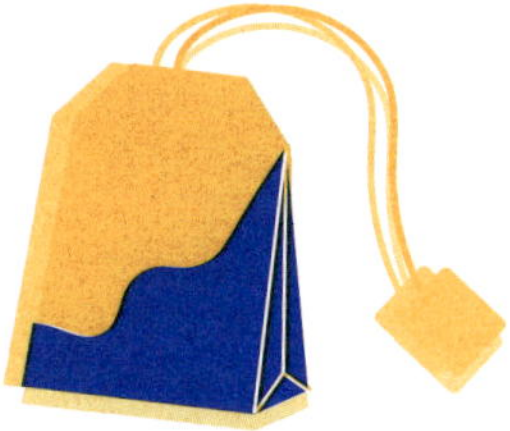

Indigestion

Too much food, overly rich food or eating too fast are the commonest causes of discomfort during or after eating. Heartburn presents as pain behind the breastbone resulting from stomach acid refluxing up into the gullet ("acid reflux"). "Acid indigestion" is a popular term covering both heartburn and indigestion suspected to result from high stomach acid.

Indigestion can also result from mild acidosis (p.62). This often results from not eating a healthy diet (p.58) and can:

- Increase stomach acid production, in turn causing heartburn, peptic ulcers and gastritis (inflamed stomach lining)
- Encourage food sensitivity, which can cause gastritis and oesophagitis (an inflamed gullet)

Indigestion can also result from gastritis or a peptic ulcer (p.257), and many people with either of these make too little stomach acid. Low stomach acid is more likely in later life (affecting one in two over-60s) and with stress or prolonged use of antacids or acid-suppressant medication. It encourages *Helicobacter pylori* bacteria to inflame stomach lining cells and hamper their production of protective bicarbonate-containing mucus. It also encourages stomach cancer. Around two in five of us are infected with *Helicobacter pylori*, though only one in ten infected people has a peptic ulcer.

Heartburn is a frequent symptom of low stomach acid. This helps explain why treating heartburn by suppressing gastric acid with antacids may do no good; it may even worsen the problem. Organic acids such as those in vinegar are weaker than stomach acid, but might help provide an acidic environment for efficient protein digestion in people with indigestion resulting from low stomach acid.

The dilemma is that people generally don't know whether they have high or low stomach acid. So it isn't clear whether either antacids, or food acids (as in cider vinegar and lemons), might help. To help identify poor stomach-acid production, try the following:

- Drink a teaspoon of sodium bicarbonate in a glass of water on an empty stomach. If you don't belch within 5–10 minutes (from acid converting sodium bicarbonate into carbon dioxide) you may have low acid, in which case antacids are unlikely to help.
- With indigestion, drink 1 tablespoon of apple cider vinegar in a glass of water. If it helps, a lack of stomach acid may have been to blame.

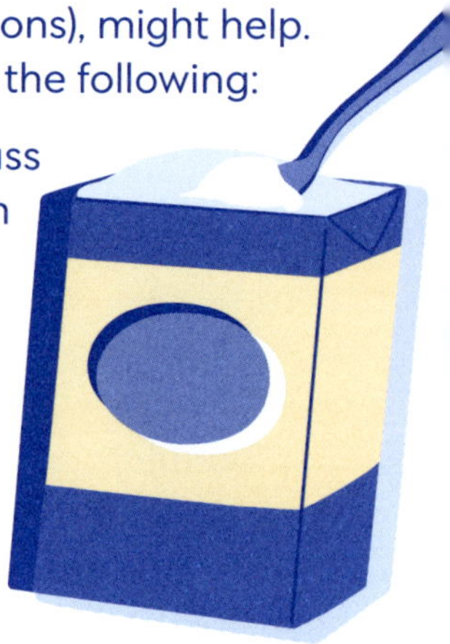

LEMONS

Lemon acids might aid protein digestion, so may be useful for people with low stomach acid. Also, lemons are metabolized to potassium carbonate, so as part of a healthy diet help prevent mild acidosis. Finally – and theoretically – their limonene might help prevent heartburn by promoting healthy stomach contractions.

+ ACTION: For heartburn, drink 1 tablespoon of lemon juice in a glass of warm water.

SODIUM BICARBONATE

This can lower stomach acidity.

+ ACTIONS: Consider taking it as an antacid if you get heartburn (p.217). If you have frequent heartburn or other indigestion, see your doctor, as it would be wise to discuss your diet, consider other treatment and, perhaps, investigate the cause.

OLIVE OIL

Olive oil stimulates the production of bile in the liver and its expulsion from the gallbladder into the intestine, so as part of a healthy diet it can help to prevent indigestion caused by the poor digestion of fats.

+ ACTION: Take 1–2 tablespoons of extra-virgin olive oil with each fatty meal.

HONEY

Honey is said to discourage indigestion but more research is needed to confirm this. Raw honey may be particularly useful as it's an alkali-producing food (p.62).

+ ACTION: Try using honey in place of sugar as a sweetener.

GARLIC

Garlic is a traditional remedy for indigestion.

+ ACTION: Include garlic in your daily diet or take a garlic supplement. You need both water- and oil-soluble sulphur compounds (pp.78–9) but stop if either worsens your indigestion.

SPICES

Antispasmodic, bitter, digestive and choline-containing spices (p.89) may help. Ginger helps heartburn by speeding stomach emptying. Chilli, cayenne and paprika kill peptic ulcer bacteria, as do kokum and mastic. Galangal helps peptic ulcers more than do the anti-ulcer drugs cimetidine and omeprazole. Black pepper can stimulate stomach acid secretion.

+ ACTION: Include these spices in your diet.

TEAS

Antispasmodic, bitter, digestive and choline-containing teas may help. In particular, try peppermint.

+ ACTION: Include these teas in your diet.

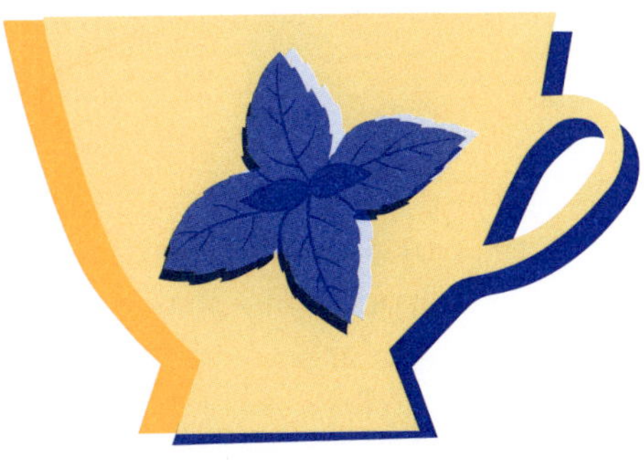

Infection

See also *Athlete's foot; Cold sores, Colds, Conjunctivitis, Flu, Laryngitis, Sore throat and sinusitis, Dandruff, Ear infection, Gastroenteritis, Nail infection, Peptic ulcer, Ringworm, Thrush, Warts.* Various micro-organisms can cause infection, including bacteria, viruses and fungi. It's been suggested that mild acidosis (p.62) encourages bacterial and viral infections.

APPLE CIDER VINEGAR

Cider vinegar's acetic, lactic and traces of malic acids are mainly responsible for its antifungal, antibacterial and antiviral actions. Laboratory studies show cider vinegar can restrict the growth of *Escherichia coli* (*E. coli*) bacteria (which can cause gastroenteritis, urinary infection and neonatal meningitis), *Staphylococcus aureus* bacteria (which can cause blood, bone, joint and skin infections, and food poisoning) and *Candida albicans* fungi (which can cause infections ranging from vaginal thrush to potentially life-threatening illness).

Indeed, a study at Middlesex University in the UK suggests cider vinegar is up to 90 per cent as effective as antibiotics for fighting certain infections in the laboratory. It is almost as effective as common antibiotics at killing *Escherichia coli* and methicillin-resistant *Staphylococcus aureus* bacteria (MRSA). However, we don't yet know how effective cider vinegar is at doing this in the human body.[154]

+ ACTION: Take 1–3 tablespoons of apple cider vinegar a day. For bacterial or fungal skin infections, try applying apple cider vinegar to the affected skin several times a day.

LEMONS

Lemon oil has some antibacterial, antiviral and antifungal action, mainly thanks to its limonene and antioxidants. The flavonoid hesperidin may help prevent serious infection.

+ ACTION: Include the zest and juice of a lemon in your daily diet.

OLIVE OIL

Extra-virgin olive oil, whether consumed or applied to the skin, has some antibacterial, antiviral and antifungal activity, thanks to its polyphenols and other antioxidants.

An extract of virgin olive oil added to mayonnaise or salad inoculated with salmonella and listeria bacteria reduced the bacterial counts. The researchers attribute this to olive oil's polyphenols and believe olive oil could help to protect against gastroenteritis from contaminated food.[155]

+ ACTION: Consume at least 2 tablespoons of extra-virgin olive oil each day.

HONEY

Honey kills many disease-causing bacteria, viruses and fungi. Honey's antimicrobials help counter wound infections. Its prebiotic sugars and probiotic bacteria help prevent intestinal infections and reduce the severity and length of colds. Honey's immunity-boosters, anti-inflammatories and antioxidants also help. Raw honey may be particularly useful as it's an alkali-producing food (p.62).

A Saudi Arabian team that tested six supermarket honeys found all retained antibacterial activity even after refrigeration for 6 months or boiling for 15 minutes.[156]

+ ACTION: Eat 1 to 2 teaspoons of raw or antimicrobial-rich honey 3 times a day.

GARLIC

This has been used for millennia to treat infections. During World War II, garlic became known as "Russian penicillin" as new antibiotics were in short supply, so Red Army physicians used garlic instead. Today, garlic remains a popular anti-infective agent worldwide.

A research review concluded that garlic can help prevent viral infections by enhancing the immune response.[157]

Also, laboratory studies show the following:

- Bacteria can become resistant to antibiotics but not to garlic.

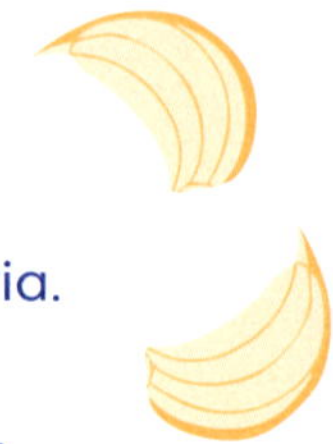

- Allicin, a component of freshly crushed garlic, has antiviral properties and is effective against a broad range of bacteria.
- Garlic has antibacterial effects against bacilli, brucellae, enterobacter, mycobacteria, pseudomonas, staphylococci, streptococci and vibrio bacteria as well as *Campylobacter jejuni, Cryptococcus neoformans, Enterococcus faecalis, Escherichia coli, Helicobacter pylori, Klebsiella pneumoniae, Neisseria gonorrhoeae, Proteus vulgaris* and *Salmonella enteritidis.*
- Allicin-containing garlic supplements may help to cure infections caused by the "superbug" methicillin-resistant *Staphylococcus aureus* (MRSA).
- Garlic has antiviral effects against coxsackie viruses and human cytomegaloviruses, as well as *Herpes simplex* types 1 and 2, human immunodeficiency virus type 1, human rhinovirus type 2, influenza virus type B, parainfluenza virus type 3, vaccinia virus and vesicular stomatitis virus.
- Garlic may enhance the efficacy of the flu vaccine.
- Garlic has antifungal effects against aspergillus, microsporum and trichophyton as well as *Cryptococcus neoformans, Pneumocystis jirovecii* and various yeasts, including the yeast-like fungus *Candida albicans.* Garlic can be more potent than certain antifungal medications, including amphotericin B, gentian violet, griseofulvin, ketoconazole and nystatin.
- Garlic has anti-protozoal effects against cryptosporidia, *Entamoeba histolytica, Toxoplasma gondii* and various types of plasmodium (which causes malaria).

Few studies of people have compared garlic with antibiotics, antiviral, antifungal or anti-protozoal drugs. However, garlic might be well worth trying along with such drugs and (for a non-serious infection) on its own.

+ ACTIONS: To help prevent or treat infection, try including garlic in your daily diet or taking a garlic supplement containing the oil-soluble and water-soluble sulphur compounds of garlic (pp.78–9).

SPICES

Antibacterial, antifungal, anti-inflammatory and antiviral spices can help.

+ ACTIONS: Include these in your diet. Also, for a boil, apply a drop of clove oil twice a day; for a fungal skin infection, apply a poultice of turmeric paste.

TEAS

Choose between antibacterial, antifungal and antiviral teas, depending on the likely infecting agent. Anti-inflammatory and astringent teas may help, too.

+ ACTIONS: Include these teas in your diet. Also, for a boil, apply a compress or poultice made with an antibacterial tea. For a fungal skin infection, use a wash or bath of an antifungal tea; for dandruff or seborrhoeic dermatitis, rinse your scalp or other affected skin with lemongrass tea.

Infertility

Before and during any medical investigations and treatment, it's wise for both the man and the woman to eat a healthy diet (p.58). And natural remedies are worth considering.

To fertilize an egg successfully, a sperm must first undergo a stage called "capacitation" which makes the surface of its head capable of sticking to an egg. This involves a compound called "fertilization-promoting peptide" that is produced by the prostate and mixes with sperms on ejaculation. Capacitation occurs in their cervix or womb only if the alkalinity is right. This happens just before ovulation, when cervical glands produce mucus that is "sperm-friendly" – meaning suitably alkaline, abundant, clear, elastic and watery, and with its "strands" aligned to encourage sperm penetration. High levels of the hormone progesterone can prevent ovulation.

Having low progesterone can also make it difficult for a woman to become and stay pregnant. This is because progesterone helps create a healthy uterine lining suitable for a fertilized egg to attach to, then remain in good condition. Low progesterone can also cause irregular or absent periods. Its levels naturally decline with age; not eating a healthy diet (p.58); ongoing stress; too much exercise; extreme weight-loss diets; and certain health problems (for example, polycystic ovary syndrome (PCOS), hypothyroidism (underactive thyroid) and autoimmune diseases.

HONEY

Early research suggests this can help increase male fertility, mainly by its antioxidant properties improving sperms' motility and form. Honey may also aid female fertility by improving egg quality. Raw honey may be particularly helpful as it's an alkali-producing food (p.62).
+ ACTION: Eat 1 teaspoon of honey 3 times a day.

SPICES AND TEAS

There's early evidence that turmeric can boost a woman's progesterone, which could help fertility problems associated with low progesterone. Progestone-boosting spices and teas may help too.
+ ACTIONS: Incorporate turmeric into your daily diet. Also, consume progesterone-boosting spices and teas.

Inflammation

This occurs when the body is trying to fight infection, deal with mild acidosis (p.62) or an unhealthy gut microbiome, or heal damage in the body. Inflammation is a normal, healing reaction in reponse to one or more of a great many acute ("short-lived") health problems, including infections, hay fever, and cuts, grazes and wounds.

Inflammation is also an important part of a very long list of chronic ("persistent") health problems called "chronic inflammatory diseases". These include Alzheimer's disease, artery disease (which can cause poor circulation, heart attacks and strokes), asthma, auto-immune disease (such as lupus and rheumatoid arthritis), cancer, chronic liver and kidney disease, chronic obstructive pulmonary disease (COPD), diabetes, eczema, inflammatory bowel disease, interstitial cystitis, irritable bowel syndrome (IBS), osteoarthritis, Parkinson's disease and psoriasis. What's more, inflammation is a key part of chronic metabolic stress and metabolic syndrome. Research suggests that inflammation associated with mild acidosis (p.62) is a possible link between all these chronic inflammatory diseases.

For more information on any of these conditions, see their relevant A–Z entry.

A healthy diet (p.58) can help prevent inflammation, partly thanks to its many antioxidants, including carotenoids, polyphenols, vitamins C and E and antioxidant enzymes. It can also help prevent inflammation arising from mild acidosis.

OLIVE OIL

This contains many anti-inflammatory compounds – including beta-sitosterol, monounsaturated fatty acids, the terpenoid called squalene and the polyphenols oleocanthal and tyrosol.

A study in Philadelphia found that oleocanthal inhibits the COX-2 enzymes that enable the formation of inflammatory prostaglandins. This action resembles that of the anti-inflammatory drug ibuprofen, though is much less powerful. Two tablespoons of olive oil have the same effect as 1/20th of the adult dose of ibuprofen.[158]

Researchers report that the antioxidants squalene, beta-sitosterol and tyrosol in olive oil discourage the production of inflammatory compounds from omega-6 fats (which we get mainly from red meat, corn oil and sunflower oil), or render them harmless.

+ ACTION: Consume 2 tablespoons of extra-virgin olive oil each day.

LEMONS

These contain anti-inflammatory substances such as flavonoids, so it could be beneficial to add them to your diet if you have a health problem involving inflammation.

+ ACTION: Include lemons in your diet.

HONEY

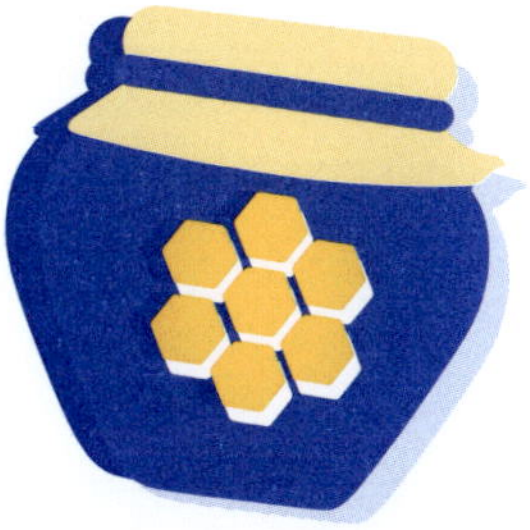

This contains various anti-inflammatory compounds. Its oligosaccharides aid the growth and activity of those probiotic gut bacteria that discourage inflammation. Raw honey reduces inflammatory prostaglandins.

Inflammation can be triggered by high blood sugar, as this encourages oxidation in blood vessels and damage ("glycation") to proteins. Honey triggers lower blood sugar spikes than does table sugar. Raw honey may be especially helpful as it's an alkali-producing food (p.62). Also consider these studies:

- Eating 70g of natural honey each day for 30 days reduced the inflammation marker C-reactive protein.[159]
- In a study in Dubai, 12 people had a blood test before and after a 12-hour fast, then consumed about a tablespoon of raw honey daily for 15 days before having another test. Honey lowered the levels of inflammatory prostaglandins in their blood.[160]

+ ACTION: Substitute table sugar with raw honey. Consume a teaspoon of honey within the hour before bedtime.

GARLIC

Many garlic constituents have antioxidant or other anti-inflammatory actions. These include its flavonoids, saponins and many of its sulphur compounds. This helps to explain its reputation for helping to treat diseases that involve inflammation, such as allergy, Alzheimer's disease, arthritis, asthma, atherosclerosis, cancer, diabetes, eczema, hay fever, heart attacks, infection, inflammatory bowel disease, metabolic syndrome, multiple sclerosis, osteoporosis, psoriasis and strokes. Consider these positive studies:

- A Canadian laboratory study found that sulphenic acid (produced from alliin by the enzyme alliinase) is the fastest antioxidant ever seen! The researchers believe this helps explain garlic's medicinal benefits.[161]
- A research review at the University of Texas notes that many inflammatory diseases have been linked with activation of an inflammation-inducing substance called nuclear transcription factor KB. The pathway activating this substance can be interrupted by substances derived from various spices and herbs, as well as by garlic's diallyl sulphide, S-allylmercaptocysteine and ajoene. This, they say, "provides reasoning for seasoning".[162]

- However, a study in people with pro-inflammatory risk factors found garlic had no effect on commonly measured biomarkers of inflammation: in a study of 90 overweight smokers, taking a daily garlic powder supplement did not reduce these biomarkers of inflammation.[163]

+ ACTION: Until we know more, include garlic in your daily diet by taking a garlic supplement. You need water- and oil-soluble sulphur compounds (pp.78–9).

SPICES AND TEAS

+ ACTION: Consume anti-inflammatory spices and teas, and note that those containing cannabinoids (pp.99 and 101) also have anti-inflammatory action.

Inflammatory bowel disease

This includes ulcerative colitis and Crohn's disease.

OLIVE OIL

Powerful drugs such as steroids can dampen the symptoms of inflammatory bowel disease, but there is no cure. Some good news is that olive oil may help to prevent ulcerative colitis from developing.

In a study at the University of East Anglia, inolving more than 25,000 people, none of whom had ulcerative colitis at first, those with the highest dietary intake of oleic-acid had a 90 per cent lower risk of developing it! The researchers suspect oleic acid helps by blocking inflammatory chemicals in the bowel. They estimate that one in two cases could be prevented by consuming 2–3 tablespoons of olive oil a day![164]

+ ACTION: Consume 2–3 tablespoons of extra-virgin olive oil a day.

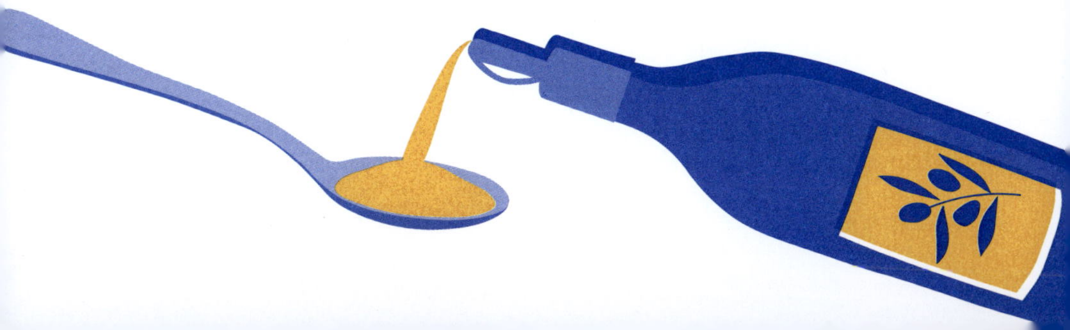

Insect bites and stings

Insect bites and stings can vary from the irritating but relatively unpainful bite of a mosquito, to a very painful wasp or bee sting. Sodium bicarbonate is alkaline, so helps neutralize the acid in bee stings, while apple cider vinegar and lemon juice are acidic, which helps neutralize the alkalinity in wasp stings.

APPLE CIDER VINEGAR OR LEMON JUICE

This may soothe the pain and itching of a wasp sting.
+ ACTION: Apply either of these to the sting.

SODIUM BICARBONATE

This may soothe the pain and itching of a bee sting or a mosquito bite.
+ ACTION: Put 1 tablespoon of sodium bicarbonate in a small bowl and mix with enough water to make a paste. Apply this paste to the sting or bite, cover with a bandage, and leave it on for at least 15 minutes.

Insomnia

This common sleep disorder makes it hard to fall asleep, or to stay asleep for the whole night.

LEMONS

Inhaling the vapour of lemon oil is said to have sedative properties.
+ ACTION: Add a few drops of lemon essential oil to your bath water, then relax in the bathtub.

HONEY

Research increasingly backs honey's reputation for aiding sleep. This may be because:

- Its sweetness stimulates serotonin production, and its tryptophan is readily converted into serotonin. Serotonin calms brain activity and enables production of the "sleep hormone" melatonin.
- Honey gently boosts insulin, which also encourages sleep.
- Honey can reduce anxiety.

+ ACTION: Take 1–3 teaspoons of honey within the hour before bedtime.

SPICES AND TEAS

Calming (pp.89 and 99), sedative and choline-containing spices and teas (pp.89 and 99) may help insomnia.

+ ACTION: Include the spices in your evening meal; drink the teas before bedtime.

Irritable bowel syndrome (IBS)

This is associated with low-grade inflammation of the gut lining. Possible symptoms include pain, constipation, diarrhoea, passing mucus, bowels never feeling empty, wind and bloating. One in three people sometimes has an irritable bowel; one in five of these has frequent trouble, known as irritable bowel syndrome (IBS).

LEMONS

Their pectin may reduce symptoms by making stools softer and easier to pass.

+ ACTION: Include the zest and juice of a lemon in your daily diet.

HONEY

Honey may help because of its prebiotic sugars, probiotic bacteria and anti-inflammatories.

+ ACTION: Eat 1 teaspoon of honey 3 times a day.

SPICES

Anti-inflammatory, antispasmodic, digestive, pain-relieving and, if necessary, laxative spices may help. In particular, try nutmeg, as its oil inhibits the production of a particular pro-inflammatory prostaglandin (PGE2) linked with certain types of IBS.

+ ACTION: Include these spices in your diet.

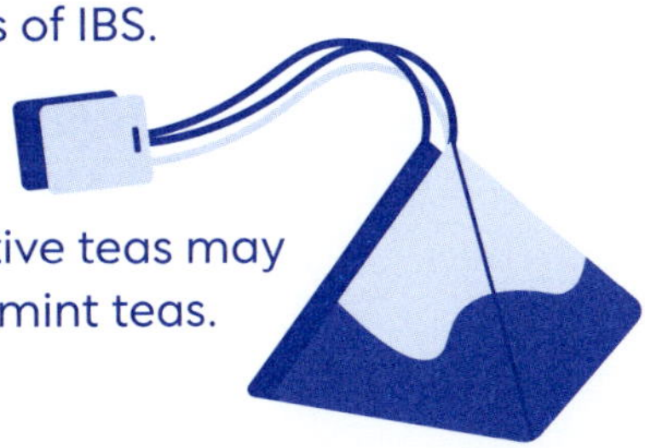

TEAS

Anti-inflammatory, antispasmodic and digestive teas may help. In particular, try chamomile and peppermint teas.

+ ACTION: Include these teas in your diet.

Kidney stones

These are more likely in people who don't eat a healthy diet (p.58). Calcium-oxalate stones are the commonest stones, while uric-acid stones can form, for example, in people with gout. Having mild acidosis (p.62) makes these two types of stone more likely. This is because it's associated with calcium being withdrawn from bones and teeth and excreted in urine to help maintain a normal acid–alkali balance in the various parts of the body.

An Italian study of 187 people with calcium-containing stones found their diet's acid-producing potential was the biggest risk factor. The researchers suggest such people should eat plenty of vegetables and fruit but relatively little animal protein.[165]

Calcium-containing stones are also encouraged by pre-diabetes, as carbohydrate raises blood sugar, which raises insulin, which makes the kidneys discharge calcium in the urine. Studies show that stones are also more likely with metabolic syndrome and obesity, each of which can be associated with mild acidosis.

APPLE CIDER VINEGAR

This is said to help dissolve common, calcium-containing stones. These are more likely when threatened over-acidity of body fluids leads to calcium being withdrawn from bones and teeth and excreted in the urine to keep the body's acid–alkali balance within its normal tightly controlled range. Apple cider vinegar, unlike other vinegars, is said to have a mild alkalinizing effect after it has been digested, so might reduce the body's need to draw calcium from bones. It might also help by reducing insulin spikes in blood after eating carbohydrate foods. The hormone insulin encourages stones by making the kidneys discharge more calcium in urine.

+ ACTION: If you have kidney stones, try including apple cider vinegar in your diet.

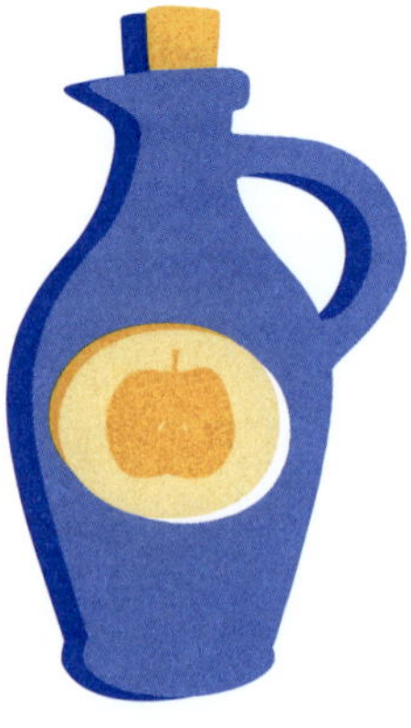

LEMONS

These can help prevent stones because:

- They provide calcium, magnesium, selenium, vitamin B and fibre.
- Their acidity discourages high blood sugar.
- The metabolism of lemon acids in the body has a mild alkalinizing effect that could help dissolve stones containing calcium or uric acid.

+ ACTIONS: Include the zest and juice of a lemon in your daily diet. To reduce pain, drink the juice of half a lemon in a glass of water every 30 minutes for 4 hours, or until the pain subsides.

SODIUM BICARBONATE
This can alkalinize urine, making it more able to rid the body of uric acid without forming stones.
+ ACTION: Discuss with your doctor whether to take sodium bicarbonate for kidney stones (p.69).

Low sex drive

This is relatively common in both men and women. It can result from smoking, not eating a healthy diet (p.58), obesity, too much or too little exercise, and various health problems, including ageing, anxiety, artery disease, depression, fatigue, high blood pressure, stress and an underactive thyroid. These reduce a person's energy, disrupt their hormone balance and impair the blood flow to their sex organs.

Erection of the penis in a man and the clitoris in a woman requires normal levels of nitric oxide in the blood, as this is needed to dilate blood vessels. (Note that the drug sildenafil – Viagra – works in the same way as nitric oxide.) We get nitric oxide when certain mouth bacteria convert nitrate in food into nitrite, which the body turns into nitric oxide. Nitric oxide is vital not only for good blood flow but also for healthy immunity, airway function, digestion, regulation of neurotransmitters (nerve message carriers), and normal energy production by mitochondria (tiny "energy factories" in each body cell).

However, nitric oxide levels fall with age. Poor production can also result from a poor diet, obesity, lack of exercise, and hormone imbalance. A sedentary lifestyle can also reduce the body's ability to distribute nitric oxide.

If you are concerned about your sex drive, encourage more nitric oxide in your blood by consuming more foods containing:

- Nitrate – leafy greens are the richest source, followed by beetroots and carrots
- The amino acids L-arginine (in high-protein foods such as meat, fish, dairy, grains, legumes, seeds) and L-citrulline (needed to make L-arginine; the richest source is watermelon)
- Foods rich in vitamin C, which help increase nitric oxide
- Garlic, as this not only increases nitric oxide in the blood but can also increase the hormone testosterone

Getting enough exercise is important too.

LEMONS

These are rich in vitamin C, which can help by increasing nitric oxide.
+ ACTION: Include lemons in your diet.

OLIVE OIL

A saying in Greece proclaims: "Eat butter and sleep tight, eat olive oil and come at night." Certainly, folklore suggests that olive oil has aphrodisiac properties!
+ ACTION: Consume 2 or 3 tablespoons of extra-virgin olive oil every day, as part of a healthy diet, to see if this helps.

HONEY

Honey is reputed to improve a low sex drive. Jasmine, marjoram and orchid honeys are especially favoured.
+ ACTION: Consume 1 teaspoon of honey 3 times a day.

GARLIC

Scientific evidence backs the belief that garlic increases libido and discourages impotence. Garlic also expands arteries, improving blood flow to the genitals and hormone-producing glands. Garlic increases nitric oxide in blood (see above). What's more, it boosts testosterone and its diallyl disulphide boosts luteinizing hormone (a pituitary hormone regulating testosterone production).

Japanese researchers found that rats fed with garlic had higher testosterone after 28 days.[166]

+ ACTION: Include garlic in your diet or take a garlic supplement. You need water- and oil-soluble sulphur compounds (pp.78–9).

SPICES

Several spices can boost libido. For men, these include black pepper (thanks to its piperine); celery seed (thanks to its androstenone); ginger (which might enhance the action of testosterone); and nutmeg (thanks to its myristicin). In both men and women, saffron has long been suggested to boost libido (thanks to its "feel-good" hormones).

+ ACTIONS: Include the appropriate spices in your diet.

TEAS

Ginseng tea may help men with their sex drive. For women, fenugreek, saffron and *Vitex agnus castus* may help libido; black cohosh, dong quai, hibiscus, red clover and rosehip teas are reputedly useful too.

+ ACTIONS: Include these teas in your diet. Inhale the fragrance of the steam from rosehip tea. The aromas of cinnamon, coriander, ginger and vanilla are said to be aphrodisiac, with ginger especially useful for women.

Memory loss

See also *Dementia*. Declining memory is usually part of the cognitive decline that may be associated with ageing. For some people, though, it is an early warning sign of impending dementia (p.170).

APPLE CIDER VINEGAR

Preliminary evidence suggests apple cider vinegar can improve memory or slow its loss.

+ ACTION: Try including it in your diet.

LEMONS

Studies of mice suggest that antioxidants such as lycopene, vitamin C, citric acid and flavonoids discourage memory loss. Lemons are also rich in antioxidants that might help.

+ ACTION: Include the zest and juice of a lemon in your daily diet.

HONEY

Honey is said to help with memory loss, possibly because it:

- Contains vitamin B and acetylcholine
- Promotes production of melatonin (a hormone that helps record long-term memories). People who have honey before bedtime report increased dream intensity and recall
- Discourages low blood sugar and therefore the production of cortisol, which can diminish short-term memory

In a study at Waikato University, New Zealand, 45 rats consumed a sugar-free diet or a diet containing sugar or honey. After 1 year, the honey group had better spatial-recognition memory.[167]
+ ACTIONS: As a sweetener, substitute honey for table sugar. Consume a teaspoon of honey within the hour before bedtime.

TEAS

Several studies have found that drinking *Camellia-sinensis* tea has beneficial effects on memory.
+ ACTION: Include this tea in your daily diet.

Macular degeneration (age-related)

This damages the macula (a small area of the retina that controls central vision). This means it is hard to recognize faces or to read or drive. It's a leading cause of vision loss in older adults, making it difficult for a person to see what they are trying to focus on. Macular degeneration is more likely in people who eat a diet high in saturated fat or have high blood pressure or cardiovascular disease. Being overweight or obese makes it more likely to be severe.

LEMONS

Dutch researchers who followed up 4,170 over-55s for 8 years found that the 560 who developed age-related macular degeneration ate less vitamin C-rich food than the others. But taking vitamin C supplements made no difference![168]

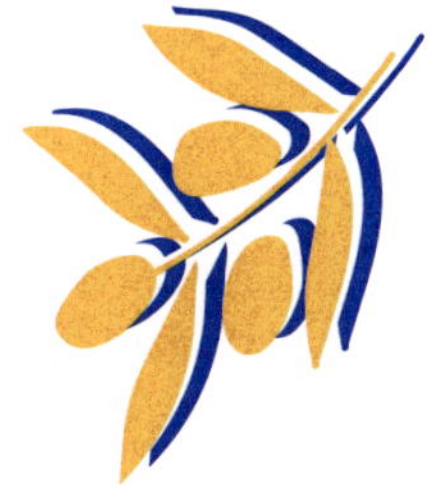

+ **ACTION:** Include the zest and juice of a lemon in your daily diet.

OLIVE OIL
This is an excellent substitute for saturated fat in the diet.
+ **ACTION:** Include olive oil as part of a healthy diet (p.58).

Menopause problems

The period of time when a woman stops having periods and fertility ends causes challenges for some women, though others sail through. The best-known challenges are hot flushes and sleep problems. Others include depression, forgetfulness, headaches, irritability, itching, joint and muscle pain, skin changes, vaginal dryness and weight gain. The lower oestrogen in the years after the menopause can encourage urine infection, an overactive bladder and osteoporosis.

SPICES
Oestrogen-containing spices may help. Also try allspice. And note that cumin reduces bone loss from osteoporosis.
+ **ACTION:** Include these spices in your diet.

TEAS
Several herb teas are traditionally used to ease menopausal symptoms, including those containing plant oestrogens, as well as dong quai, passionflower and *Vitex agnus castus*.
+ **ACTION:** Consider including these teas in your diet.

Mouth ulcers

Also called aphthous ulcers and canker sores, these can be extraordinarily painful.

One cause is injury – for example, from overly enthusiastic tooth brushing, or from biting the inside of your cheek, or wearing poorly fitting dental braces. Other causes include acidic foods; dietary deficiency of iron; vitamin B12, folate or zinc; stress; poor immunity; and certain drugs – including beta-blockers (for high blood pressure,

or anxiety), calcium channel blockers (such as amlodipine, for high blood presssure), nonsteroidal anti-inflammatory drugs (NSAIDs, for pain) and alendronate (for osteoporosis).

LEMONS

Lemon oil can help heal mouth ulcers, thanks to its anti-inflammatory action.

+ ACTION: Mix 3 drops of lemon essential oil with 1 tablespoon of sweet almond or other carrier oil. Apply a few drops to the ulcer every 2 hours.

SODIUM BICARBONATE

This can be soothing and can aid healing.

+ ACTION: Dissolve 1 teaspoon of sodium bicarbonate in a glass of water and swirl a mouthful around your mouth every 2–3 hours.

HONEY

This reputedly helps soothe mouth ulcers.

+ ACTION: Coat the ulcer with honey every 2 hours. Ideally, choose a honey with high anti-inflammatory action, such as manuka honey with a UMF of at least 10 or more.

GARLIC

Garlic can help with mouth ulcers in various ways.

+ ACTIONS: Dab the ulcer with the cut end of a garlic clove several times a day. But don't repeat if the pain worsens the first time. Include raw garlic in your daily diet or take a garlic supplement. You need water- and oil-soluble sulphur compounds (pp.78–9).

Muscle fatigue and aching

Muscle fatigue and burning pain (the "burn") during intense exercise result from the build-up in muscles of acidic substances such as phosphate and hydrogen ions. These signify that the muscle has exhausted its sugar stores and must switch to using lactate as a fuel instead. They also signal that the local acidosis is over-exciting the muscle's nerve receptors.

In contrast, aching the next day results from muscle damage and exercise-induced inflammation. Muscle fatigue and aching that are not related to exercise can result from a slow-onset immune reaction associated with a food sensitivity enabled by mild acidosis.

LEMONS

Inflammation-induced pain and stiffness after exercise might respond to anti-inflammatories such as nobiletin in lemon oil.
+ ACTIONS: Put 1 teaspoon of lemon oil in your bathwater and relax for half an hour. Or add 3 drops of lemon oil and a few drops of ginger oil (a pain reliever and local circulation-booster) to 3 tablespoons of sweet almond or other carrier oil, and use this to massage the muscles.

SODIUM BICARBONATE

Taking this can buffer acidosis in muscles, enabling more prolonged exercise. This "soda loading" can reduce muscle fatigue and enhance recovery. But the large amounts (for example, about 0.3g per kg body-weight) often recommended by sports coachs can cause symptoms such as nausea and diarrhoea. And it shaves only seconds off performance time. So its use is controversial.

A research review noted that taking sodium bicarbonate 60–180 minutes before the event improved performance for 400–800m runners, 200m swimmers, cyclists and boxers.[169]
+ ACTION: Consider taking this before high-intensity, short-duration exercise, but consult a qualified coach or a doctor first.

HONEY

This may help as it contains compounds that improve glucose uptake, and burning, in muscles, which reduces lactic-acid production. These compounds include certain acids, flavonoids, glucose-metabolizing principles, minerals and vitamins, as well as hydrogen peroxide and nitric oxide.
+ ACTION: Take 1 teaspoon of honey before, during and after exercise.

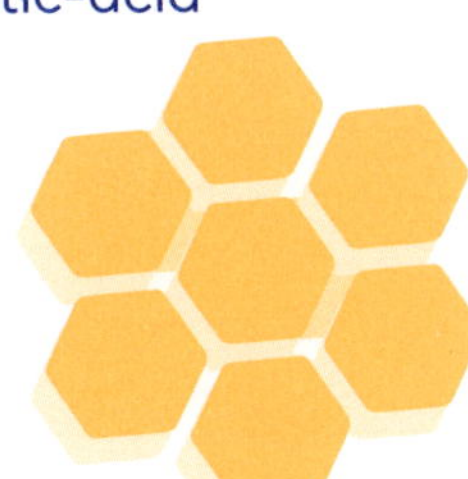

SPICES

Anti-inflammatory, pain-relieving, vasodilatory and warming spices may help. In particular, try ginger. Counter-irritant spices applied to the skin over the sore muscle may help.

+ ACTIONS: Include your chosen spices in your diet. Or apply such a spice externally in a compress, cream, massage oil, or poultice, or as tea added to your bathwater.

TEAS

Anti-inflammatory, antispasmodic and pain-relieving teas may help.

+ ACTIONS: Include these teas in your diet. Also choose one or more of them to use in a compress or poultice, or in your bathwater.

Nail infection

Fungal nail infections manifest as discoloured, thickened nails, and can be difficult to get rid of. The following may help.

SODIUM BICARBONATE

This white powder can help absorb moisture that may cause toenail fungus.

+ ACTIONS: Rub a paste of sodium bicarbonate and water over affected toenails or fingernails and leave it on for 20 minutes. And sprinkle sodium bicarbonate between toes each day.

GARLIC

Due to possible antifungal properties, garlic may provide some benefit when trying to treat a fungal nail infection

+ ACTION: First, do a patch test on the adjacent skin (p.82). If this shows no problem, apply garlic oil (for example, from a garlic perle – a capsule of garlic oil) to the infected nail and adjacent skin 2 or 3 times a day for 6 months for fingernails, or a year for toenails. Or use the oil from garlic oil macerate (p.80). Include garlic in your daily diet or take a garlic supplement. You need water- and oil-soluble sulphur compounds (pp.78–9).

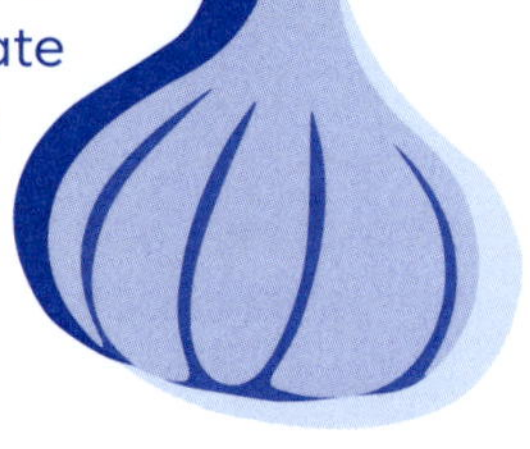

Nausea and vomiting

The many possible triggers include gastroenteritis (p.194), infections in general (p.220), mild acidosis (p.62) and a slow-onset immune reaction associated with a food sensitivity enabled by such acidosis. Other triggers include anxiety (p.123) and pregnancy.

SPICES

Cinnamon, cloves, ginger and nutmeg are potentially useful. In particular, ginger reduces motion sickness, as well as pregnancy nausea and vomiting. Dried ginger is more effective than antihistamine medication.

+ ACTIONS: Aim to work out the cause of your nausea and vomiting then treat it appropriately. Try including anti-nausea spices in your diet. Ginger is traditionally used to counter nausea, so try eating ginger biscuits, drink fresh ginger tea or ginger beer, chew crystallized ginger or take ginger capsules.

TEAS

Butterfly pea tea is reputed to help nausea.

+ ACTION: Consider drinking this tea to help with nausea and vomiting.

Neuralgia

This is a sharp, shocking pain from an irritated nerve.

LEMONS

The cooling and anti-inflammatory properties of lemon juice may ease neuralgia.

+ ACTIONS: Apply warmed lemon juice over the painful area and repeat each hour for half a day. Alternatively, add 3 drops of lemon oil to 2 tablespoons of sweet almond or other carrier oil, and smooth over the affected area. You can also add a few drops of lemon oil to the water in an aromatherapy diffuser, or put them in a bowl of just-boiled water and lean over it with a towel over your head, to inhale the vapour for a few minutes.

GARLIC

Some people with trigeminal neuralgia (severe pain in one side of the face from irritation of the trigeminal nerve) report that repeated applications of garlic to the painful area are helpful. Garlic might work by producing hydrogen sulphide and nitric oxide, both of which expand arteries, so improving the blood supply to nerves. Its anti-inflammatory compounds can also help. In addition, its allixin is said to encourage nerve growth and wellbeing.

However, if pain results from pressure on a nerve, as with sciatica pain in the back, hip and outer side of the leg, garlic is unlikely to help.

+ ACTION: First, do a patch test (p.82). If this shows no problem, apply garlic oil macerate or the oil from a garlic perle (p.80) to the painful area several times a day. Include garlic in your daily diet or take a garlic supplement. You need oil-soluble sulphur compounds (p.79).

SPICES

Pain-relieving spices may be useful, as may, depending on the cause, antibacterial, anti-inflammatory or antiviral spices. Counter-irritant spices could help, too.

+ ACTIONS: Include the spices in your diet. Apply a counter-irritant or other chosen spice to the overlying skin in a compress, cream, massage oil or poultice, or apply capsaicin cream (available from a pharmacy or the internet).

TEAS

Pain-relieving teas may be useful, as may, depending on the cause, antibacterial, anti-inflammatory, antispasmodic and antiviral teas.

+ ACTIONS: Include these teas in your diet. Also apply them in a compress or in a wash for the affected area.

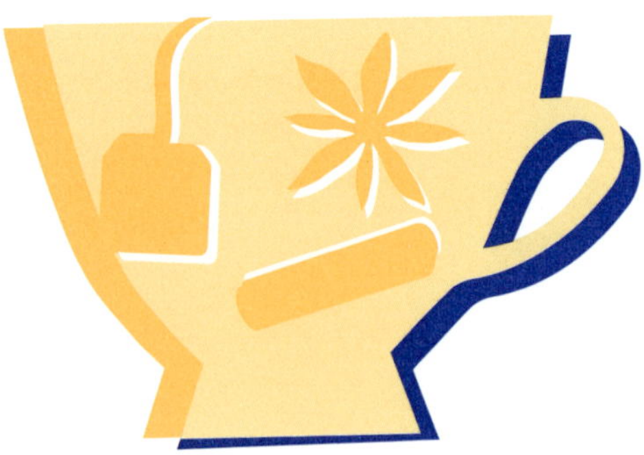

Nosebleed

Nosebleeds most often result from the burst blood vessel in the lining of the nose. They are usually not serious and often appear worse than they are. They are more common in children.

They can result from nose-picking; a foreign body in the nose; a cold; hay fever (allergic rhinitis); high blood pressure; nasal polyps; certain medications – for example, aspirin or other non-steroidal anti-inflammatories, decongestants or blood thinners (anticoagulants); a bleeding disorder; or a cancer. If you have repeated nosebleeds, consult a doctor.

APPLE CIDER VINEGAR

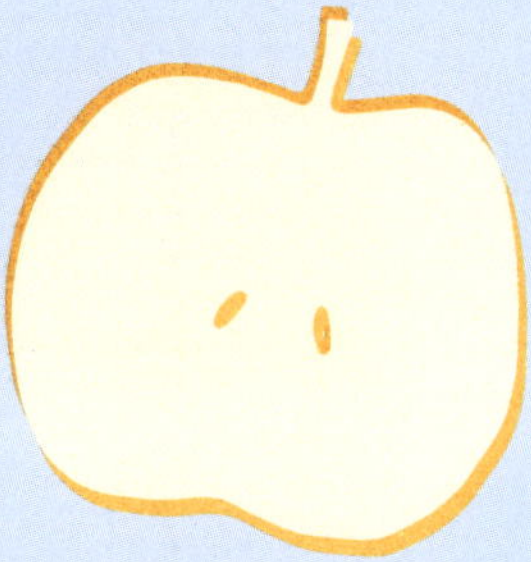

There are isolated reports that apple cider vinegar helps stem a nosebleed. This is also a traditional remedy for nosebleeds.

+ ACTIONS: To see if apple cider vinegar helps, soak a ball of cotton wool in the vinegar, lean your head back, then gently put the ball in the affected nostril, making sure not to stick it in too far! If you have frequent nosebleeds, try drinking 2 teaspoons of apple cider vinegar in a glass of water 3 times a day for, say, 3 months.

LEMONS

Lemon juice has astringent properties, and a lemon's peel, pith and core are rich in rutin and other flavonoids that can strengthen blood vessels.

+ ACTIONS: Soak a cotton-wool ball in lemon juice, lean your head backwards, then put the ball in the affected nostril and leave for 10 minutes. If you have frequent nosebleeds, try including the zest and juice of a lemon in your daily diet.

Overweight and obesity

Huge numbers of people carry too much weight in their body – for example:

- In the US, 74 per cent of adults are either overweight (body mass index/BMI 25–29) or obese (BMI 30 or higher), with 42 per cent of the whole group obese.
- In the UK, 64 per cent of adults are either overweight or obese, with 26 per cent of the whole group obese.

The main reason is not eating a healthy diet (p.58). Such a diet is overladen with meat, refined grain, sugar, carbonated drinks and ultra-processed foods, but low in vegetables (including beans), nuts, seeds and fruits.

An unhealthy diet promotes overweight and obesity partly by encouraging low stomach acid and mild acidosis (p.62).

People who don't eat meat – and are therefore less likely to have mild acidosis – are also less likely to be obese: a study of 37,875 people concluded that meat eaters are more likely to be obese.[170]

Low stomach acid affects one in two over-60s. It reduces absorption from the stomach and gut of many vital nutrients (including protein, vitamins B and C, calcium, copper, chromium, iron, magnesium, manganese, selenium, zinc). And it can encourage an imbalance in the numbers and proportions of gut bacteria and other micro-organisms that affects appetite regulation and subsequent calorie intake. Note that low stomach acid can also result from stress, or prolonged use of antacid or acid-suppressant medication.

The body's response to an unhealthy diet is often to demand more food in an attempt to achieve good nourishment. But eating more of the same encourages more weight gain; it does not achieve good nourishment!

Most obese people are in fact malnourished, as they lack the foods they need but consume a surplus of those that supply little good nourishment. Severe malnutrition decreases the bicarbonate content of pancreatic juice, encouraging mild acidosis (p.62).

Scientists in Germany say the mild acidosis experienced by many obese people can produce a constant "pro-inflammatory" state that could be the link between obesity and the diseases commonly associated with it.[171]

Avoid a high-protein, low-carbohydrate diet, as this encourages mild acidosis. An added bonus of an alkali-producing diet is that you can eat more yet still lose weight, because eating more vegetables and fruit can turn a fat-storing tendency into a fat-burning one.

APPLE CIDER VINEGAR

This has been reputed for thousands of years to promote weight loss. Research suggests it does so by:

- Helping to compensate for any lack of stomach acid. This improves nutrient absorption, which in turn helps because absorbing a good balance of different nutrients helps prevent a person feeling so hungry that they overeat
- Aiding satiety after eating
- Slowing the rise in blood sugar after a meal. This helps prevent a high blood sugar spike and the resulting low blood sugar dip that can trigger hunger
- Helping the body burn calories faster

The evidence isn't strong and the studies are short but consider these:

- Researchers in Lebanon found that drinking 1 tablespoon of apple cider vinegar early each morning was associated with falls in body weight, waist and hip measurements, body fat, body mass index (BMI), and blood sugar and blood fats.[172]
- Japanese researchers report that for mice on a high-fat diet, those given daily acetic acid for 6 weeks gained a lot less body fat than those given no vinegar. The acetic acid group had increased activation of genes that produce proteins which break down fats.[173]
- A study of 18 people at Southern Utah University examined how acids in vinegar, pickle juice, acetic acid, lemon and lime juice affect blood sugar after a carbohydrate snack. Only vinegar lowered it

significantly, suggesting that compounds in vinegar other than acetic acid contribute to its blood sugar-lowering effect.[174]

- When 12 volunteers drank 2 tablespoons of vinegar before a carbohydrate-rich meal, they had lower than expected levels of glucose and insulin, and their feeling of fullness more than doubled.[175]

+ ACTIONS: Try including apple cider vinegar in your diet to help with weight loss or avoid putting on too much weight.

LEMONS

Lemon juice has similar acidity to vinegar, so could be equally beneficial for overweight and obesity. Lemons contain pectin, which forms a gel in the digestive tract. This gel mops up triglyceride fats and reduces their absorption; it also increases satiety (feeling "full"). Consider the following studies:

Researchers in Texas found that pectin increased satiety. Lemon acids and pectin slow the absorption of sugar after a meal with a high glycaemic index (blood sugar-raising effect), which in turn slows the rise in blood sugar. This helps prevent low blood sugar dips, which can trigger overeating.[176]

Women in their 50s gained 2.25kg (5lb) less over 10 years when they took calcium supplements. This suggests many were previously short of calcium – possibly because they lacked stomach acid, as is the case in 40 per cent of women of this age. Taking vinegar with meals would improve their calcium absorption.[177]

Lemons' vitamin C might aid weight loss, too, as this study at Arizona Stage University suggests. It found that volunteers with adequate vitamin C burnt 30 per cent more fat during exercise than those with low levels. Also, when obese women who were trying to lose weight took vitamin C, they lost twice as much. We need adequate vitamin C to produce enough carnitine – an amino acid that helps our body burn fat well.[178]

+ ACTION: Include the zest and juice of a lemon in your daily diet.

OLIVE OIL

A high consumption of fat often used to be blamed for obesity, but studies show this may not be true. In the 1960s, Americans obtained 45 per cent of their calories from fats, and 13 per cent were obese. But in 2010, Americans obtained only 33 per cent from fats, yet 34 per cent were obese. Of course, fat can contribute to obesity if your diet contains too many calories from fat. But you can eat any amount of fat without it making you fat if this fits into a healthy balanced diet and provides the necessary calories.

There are several reasons why olive oil as part of a healthy diet could help to prevent or treat obesity, or discourage related diseases:

- Including olive oil in each meal helps to suppress hunger because its fat stimulates the release of cholecystokinin. This hormone, made in the lining of the small intestine, decreases hunger by signaling satiety, so making a person feel full.
- Olive oil's slight acidity, provided it is not neutralized by other foods, can slow sugar absorption, keeping your blood sugar level steadier for longer and helping to prevent hunger and therefore overeating when snacking between meals.
- Acidic foods help to compensate for any lack of stomach acid (which affects one in two over-60s). Low stomach acid leads to poor absorption of protein and certain other nutrients, which can encourage hunger and overeating. Olive oil is only slightly acidic but it helps a little.
- Olive oil's omega-3 polyunsaturated fats "switch on" fat-burning genes.
- Olive oil partially inhibits stomach contractions. This means that the stomach empties its contents into the gut more slowly after a meal, which prolongs the feeling of fullness.
- Obesity encourages inflammation in various parts of the body; extra-virgin olive oil contains several anti-inflammatory agents.

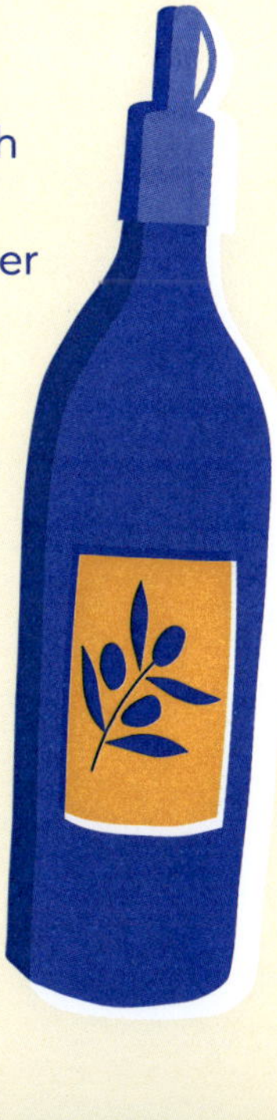

- Oleuropein – one of olive oil's polyphenols – can encourage weight loss in several ways: it boosts the body's heat production and thus its use of calories; it helps the body produce insulin, a hormone that helps regulate metabolism; it is thought to help prevent overeating; and laboratory tests have found that it lowers body fat and weight gain in animals fed high-cholesterol and high-fat diets.

A study in mice suggests elenolic acid (a compound present in mature olives and extra-virgin olive oil) can lower blood sugar and promote weight loss. This is interesting because olive oil contains elenolic acid.

Another study found that obese mice with diabetes given elenolic acid had a 10.7 per cent reduction in obesity after 4–5 weeks, as well as blood sugar levels and insulin sensitivity comparable to those of healthy lean mice. The blood sugar-lowering effect was similar to that of the injected diabetes drug liraglutide and better than that of the diabetes drug metformin. Elenolic acid reduced food intake and promoted weight loss by increasing levels of the hormones PYY (peptide YY) and GLP-1 (glucagon-like peptide-1) which help people feel full, prevent overeating and control blood sugar levels.[179]

Note that one of the popular weight-loss drugs, semaglutide, acts like the hormone GLP-1. It is used as Ozempic and Rybelsus for diabetes, and as Wegovy for weight loss and weight management. While olive oil has only a very low concentration of elenolic acid, there's reason to believe it may have similar, though smaller, effects in humans.

- A Spanish study of 613 people found that consuming monounsaturated fat-rich olive oil reduced the risk of obesity compared with consuming sunflower oil, which is rich in polyunsaturated fat.[180]
- A Japanese study in rats found that oleuropein (one of olive oil's polyphenols) decreased body weight. It did this by encouraging a particularly metabolically active type of body fat called "brown fat" to burn calories. Note that brown fat is a type of fat between the shoulderblades that stimulates the breakdown of triglyceride blood

fats. Brown fat also helped decrease body weight by encouraging the production of the hormones noradrenaline and adrenaline.[181]

Olive oil contains a monounsaturated fat called oleic acid. When olive oil is consumed, cells in the small intestine convert oleic acid into a substance called oleoylethanolamide, which curbs hunger.[182] Substituting olive oil for saturated fat in the diet was associated with a small loss of body weight and fat mass.[183]
+ ACTION: Take at least 2 tablespoons of extra-virgin olive oil each day as part of a healthy diet that provides the calories needed to maintain your goal weight.

HONEY
Substitute honey for some or all of the sugar in your diet. This is because honey is sweeter than table sugar, so we can use less of it. It also has a lower glycaemic index, so doesn't raise our blood sugar so much. And its flavour is more characterful than that of sugar.

During sleep, most of our body's cells burn more fat than glucose. But chronic metabolic stress (p.152) reduces night-time fat-burning. It also discourages sleep, thus reducing the "sleep" hormone melatonin that encourages fat-burning. And it encourages blood sugar and blood fats to be laid down as fat around the waist. Honey before bedtime helps prevent metabolic stress, optimizing the burning of fat to provide energy at night. Choose raw honey if you can; this may be particularly useful as it's an alkali-producing food (p.62).

- In a study at Waikato University, New Zealand, 45 rats were fed a sugar-free diet or a sugar- or honey-containing diet. After a year, the honey group had gained less weight.[184]
- In a study at the Mashhad University of Medical Science, Iran, volunteers who consumed 70g (2½oz) of honey daily for 4 weeks had a 1.3 per cent weight reduction compared with those who consumed sucrose.[185]

+ ACTIONS: Substitute honey for some or all of the added sugar in your diet. Take 1 teaspoon of honey within the hour before bedtime.

GARLIC

Garlic is reputed to aid weight loss. Early research suggests it might help by:

- Reducing appetite
- Encouraging heat production by brown fat (see "Olive oil", above)
- Inactivating gastric lipase, the enzyme that breaks down fat so it can be absorbed into the blood
- Making pre-adipocytes (fat-cell precursors) less likely to develop into adipocytes
- Reducing the fat absorbed from a meal

For example:

- In an Indian study, rats were either fed a diet that was 65 per cent fruit sugar (too much of which encourages type 2 diabetes), or a diet that was 65 per cent fruit sugar but also with raw garlic, or a "control" diet of 65 per cent cornflour. Those given fruit sugar and garlic gained less weight over 8 weeks.[186]
- French researchers reported that vinyl dithiin formed during allicin breakdown made pre-adipocytes (cells that develop into adipocytes – meaning fat cells) less likely to accumulate fat inside them, or to produce inflammatory molecules (such as interleukin-6).[187]
- Japanese researchers found that rats on a high-fat diet given a garlic powder supplement for 28 days lost weight. The garlic increased their adrenaline and noradrenaline – hormones that stimulate triglyceride metabolism and are thought to boost heat production in brown fat. Garlic also increased uncoupling protein – which similarly increases heat production in brown fat. The researchers also found that alliin, diallyl disulphide and diallyl trisulphide increased adrenaline and noradrenaline.[188] Also, garlic's ajoenes inactivate gastric lipase, the enzyme needed for digestion of fats.[189]

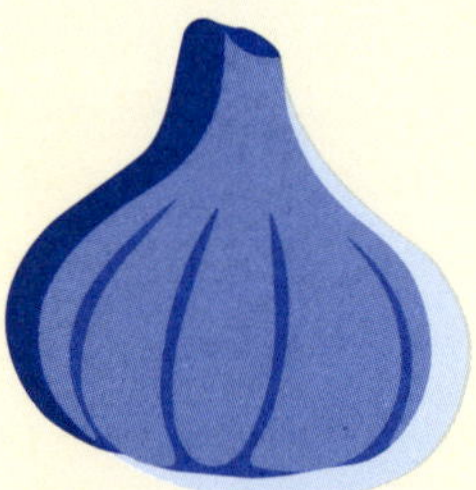

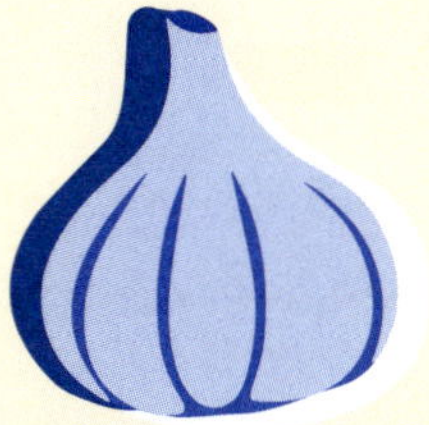

+ ACTION: Until we know more, include garlic in your daily diet or take a garlic supplement. You need water- and oil-soluble sulphur compounds (pp.78–9).

SPICES

Warming spices may help. The outer layer of pepper – particularly black pepper – contains a compound called piperine that can inhibit the formation of new fat cells. Chilli, cayenne and paprika reduce appetite. Also, use kokum and nigella.

+ ACTION: Include these spices in your diet.

TEAS

Several compounds in *Camellia-sinensis* tea can help, including its catechins, L-theanine, theaflavin, thearubigin and theabrownin. Tea extracts have been found to prevent obesity by increasing brown-fat cells, inhibiting fat cell production, increasing energy expenditure, and inhibiting lipid synthesis. Metabolism-boosting teas may help too (though see "Warming", p.103). Also, try appetite-reducing teas such as chickweed, dandelion, nettle, peppermint (whose scent alone reduces appetite) and red clover. Teas rich in beta-sitosterol can reduce fat absorption from the gut. The phaseolamin (a protein that inhibits starch breakdown) in hibiscus tea could help by reducing starch absorption from the gut. And ginseng tea can promote weight loss. Butterfly pea tea is said to help too, possibly because of its caffeine, epigallo-catechin and epigallocatechin gallate.

+ ACTION: Include these teas in your diet.

Osteoporosis

Osteoporotic bone is light and fracture-prone, partly because its cells are being destroyed faster than they are being created. The lifetime risk of a fracture associated with osteoporosis is 30–40 per cent for a woman, 13 per cent for a man. Risk factors include not eating a healthy diet (p.58). Unhealthy diets include those with insufficient calcium, magnesium, zinc, vitamins C, D and K, plant oestrogens and fibre, or too much diet cola (because of its phosphoric acid). Osteoporosis is also more likely with obesity; advancing age; a family history of the condition; too much or too little exercise; smoking; too little bright outdoor light; an early menopause; too much alcohol; a history of anorexia or bulimia; various medications (such as anti-epilepsy drugs, aluminum-containing antacids. and glucocorticoid steroid hormones) and certain illnesses (including gut and thyroid disorders).

Another culprit is high blood levels of the amino acid homocysteine. Possible causes of this include an inborn tendency; a lack in the diet of vitamins B6 and B 12 and folic acid; kidney disease; psoriasis; an underactive thyroid; and certain medications.

Also, research increasingly points to the involvement of inflammation. This can result from an unhealthy diet. Studies suggest mild acidosis (p.62) can encourage osteoporosis by:

- Causing inflammation
- Drawing calcium from bones to partner acidic anions in urine
- Encouraging dehydration

Decreasing the activity of bone-building cells ("osteoblasts") and increasing that of bone-destroying cells ("osteoclasts").

Finally, a lack of stomach acid can reduce calcium absorption by 80 per cent. This affects one in two over-60s and is more common in people who are stressed, habitually take antacids or acid suppressants, or eat an acid-producing diet high in meat, grain, sugar and carbonated drinks, and low in fruit and vegetables.

APPLE CIDER VINEGAR

First, this makes calcium from food or supplements more soluble and so better absorbed. Second, its acidity is useful for people – including around one in two over-60s – who have low stomach acid and thus poor absorption of calcium and certain other minerals. Apple cider vinegar can increase stomach acidity. Third, even though it is acidic, the net result in the body after it has been digested and metabolized is mildly alkaline.

+ ACTION: Include apple cider vinegar in your diet, as this may help prevent or treat osteoporosis.

LEMONS

Lemons contain a wide variety of antioxidant and therefore anti-inflammatory substances, including the polyphenols nobiletin and hesperidin; research has proven that hesperidin decreases bone density loss in mice.[190]

Lemon pectin may be useful, too, as gut bacteria break it down, releasing short-chain fatty acids (such as butyric acid), which raise acidity in the colon. This boosts the absorption of bone-friendly minerals such as calcium and magnesium.

The digestion and metabolism of lemons produces alkaline end-products in the body. This helps prevent any need for the body to extract calcium and other minerals from bones to accompany acid that has to be excreted in urine.

Finally, lemon acids help those who lack enough stomach acid for good calcium absorption.

+ ACTION: Include the zest and juice of a lemon in your daily diet.

SODIUM BICARBONATE

A review in Brazil strongly suggests that diet-induced mild acidosis has adverse effects that might be counter-balanced by a healthy (and therefore alkali-producing) diet.[191]

Studies on taking sodium bicarbonate for osteoporosis have had mixed results. But

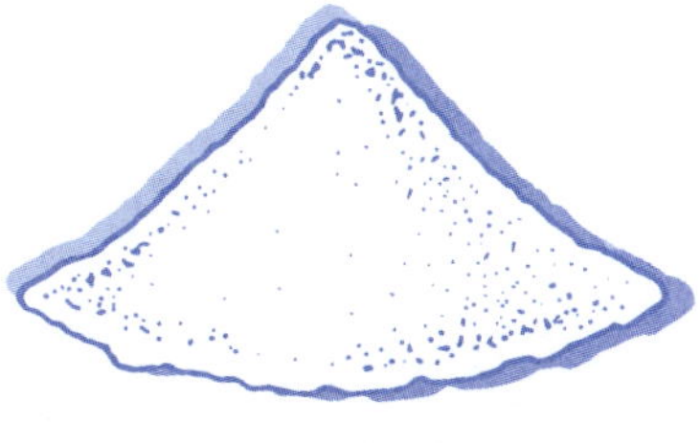

long-term randomized controlled trials have generally not confirmed a positive effect on bone mineral density.

+ ACTION: Eat a healthy diet, with plenty of vegetables and fruit. Consider taking ½–1 teaspoon of sodium bicarbonate each day, though discuss this with your doctor first, and note the tips and warnings on page 67.

OLIVE OIL

Olive oil might help for the following reasons:

- Extra-virgin olive oil contains a variety of antioxidants and anti-inflammatory agents.
- Olive oil aids calcium absorption.
- Increased olive oil consumption is associated with increased bone mineralization.
- Good bone mineralization is dependent on consuming enough oleic acid (the main fatty acid in olive oil) and essential fatty acids.
- The Mediterranean diet discourages osteoporosis.

Studies at the National Institute for Agricultural Research in France found that two olive oil polyphenols – oleuropein and hydroxytyrosol – greatly reduce inflammation-induced bone loss in osteoporosis. (So dramatic is this effect that the Belgian firm BioActor has patents to use these polyphenols in foods, food supplements and herbal medicines for osteoporosis prevention.[192])

The lowest incidence of osteoporosis in Europe is around the Mediterranean. The beneficial effect is attributed mainly to the Mediterranean diet.[193]

+ ACTION: Consume at least 2 tablespoons of extra-virgin olive oil each day.

GARLIC

Garlic's anti-inflammatory antioxidants might help (see above).

+ ACTION: Include garlic in your daily diet or take a garlic supplement. You need water- and oil-soluble sulphur compounds (pp.78–9).

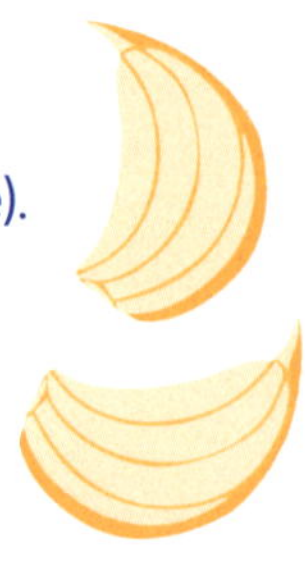

SPICES AND TEAS

The plant oestrogens in certain spices and teas may help.

+ ACTION: Consume oestrogen-balancing spices (p.92) and teas (p.102).

Pain

Damaging factors such as inflammation, injury, heat, cold and lack of oxygen can trigger pain receptors. They do this by releasing agents that include hydrogen ions (protons) and adenosine triphosphate (from damaged cells), serotonin and prostaglandins (from mast cells) and cytokines and nerve growth factor (from particular white blood cells called macrophages). Hydrogen ions cause local acidosis. Then the above agents act on pain receptors that send nerve signals to the spinal cord and brain, causing pain.

Pain is sensed when damaged body tissue has a pH (acid–alkali balance) of 7 or below (depending on its site). This is slightly acidic.

The pH of undamaged tissue is between 7.35 and 7.45, which is slightly alkaline.

It's likely that mild "whole-body" (as opposed to local) acidosis (see "Mild acidosis") encourages pain, too. And not eating a healthy diet (p.58) encourages mild acidosis. So anyone troubled with pain of any sort, including headaches, period pain, sciatica and tendonitis, might benefit from eating a healthy diet.

SODIUM BICARBONATE

This may relieve pain associated with inflammation. It is thought to do this by activating a signalling pathway in the body that makes immune cells called macrophages produce fewer pro-inflammatory cytokines and more anti-inflammatory ones.

+ ACTIONS: Try taking sodium bicarbonate (p.69) but consult a doctor first if your pain is severe or you don't know its cause.

OLIVE OIL

Anti-inflammatory compounds in extra-virgin olive oil might ease pain from inflammation (p.224).

+ ACTION: Take at least 2 tablespoons of extra-virgin olive oil each day.

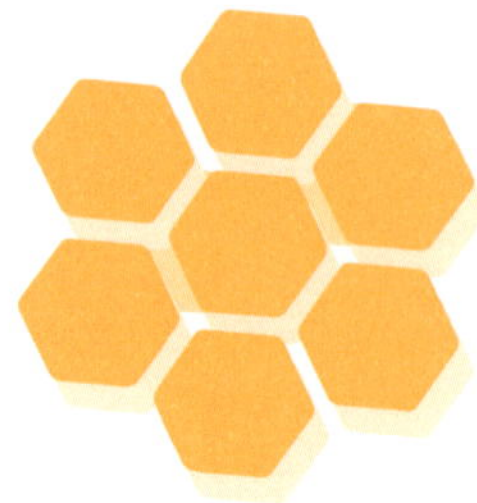

HONEY

Anecdotal reports suggest this eases pain. If so, it may be because:

- Its sweetness encourages the pituitary gland to release soothing morphine-like endorphins.
- Its sweetness stimulates the production of serotonin – a nerve message carrier that can reduce pain.
- It contains tryptophan – the passage of tryptophan into the brain for conversion into serotonin decreases sensitivity to pain.
- It discourages pain related to mild acidosis (p.62) or to high homocysteine, because it contributes to a more alkaline environment in the body (p.62).
- Certain honeys contain quinoline alkaloids, thought to have a pain-relieving effect.

+ ACTIONS: Take 1 teaspoon of raw honey 3 times a day. Massage honey into the skin over painful muscles and joints.

SPICES

Pain-relieving and salicylate-containing spices can help, as may those with cannabinoids (p.91). Juniper's effects resemble those of the non-steroidal, anti-inflammatory drug indomethacin.
+ ACTION: Include these spices in your diet.

TEAS

Pain-relieving teas can help, as may those with cannabinoids.
+ ACTION: Include these teas in your diet.

Parkinson's disease

This chronic brain disease causes a tremor, slow movements, muscle stiffness and poor balance and coordination. It makes a person walk with small shuffling steps and they find it difficult to start moving.

The key cause of Parkinson's is inflammation in the brain, often due to oxidative damage. This causes low levels of several neurotransmitters (nerve message carriers). The main result is low dopamine, due to a reduction in the number of dopamine-producing brain cells in the part of the brain called the substantia nigra. There are also low levels of acetylcholine, gamma-amino-butyric acid (GABA), noradrenaline (norepinephrine) and serotonin.

Medical therapy focuses on supplying dopamine, mimicking its effects, or slowing its breakdown. Monoamine oxidase inhibitor (MAOI) drugs inhibit monoamine oxidase, the enzyme responsible for dopamine breakdown. They also slow the breakdown of serotonin and noradrenaline.

A hallmark of Parkinson's is the abnormal build-up in brain cells of the protein alpha-synuclein. This is mainly due to "misfolding" of this protein's molecules, making it cluster in clumps called "Lewy bodies". There may be poor clearance of this damaged protein, as well as oxidative stress, poorly functioning mitochondria (the cells' energy-producing "factories") and genetic mutations affecting its structure and stability.

Factors that can be associated with the development of Parkinson's include:

- Age: the risk increases with age, usually starting around age 50 or older
- A family history of Parkinson's
- A low level of vitamin D; this is associated with higher levels of the inflammation marker C-reactive protein. A study of 3,000 people in Finland reports that those with the lowest vitamin D levels had a three-fold risk of Parkinson's![194]
- Exposure to toxins such as pesticides, herbicides, solvents and certain heavy metals (for example, lead and manganese)
- Working with detergents
- A history of having had repeated blows to the head
- Taking certain medication, such as antipsychotics, anti-nausea medications, and drugs for hyperkinetic movement disorders
- Taking certain illicit drugs, including amphetamine and methamphetamin, and synthetic heroin contaminated with the neurotoxin MPTP

Researchers believe that Parkinson's often results from a combination of factors.

Taking certain medical drugs can trigger the Parkinson's-like state called "parkinsonism". This usually stops or improves within weeks to months of stopping the drug. One potential culprit is prochlorperazine, used for nausea, dizziness, giddiness and psychosis. Others include certain anticonvulsants (for example, sodium valproate); anti-nausea drugs (such as metochloproamide); antidepressants (such as fluoxetine and venlafaxine); antipsychotics (such as chlorpromazine and prochlorperazine); and blood pressure drugs (calcium channel blockers, such as amlodipine). Consult your doctor if you suspect drug-induced parkinsonism.

LEMONS, GARLIC AND HONEY

These are rich in antioxidants, which discourage inflammation.

+ ACTION: Include lemons, garlic and honey in your diet.

OLIVE OIL

The Mediterranean diet – of which olive oil is an important part – is associated with a lower risk of Parkinson's.

An overview of 12 studies involving more than 1.5 million people shows that strict adherence to the Mediterranean diet is associated with a 13 per cent reduction in the risk of Parkinson's.[195]

+ ACTION: Take at least 2 tablespoons of extra-virgin olive oil each day.

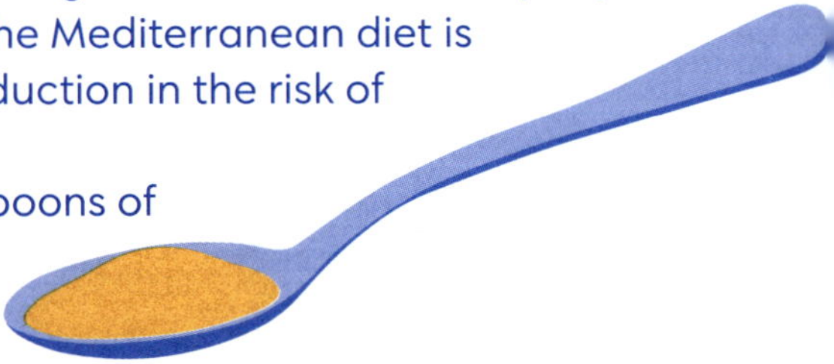

SPICES AND TEAS

Antioxidant, cholinergic and monoamine-oxidase-inhibiting spices and teas might help, as may those that boost the action of GABA and serotonin.

+ ACTION: Include these spices and teas in your diet.

Peptic ulcer

The main cause of peptic ulcers is *Helicobacter pylori* infection. Of the two in five people in the UK infected with these bacteria, one or two gets an ulcer. The bacteria are becoming increasingly resistant to antibiotics. Another cause is long-term use of non-steroidal anti-inflammatory painkillers such as aspirin and ibuprofen.

Several factors make the lining of the stomach, or duodenum, more vulnerable to ulceration. First is damage to the lining. Second is thinning of the mucus protecting against stomach acid and the digestive enzyme pepsin. Third is disrupted stomach-acid regulation.

Duodenal ulcers are four times as common as gastric ones. Most duodenal ulcers are associated with higher than normal stomach-acid levels, most gastric ulcers with normal or low levels. People with too little stomach acid include one in two over-60s and many of those who are stressed, or habituated to antacids or acid suppressants, or who eat an acid-producing diet rich in meat, grain, sugars and carbonated drinks and low in fruit and vegetables.

Having mild metabolic acidosis (p.62) can play a role in the development of erosive stomach ulcers.

APPLE CIDER VINEGAR

It's possible, but not proven, that if someone with peptic ulcer symptoms has tested positive for the presence of *Helicobacter pylori* and suspects a lack of stomach acid (for example, because acid-suppressants don't relieve their symptoms), then cider vinegar's acidity might discourage the infection. Note, though, that it might temporarily worsen ulcer pain.

+ ACTIONS: If you want to try it, try either drinking a glass of water containing 2 teaspoons of cider vinegar each day, or using cider vinegar as a condiment or adding it to recipes.

LEMONS

If someone with peptic ulcer symptoms tests positive for *Helicobacter pylori* and suspects a lack of stomach acid (for example, because antacids don't relieve their symptoms), the acidity of lemon juice might discourage the infection.

An Italian review mentioned several studies showing that citrus fruits and their bioactive compounds, along with antibiotics, could help eradicate *Helicobacter pylori* and avoid peptic ulcer relapse.[196]

+ ACTIONS: Drink a glass of water containing 2 teaspoons of lemon juice with each meal, or add lemon juice to some of your everyday recipes.

OLIVE OIL

Including this in your diet may help a peptic ulcer, thanks partly to its polyphenols (p.20).

A Spanish laboratory study found that olive oil's polyphenols diffuse into stomach acid, where they exert strong activity for several hours against *Helicobacter pylori* (even antibiotic-resistant types). One olive oil polyphenol (called Ty-EDA) was so effective that only 1.5μg/ml was needed to kill the bacteria. To put this into perspective, most virgin olive oils contain up to 240μg/ml of Ty-EDA. The researchers note that the concentration of olive oil polyphenols needed to kill the bacteria was much lower than the concentration of polyphenols we get from consuming tea or wine.[197]

A Russian study found that when people with a peptic ulcer replaced dietary animal fat with olive oil, the ulcer size greatly decreased and healing improved.[198]

+ ACTION: Take at least 2 tablespoons of extra-virgin olive oil each day.

HONEY

Methylglyoxal in manuka honey with a UMF of 10 or more kills the *Helicobacter pylori* bacteria responsible for most peptic ulcers.

Helicobacter pylori is 5–10 times more sensitive to manuka than to other honeys; a 5 per cent solution of manuka honey completely inhibits its growth.[199]

+ ACTION: Consume two teaspoons of manuka or jellybush honey, UMF 20, 2 to 3 times daily for several weeks.

Period problems

These include heavy periods, irregular periods, period pain (see *Cramps* and *Premenstrual syndrome*).

SPICES AND TEAS

Astringent, oestrogen-containing and tannin-containing spices and teas may help with heavy periods. Progesterone-balancing spices and teas might help with irregular periods.

+ ACTION: Add these spices and teas to your diet.

Piles (haemorrhoids)

Spongy "pads" in the walls of the anus normally prevent leaking of the bowel's contents. In some people, though, they become bulky and readily inflamed. They are then known as "piles". Several things can make the pads swell and make the veins in them engorged. These include high pressure on them in someone who is constipated, pregnant, or doing heavy lifting. Any fragility of the walls of the veins in piles encourages leaking. Piles may cause discomfort and itching and, perhaps, bleeding. A healthy diet helps by making it easier to empty the bowel. It also provides vitamin C, rutin and several other flavonoids that can help strengthen veins.

LEMONS

Their vitamin C and certain flavonoids, including rutin, can strengthen veins; their fibre helps prevent constipation; and their antioxidants reduce inflammation.

+ ACTION: Include the zest and juice of a lemon in your daily diet.

OLIVE OIL

This too contains rutin, to help strengthen veins.

+ ACTION: Include 2 tablespoons of olive oil in your daily diet.

GARLIC

This might help because of its fibre, flavonoids and vitamin C: all of these are anti-inflammatory.

+ ACTION: Include garlic in your diet or take a garlic supplement. You need water- and oil-soluble sulphur compounds (pp.78–9).

Polycystic ovary syndrome (PCOS)

This often begins after sudden weight gain, or after stopping oral contraception. In adolescents and young adults it can cause acne, excess facial and body hair and period problems. Each polycystic ovary may have as many as 10 or more cysts, all of which are immature follicles that haven't developed to release an egg, whereas a normal ovary would have fewer but larger follicles.

Without treatment, the menopause usually arrives early. Around this time metabolic disorders and cardiovascular diseases become more likely – with, for example, an increased risk of diabetes, high blood pressure, high LDL cholesterol (which if oxidized is "bad") and low HDL cholesterol (the "good" sort), strokes and womb cancer.

Women with PCOS are particularly likely to have high blood sugar. This is associated with eating an unhealthy diet – in particular, having too much blood sugar-raising food (such as white bread, white rice, pasta, sugary cereals, biscuits, cakes, crisps, sweets, fruit juice and sweetened drinks, including energy and sports drinks).

High blood sugar encourages resistance to insulin (a hormone that regulates blood sugar and fat metabolism). Insulin resistance, in turn, encourages pre-diabetes and type 2 diabetes. So high blood sugar is a big risk factor for these conditions in women with PCOS.

Researchers consider that high insulin is a key factor in causing PCOS; mild acidosis (p.62) may also be to blame.

OLIVE OIL AND LEMONS

As part of a healthy diet these can aid weight loss and help return the body's metabolic profile to normal, thus lowering the risk of developing this syndrome.

An Italian study found that substituting olive oil for saturated fat in the diet helps to lower blood sugar.[200]

+ ACTION: Consume 2 tablespoons of extra-virgin olive oil a day and include lemons in your diet.

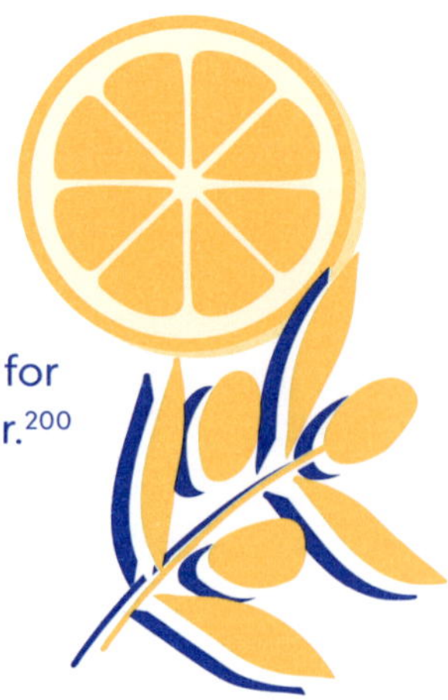

Poor appetite

This is common with certain short-term illnesses (for example, infections). It can also result from depression, anaemia, certain medications (eg, certain antibiotics and anti-cancer drugs) and certain long-term illnesses, such as diabetes, dementia, an underactive thyroid and cancer.

SPICES

Digestive spices can boost appetite and include coriander, ginger and turmeric.

+ ACTION: Include these spices in your diet.

TEAS

Digestive teas can boost appetite and include chamomile and fennel.

+ ACTION: Include these teas in your diet.

Poor circulation

See also *Artery disease*. Possible symptoms include feeling uncomfortably cold, poor memory, male impotence and slow wound healing (especially on legs, ankles and feet). The possible causes include:

- Abnormal sensitivity to cold – including Raynaud's phenomenon: abnormal narrowing of arteries in fingers and toes that can make them temporarily white, blue, red or purple
- Ageing
- High blood fats – which encourage atherosclerosis
- High blood pressure – slows blood flow by making artery walls thinner and less elastic
- High blood sugar – impedes blood flow by narrowing arteries and making them less elastic
- Lack of exercise – as exercise increases the rate of blood flow
- Obesity – encourages high blood pressure, diabetes and high cholesterol
- Smoking – nicotine in cigarettes and vapes damages artery walls and thickens blood

OLIVE OIL AND LEMONS

As part of a healthy diet (p.58) these may help with poor circulation.
+ ACTION: Consume a lemon and 2 tablespoons of extra-virgin olive oil each day.

GARLIC

Garlic is known as a "warming" herb as it dilates arteries, which boosts circulation. It may also help to prevent or treat artery disease. And it makes blood less sticky, which aids blood flow.
+ ACTION: Include garlic in your daily diet or take a garlic supplement. You need water- and oil-soluble sulphur compounds (pp.78–9).

SPICES

Warming spices may help.
+ ACTIONS: Include these in your diet. For cold hands and feet, put 1 tablespoon of mustard powder into a basin of comfortably hot water and soak your hands or feet in it for 15 minutes.

TEAS

Warming teas may help.
+ ACTION: Include these in your diet.

Poor immunity

See also *Autoimmune disease*. Poor immunity makes the body less able to fight infection and other disease. It is also associated with autoimmune diseases.

APPLE CIDER VINEGAR

This contains antioxidant polyphenols that can boost immunity.

Cider vinegar that is raw, meaning unpasteurized, and is also unfiltered, has a cloudy part to it called the "mother". This contains strands of enzymes and proteins, as well as bacteria that are probiotic, meaning they aid a healthy balance of bacteria and other micro-organisms in the gut. A healthy gut microbiome in turn aids the body's immunity (p.61).
+ ACTION: Add apple cider vinegar to foods such as soups, stews and salads.

LEMONS

Their vitamin C aids immunity. And their pectin fibre is fermented by "good" micro-organisms in the gut. This frees certain short-chain fatty acids (such as butyric acid) that aid immunity and reduce inflammation by stimulating production of certain antibodies and lowering production of auto-antibodies, white blood cells and cytokines.

+ ACTION: Include the zest and juice of a lemon in your daily diet.

HONEY

Honey's polyphenols have antioxidant ability, and its antimicrobial contents can also aid immunity.

Its polyphenols boost immunity thanks to their:

- Antioxidant action – this prevents oxidative stress in the body by neutralizing free radicals that could otherwise impair immune function
- Anti-inflammatory action – this suppresses the production of pro-inflammatory cytokines and also promotes anti-inflammatory cytokines
- Immune-cell modulation – this, for example, aids natural killer cells which help fight bacteria and viruses in cells
- Promotion of a healthy gut microbiome, which enhances the body's immune function

When 10 volunteers in Dubai consumed a daily 1.2g of honey per 1kg bodyweight, blood tests revealed a 50 per cent increase in white cells called monocytes and a slight increase in white cells called lymphocytes and eosinophils. These white cells are known to help the body fight infection and inflammation.[201]

+ ACTION: Substitute honey for table sugar in your diet.

GARLIC

This boosts immunity by influencing several sorts of white cells. For example, it:

- Stimulates the ability of natural killer cells to destroy virus-infected and cancer cells
- Increases the activity of macrophages (which engulf and destroy foreign bacteria)
- Activates helper T cells which detect an infection – and the type of infection – then signal other immune cells to fight it
- Maximizes the bactericidal (bacteria-killing) activity of certain types of white cells called macrophages

+ **ACTION**: Include garlic in your daily diet or take a garlic supplement. You need oil-soluble sulphur compounds (p.79).

SPICES

Immunity-enhancing spices (p.90) can boost white cell production.
+ **ACTION**: Include these spices in your diet.

TEAS

Immunity-enhancing, circulation-boosting (see warming teas) and tonic teas may help. Rooibos tea, for example, enhances immunity by boosting natural body substances called interleukins.
+ **ACTION**: Include these teas in your diet.

Poor memory

See also *Memory loss; Dementia*. This is most often due to being busy, stressed or having ageing-related deterioration. It may also be associated, for example, with poor circulation (p.261) reducing the blood flow to the brain. At worst, it is a feature of dementia. A healthy diet (p.58) and lifestyle may help prevent memory loss.

SPICES

Cholinergic and memory-boosting spices may help (p.89).
+ **ACTION**: Include these spices in your diet.

TEAS

Cholinergic and memory-boosting teas may help, as may circulation-boosting teas and teas containing ginseng or rutin.
+ **ACTION**: Include these teas in your diet.

Premature ageing

Scientists have long searched for lifestyle factors that encourage a long health span by discouraging ageing-related conditions. These include age spots, Alzheimer's disease, age-related macular degeneration, arthritis, atherosclerosis, cancer, cataracts, diabetes, heart disease, high blood pressure, osteoporosis, poor memory and wrinkled skin.

As they get older, some people opt for a diet that is easier to eat but is often less than healthy. And they may not absorb as much nourishment from their food. Both factors encourage premature ageing. A less than healthy diet (p.58) encourages many health problems. These include mild acidosis (p.62), which has damaging effects on cells and metabolism in general, some of which – for example, structural changes in proteins, oxidation of fats and a lower oxygen supply to cells – encourage premature ageing.

A US research review concludes that a healthy diet (which has a lower acid load than an unhealthy diet) and, perhaps, taking alkaline salts (such as sodium bicarbonate), might mitigate the ageing process by:

- Increasing the activity of telomerase, an enzyme that helps maintain telomere length and is associated with longer lifespan. Telomeres are protective caps on chromosomes (strands of genes in each cell nucleus that carry our body's "blueprint"). Telomeres help prevent chromosomes sticking together or unravelling. They also limit cell divisions. This protects DNA from damage, so making cells less likely to grow uncontrollably and become cancerous. Telomeres shorten each time a cell divides, eventually becoming so short that cells can no longer divide. This shortening is considered a major factor in cell ageing
- Reducing the body's own acid production, thereby slowing the accumulation of excess fibrous connective tissue known as fibrosis
- Maintaining the action of the anti-ageing protein klotho, made mostly by the kidneys

The researchers conclude that eating a healthy diet, or neutralizing mild acidosis associated with age-related poor kidney function, might lead to a longer, healthier lifespan.[202]

Flavonoids in vegetables, fruits, spices and teas can stimulate collagen production and improve skin elasticity, for example:

- Apigenin – increases collagen
- Cocoa flavanols – improve skin elasticity; reduce wrinkles
- Epicatechin, quercetin and rutin are antioxidants, so enhance collagen synthesis, scavenge potentially damaging free radicals, and help prevent the breakdown of skin's hyaluronic acid, elastin and collagen
- Genistein – thickens collagen fibres; is anti-inflammatory; and promotes DNA repair in the skin's fibroblasts

Certain groups of the world's particularly long-lived peoples drink mountain water rich in alkaline minerals such as calcium, which help prevent mild acidosis (p.62). Fermented foods (including vegetables, fruit, milk, cereal grains, meat or fish) are a traditional part of their diet. These contain fermentation acids (such as lactic, acetic and malic) that are metabolized to alkali in the body.

In contrast, mild acidosis is very common in peoples eating a typical Western diet. Ageing exaggerates acidosis because declining kidney function reduces the excretion of excess acid. Clearly it's wise in later life to opt for a healthy diet that will help us be fit and well during our remaining years.

OLIVE OIL

Damage by excessive oxidation encourages premature ageing. It is more likely in people who smoke, eat an unhealthy diet or are stressed. Extra-virgin olive oil's monounsaturated fat and antioxidants help prevent excessive oxidation. And it's possible that including olive oil in a healthy diet might help prevent premature ageing.

I once heard of a village in Lebanon where the people drank a glass of olive oil each morning and evening, and their average lifespan was 98 for the women, 97 for the men. Sadly, I can now find no reference to where and when this happened.

US researchers have found that mineral and vitamin deficiencies speed the age-related decay of the cells' mitochondria (energy-producing structures).[203]

Australian researchers suggest that people with a high intake of vegetables and olive oil, but a low intake of dairy products, margarine and sugar, had the youngest-looking skin.[204]

+ ACTION: Take at least 2 tablespoons of extra-virgin olive oil each day.

GARLIC

Garlic's vitamin C and other antioxidants help counter early ageing of skin, joints and arteries and reduce inflammation associated with heart disease, arthritis and Alzheimer's disease. Garlic may also discourage certain cancers and strokes. Finally, pectin in the garlic clove skin helps to eliminate from the body the heavy metals (such as aluminium and lead) that encourage cells to age prematurely.

In mice prone to early ageing, aged garlic extract increased lifespan.[205]

+ ACTION: Include garlic in your daily diet or take a garlic supplement. You need water- and oil-soluble sulphur compounds (pp.78–9).

SPICES AND TEAS

Antioxidant spices and teas may help with premature ageing. Rosemary tea and green tea are traditionally associated with longevity.

+ ACTION: Include these teas in your diet.

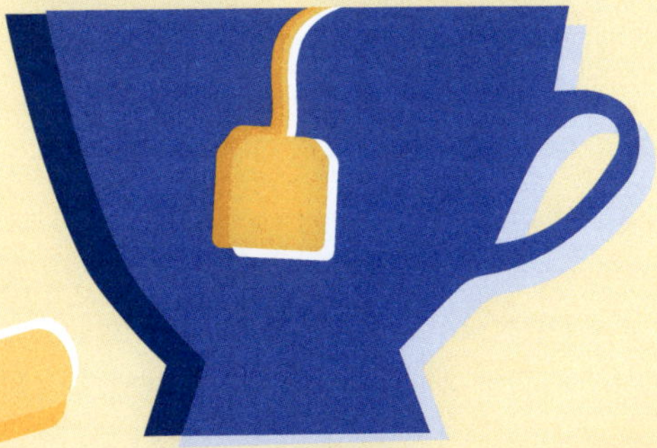

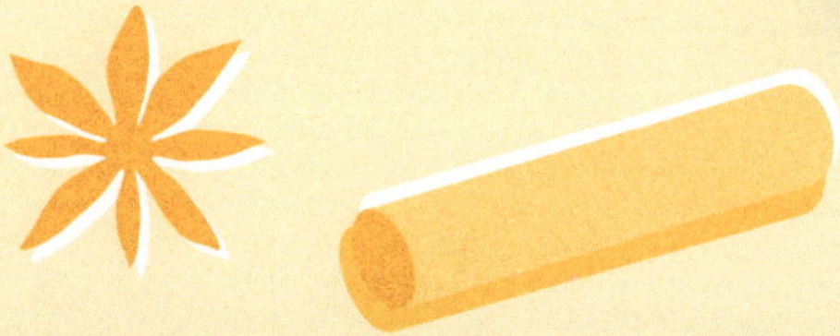

Premature death

Such a death occurs before the average or expected age of death in a population. The commonest causes are cancer, heart disease, Alzheimer's disease, Parkinson's disease and type 2 diabetes.

OLIVE OIL

The Mediterranean diet, which contains olive oil, may help prevent premature death. An overview of 12 studies involving more than 1.5 million people found that strict adherence to the Mediterranean diet cut the risk of all-cause early death by 9 per cent.[206]

+ ACTION: Consume at least 2 tablespoons of extra-virgin olive oil each day.

Pre-menstrual syndrome (PMS)

The many possible symptoms generally occur in the two weeks before a period. They can include changes in appetite; food cravings; breast tenderness, pain, swelling and lumpiness; acne; greasy hair; fluid retention; leg cramp; headaches; constipation or diarrhoea; sleep problems; fatigue; loss of interest in sex; mood swings; depression; irritability; anxiety; confusion; difficulty concentrating; forgetfulness; clumsiness; and intolerance of loud noise and bright light.

PMS probably results from changes in the levels of certain neurotransmitters (nerve message carriers), such as serotonin and GABA (gamma-amino butyric acid). These result from particular sensitivity to the changing balance of progesterone and oestrogen during this part of the menstrual cycle. Research suggests that glucaric-acid salts may help PMS by suppressing the enzyme beta-glucuronidase. This suppresion enables a process called glucuronidation in the liver which makes oestrogen more water-soluble, so aiding its elimination in urine. This can improve the body's balance of oestrogen and progesterone.

LEMONS

Limonene encourages glucuronidation.

+ ACTION: Include the zest and juice of a lemon in your daily diet during the 2 weeks before you expect a period.

GARLIC

This could help relieve PMS symptoms, thanks to certain compounds that improve hormone balance and reduce inflammation.

A study found that women who took a garlic supplement each day for three menstrual cycles reported – in contrast with those who took a placebo (dummy supplement) – a reduction in severity of their PMS symptoms.[207]

+ ACTION: Include garlic in your daily diet.

TEAS

Certain herb teas are reputed to help.

+ ACTION: Try calming teas; also fennel, *Ginkgo biloba*, St John's wort and *Vitex agnus castus* may be helpful.

Prolapsed uterus

This means that a woman's uterus (womb) is not properly supported within the body, resulting in it sagging down through the vagina. Among the many causes are obesity, straining with constipation, a chronic cough and weak pelvic muscles and ligaments.

LEMONS

Lemons may help prevent a prolapse, or stop it getting worse. This is because they can help cure constipation or a cough and their vitamin C, rutin and other flavonoids promote healthy muscles and ligaments.

+ ACTION: Eat a liquidized lemon several times a week.

Psoriasis

This is characterized by patches of red, thick, itchy, flaking skin overlying inflammation on the knees, elbows, scalp or elsewhere.

SODIUM BICARBONATE

When 31 people with mild-to-moderate psoriasis had sodium bicarbonate baths (p.69), almost all reported improvement. Indeed, the baths reduced itchiness and irritation so well that the volunteers continued their baths after the study.[208]

+ ACTION: Try a daily sodium bicarbonate bath.

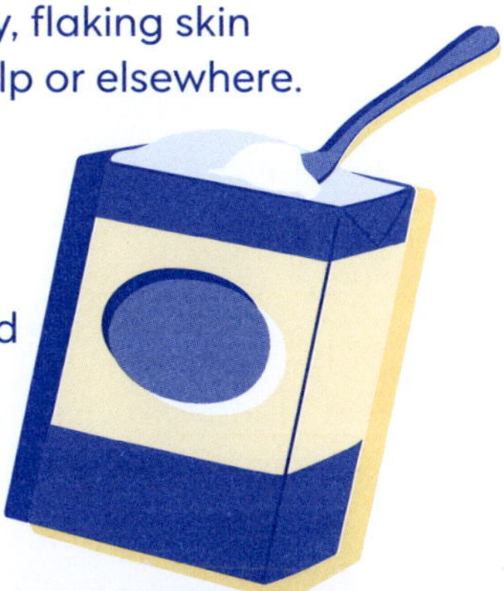

LEMONS

Citric acid in lemon juice can ease dryness and flaking. And sunshine's ultraviolet-A rays act on psoralens in lemon juice to mimic the PUVA (psoralen-UVA) therapy used for psoriasis by dermatologists. A lemon's carotenoids, coumarins and certain flavonoids (such as hesperidin) may soothe inflammation.
+ ACTIONS: Smooth lemon juice over psoriasis several times a day. Treat patches with juice, as above, then expose them to sunlight for a few minutes a day, increasing the time over several weeks. Include the zest and juice of a lemon in your daily diet.

OLIVE OIL

Applying this oil may soothe the inflammation, thanks to its monounsaturated fats, and its oleocanthal and other antioxidants.
+ ACTION: Consume at least 2 tablespoons of extra-virgin olive oil each day. Apply a film of extra-virgin olive oil to affected skin twice a day.

HONEY

Anecdotal evidence suggests honey can help. If so, this could be because of its anti-inflammatories.
+ ACTIONS: Include it in your daily diet. Add two tablespoons of raw honey to bathwater, then soak in it for 30 minutes. Apply medical-grade honey cream 3 times a day.

GARLIC

Garlic's anti-inflammatory constituents may soothe the inflammation caused by psoriasis.
+ ACTIONS: First, do a patch test (p.82) to check garlic is safe for your skin. Apply garlic oil macerate or garlic oil (p.80) to affected areas twice a day. Alternatively, bathe infected areas with garlic water (p.81). Include garlic in your daily diet or take a garlic supplement. You need water- and oil-soluble sulphur compounds (pp.78–9).

SPICES

Anti-inflammatory spices may help, as may coumarin-containing ones (p.90). In particular, try turmeric.

+ ACTIONS: Include these in your diet. Apply a compress or poultice of powdered turmeric to affected skin each day, or apply capsaicin cream – available from a pharmacy or the internet.

TEAS

Anti-inflammatory teas may help, as may coumarin-containing ones.
+ ACTION: Include these in your diet. Use these teas and emollient teas as a wash or in a bath, or apply them to affected patches of skin in a compress or poultice.

Ringworm

This rash of red, ring-shaped patches results from a fungal skin infection.

SODIUM BICARBONATE

The antifungal effect of sodium bicarbonate may help.
+ ACTIONS: Either apply dry sodium-bicarbonate powder directly to the affected skin, or apply a paste made by putting 1 tablespoon of sodium bicarbonate into a bowl and stirring in a few drops of water.

GARLIC

There is good evidence that garlic, particularly its ajoene compound, can help:

In a Venezuelan study, 60 soldiers with ringworm presenting as "jock itch" were treated with ajoene gel, or cream containing terbinafine (an antifungal drug), for 2 months. Healing occurred in 73 and 71 per cent of the two groups respectively. The researchers concluded that ajoene is useful.[209]

+ ACTIONS: Ajoene gel isn't available commercially, so apply garlic macerate or garlic oil, (p.80), twice a day until 14 days after the skin has healed. Alternatively, bathe the infected area with garlic water (p.81).Include garlic in your daily diet or take a garlic supplement. You need oil-soluble sulphur compounds (p.270).

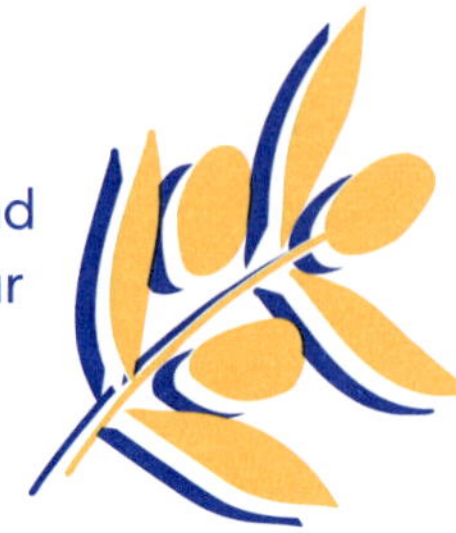

Scars

As skin heals, scar tissue generally flattens and fades, and there's some evidence that smoothing olive oil into a scar will aid this process.

OLIVE OIL

This may help to fade scars – including the stretch marks of pregnancy – by helping skin cells to regenerate.

+ ACTION: Once the skin has healed, smoothe a little extra-virgin olive oil into the scar each day.

Seborrhoeic dermatitis

This skin inflammation affects areas with the most sebaceous glands, such as the scalp, behind the ears, between the eyebrows, along the eyelashes and around the nose. It is often caused by an overgrowth of *Malassezia furfur* – a yeast and a normal inhabitant of skin. Many sufferers also have dandruff – see *Dandruff*).

OLIVE OIL

Extra-virgin olive oil makes a gentle cleanser, has antifungal properties and softens scaly areas.

+ ACTION: Smooth extra-virgin olive oil into the affected skin twice a day. If your scalp is affected, apply extra-virgin olive oil. Put a shower cap or plastic carrier bag over your hair and cover with a towel wrapped turban-style. Relax for 1 hour, then shampoo your hair. Repeat twice a week. Consume at least 2 tablespoons of extra-virgin olive oil each day.

Shingles

This painful, itchy skin rash results from varicella-zoster virus infection. When a person has chickenpox (usually many years before), the viruses lie dormant in a particular nerve's sensory cells until some trigger reawakens them. This causes shingles in the area supplied by that nerve.

HONEY

Applying honey excludes air, so reducing pain. It also provides antiviral and anti-inflammatory agents.

+ ACTION: Apply a light coating of highly antioxidant and anti-infective honey, such as manuka honey with a UMF of at least 10 or even 20 or more.

GARLIC

This can increase immunity. It also inactivates the related viruses *Herpes simplex* 1 and 2. I can find no evidence that garlic acts against varicella-zoster viruses, but folk wisdom has it that applying garlic reduces the pain and itching. It might be worth a try.
+ ACTIONS: First, do a patch test (p.82). Apply garlic oil macerate or garlic oil (p.80) twice a day. Or bathe the infected area with garlic water (p.81). Include garlic in your daily diet or take a garlic supplement. You need oil-soluble sulphur compounds (p.79).

Sinusitis

This inflammation of the lining of the sinuses (spaces within the bones of the face) generally results from infection.

HONEY

Honey's soothing, anti-inflammatory and antimicrobial properties may help, as may its oligosaccharides.
+ ACTION: Consume 1–2 teaspoons of raw honey 3 times a day, or chew some honeycomb (from a beehive, not the confectionery sort!) for 15 minutes every few hours. Also, gargle with 1 teaspoon of honey in half a glass of warm water.

Skin problems

Mild acidosis (p.62) can trigger or worsen various skin conditions by encouraging allergy, infection, inflammation, itching, and pain from broken or inflamed skin. A healthy diet (p.58) helps prevent and treat many skin problems.

SODIUM BICARBONATE

Applying this to affected skin may help cuts and grazes, eczema, fungal skin infection, heat rash, insect bites and stings, itching, psoriasis, ringworm, small burns, a splinter and sunburn.
+ ACTION: Apply to affected skin (p.69).

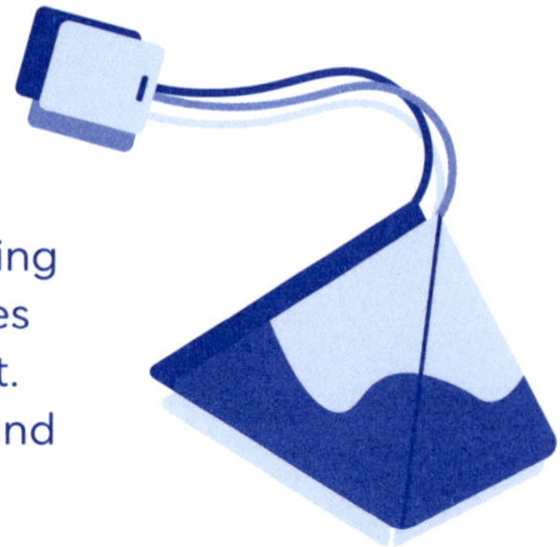

Sprains

These result from an injury stretching or tearing a ligament – the band of strong, flexible fibres connecting the bones on either side of a joint. A sprain causes pain, swelling and stiffness and limits the movement of the affected area.

TEAS

Applying cold calendula, lavender, nettle or rosemary tea may help.
+ ACTION: Apply one or more of these in a compress or poultice.

Splinter

This is a small, sharp piece of a foreign body that penetrates the skin. It can be painful and, if not removed, it encourages infection.

SODIUM BICARBONATE

Certain pastes attract water from the skin around the splinter. This osmotic effect can help draw out the splinter.
+ ACTION: Apply a paste of sodium bicarbonate and water over the splinter. Cover with a sticking plaster and leave overnight. Repeat as necessary.

HONEY

Honey, used in the same way as sodium bicarbonate paste (see above), may help draw out the splinter.

Strokes

A stroke is damage in the brain from blocking or bleeding from an artery. Nearly 9 in 10 strokes are ischaemic strokes (resulting from interrupted blood flow in an artery, so damaging local tissues); the others are haemorrhagic strokes (resulting from local bleeding from an artery).

An ischaemic stroke may be either a thrombotic stroke (resulting from a blood clot blocking an atherosclerotic artery – see *Artery disease*), or an embolic stroke (resulting from a blood clot or a dislodged piece of arterial plaque that has developed further away and travelled in the bloodstream to the site of the stroke).

The less likely sort of stroke, responsible for just over 1 in 10 strokes, is the haemorrhagic stroke, resulting from bleeding into the brain from an unhealthy artery (usually an atherosclerotic one).

Ischaemic and haemorrhagic strokes have many risk factors in common. These include air pollution, anxiety, atherosclerosis, cocaine use, contraceptive pills, depression, diabetes, genetic factors, high cholesterol, high blood pressure, kidney disease, smoking and poorly managed stress.

A thrombotic stroke's main cause is artery disease. Such a stroke can be encouraged by ageing, atrial fibrillation, chronic inflammation (as in rheumatoid arthritis and lupus), chronic infection, dehydration, heart valve disease, hormone-replacement therapy, migraine, more than nine hours' sleep a night, sleep apnoea ("stop-breathing attacks") and viral infection.

A haemorrhagic stroke's main cause is high blood pressure that has damaged an artery so much that it tears and bleeds. Such strokes can also arise from too much alcohol, and blood-thinner (anticoagulant) medication.

Doctors sometimes recommend low-dose aspirin (acetyl salicylic acid) to discourage a thrombotic stroke, partly because of its anti-inflammatory and anti-blood-clotting actions.

Transient ischaemic attacks (TIAs, or "mini strokes") are almost always thrombotic strokes.

An analysis of eight studies involving 257,551 people found a lower risk of a stroke in those with a higher vegetable and fruit intake.[210]

OLIVE OIL

Making extra-virgin olive oil your main dietary fat can help counter many of the risk factors for artery disease. Consider the following studies:

- A five-year study of 7,625 people aged 65 and over in France, reported a 41 per cent lower risk of a stroke in those who regularly consumed olive oil compared with in those who never did.[211]

- An overview of 12 studies involving more than 1.5 million people found that strict adherence to the Mediterranean diet – whose major fat is olive oil – cut the risk of dying from a stroke or a heart attack by 9 per cent.[212]
- One study found that one of virgin olive oil's polyphenols, hydroxytyrosol acetate, inhibited clotting, suggesting that olive oil might help prevent a thrombotic stroke.[213]
- A review at Boston University found that flavonoids (such as in olive oil) discourage blood clots by making artery walls more flexible.[214]

+ ACTION: Take at least 2 tablespoons of extra-virgin olive oil each day.

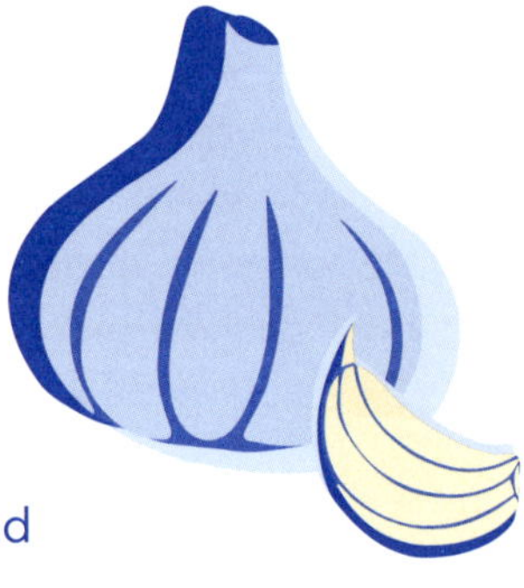

GARLIC

This may help prevent various risk factors. For example, it helps reduce high blood pressure, lower high blood fats, thin overly thick blood and improve blood sugar levels

+ ACTION: Include garlic in your daily diet or take a garlic supplement. You need water- and oil-soluble sulphur compounds (pp.78–9).

SPICES AND TEAS

Certain spices and teas contain salicylic acid salts called salicylates, which have blood-thinning and anti-inflammatory effects.

Anti-inflammatory, antioxidant, anticoagulant, blood sugar-lowering, and cholesterol-lowering spices and teas may help.

+ ACTION: Include these spices and teas in your diet.

Sunburn

It is strongly advised to prevent sunburn by keeping your skin shaded or covered, and by applying a suitable sunscreening product when in the sun.

If you do get sunburnt, applying extra-virgin olive oil to the burnt skin may be soothing. This is because it contains oleocanthal – a polyphenol with anti-inflammatory properties.

CAUTION: If badly burnt by the sun, seek medical help.

OLIVE OIL

Topical olive oil may reduce the "bubbling" and peeling of mild sunburn by locking in moisture. And its antioxidants may be soothing and aid faster healing.

+ ACTION: Apply olive oil to burnt skin twice a day.

LEMONS

The antioxidants from lemons in your diet could make getting sunburnt less likely.

+ ACTION: Include the zest and juice of a lemon in your diet.

Thrush

This is an infection of the mouth, skin or vagina with the yeast-like fungus *Candida albicans.*

GARLIC

Laboratory studies show that garlic's allicin is a highly effective remedy and its ajoene inhibits the fungal growth.

+ ACTIONS: Include garlic in your daily diet or take a garlic supplement. You need oil-soluble sulphur compounds (p.79). If you have a mouth infection, chew then spit out a raw garlic clove several times a day, though stop if this causes irritation. If you have a skin infection, first do a patch test (p.82): if this shows no problem, apply garlic oil macerate or garlic oil, (p.80), several times a day.

Alternatively, bathe the infected area with garlic water (p.81). For vaginal thrush, take garlic as above but don't be tempted to follow the sometimes-given advice to insert a raw garlic clove in the vagina as it might become stuck, which could encourage other infections.

Tooth decay and gum disease

When mouth bacteria feed on food debris in the mouth, they form a sticky and colourless coating called dental plaque on and between teeth and at the gum margins. Refined carbohydrates (in foods made with refined flour and table sugar) are the main culprits in the food debris.

Plaque is a "biofilm" of micro-organisms. If not cleaned away by brushing or flossing, or with a dental pick, calcium and other minerals from saliva infiltrate it, turning it into tartar ("calculus"). Tartar is hard, whitish, pale-yellow or brown; it can cause gingivitis (inflamed gums) and make gums bleed. Plaque bacteria also produce acids that corrode tooth enamel, encouraging tooth decay and gingivitis.

To avoid tooth decay and gum disease, it's important to look after your teeth by brushing and flossing (and using an interdental brush) twice a day and seeing a dentist and a dental hygienist regularly.

LEMONS

The antioxidants and other anti-inflammatories in lemons may relieve the pain and swelling of gingivitis.

+ ACTION: Massage unhealthy gums twice a day with lemon juice, or use an antiseptic and astringent mouthwash made with half water and half lemon juice, or with 1 drop of lemon essential oil in a cup of warm water.

SODIUM BICARBONATE

The mild abrasiveness of sodium bicarbonate powder helps remove plaque from teeth. The alkalinity of sodium bicarbonate inhibits dental-plaque formation by neutralizing acids produced by mouth bacteria. Also, sodium bicarbonate increases calcium uptake by enamel. Finally, by removing stains it helps whiten teeth.

+ ACTION: Clean teeth with toothpaste that contains bicarbonate, or with bicarbonate of soda powder.

HONEY

Honey's antimicrobials and anti-inflammatories help prevent gingivitis. Honey can also reduce tartar deposition. Although certain honeys, like sugar, encourage tooth decay, others inactivate the plaque bacteria responsible for tooth decay. This stops them producing acid from sugar. This, in turn, prevents the production of dextrans – the gummy polysaccharides that stick plaque to teeth – and reduces demineralization of tooth enamel.

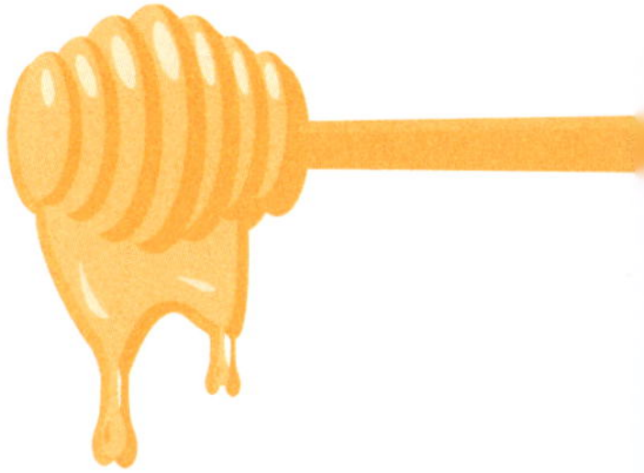

In a study at the University of Otago, New Zealand, 30 volunteers chewed a piece of manuka-honey-impregnated leather or sugarless chewing gum, for 10 minutes 3 times a day, after eating, for 21 days. The honey group had highly significant reductions in plaque. Gingivitis was reduced by 48 per cent in the honey group; the others had only a 17 per cent reduction.[215] Manuka honeys are particularly helpful for plaque.

+ ACTIONS: Choose manuka honey with a UMF of at least 10, and rub it into inflamed gums 3 times a day. Eat 1 teaspoon of honey 3 times a day.

GARLIC

The allicin in crushed, chewed, sliced or chopped garlic may reduce toothache. This may be because it kills infecting bacteria and reduces inflammation.

+ ACTIONS: Apply garlic oil macerate or garlic oil (p.80). Limit the first application to 10 minutes and stop if it irritates your gums. Repeat 4 times a day. Include garlic in your daily diet or take a garlic supplement containing oil-soluble sulphur compounds (p.79).

SPICES

Analgesic spices and local anaesthetic spices (allspice, cinnamon and cloves) may help.

+ ACTIONS: Include analgesic spices in your diet or chew some fresh ginger. Rub 2 drops of a local-anaesthetic spice oil (p.91) around the affected tooth, or chew an allspice berry, a piece of cinnamon or a clove on the side of your mouth with the toothache.

TEAS

Analgesic, antibacterial and anti-inflammatory teas may help. Barley tea, corn tea and *Camellia-sinensis* tea help prevent decay.

+ ACTION: Include these teas in your diet. Use antibacterial teas and green tea as a mouthwash after eating.

Ulcerative colitis

This autoimmune disease means the body's usually defensive immune system acting out of character by inflaming and ulcerating the colon's lining.

OLIVE OIL

As part of a healthy diet (p.58), extra-virgin olive oil's polyphenols might help soothe the inflammation.

+ **ACTION:** Take 1–2 tablespoons of extra-virgin olive oil each day.

Underactive thyroid

This butterfly-shaped gland in the neck produces several hormones that regulate many of the body's most important functions. They increase cells' oxygen consumption and body temperature. They increase the heart rate and the amount of blood the heart pumps out. They help keep bones strong by depositing calcium and phosphate in them. They aid cell growth, development and differentiation. Finally, they influence mood and behaviour, stimulate gut motility and increase your body's oxygen levels. Underactivity of the thyroid depresses all of these actions. Mild acidosis (p.62) may depress thyroid function.

SODIUM BICARBONATE

Avoid taking sodium bicarbonate as it can make medication for an underactive thyroid less effective.

+ **ACTION:** Eat an alkali-producing diet.

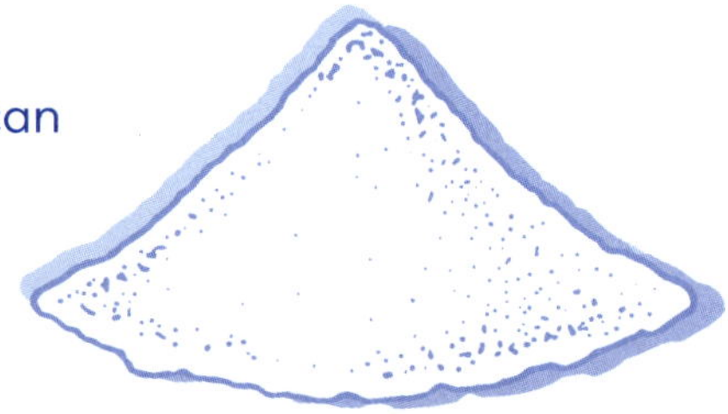

Varicose veins

These abnormally distended veins in the legs may ache or itch, and the overlying skin is more prone to eczema than is other skin. To help prevent varicose veins, a person needs a healthy diet (p.58) – one reason being that this contains vitamin C, rutin and several other flavonoids that help strengthen veins. Other factors that encourage varicose veins include being female, overweight or obese, inactive, a smoker, pregnant or on oral contraception or hormone replacement therapy (HRT), and advancing age.

To manage varicose veins, address relevant risk factors. When sitting to relax, raise your legs at a 45-degree angle to the rest of your body. This helps to prevent blood "pooling" in leg veins. Compression tights or stockings can ease aching. A healthy diet (p.58) makes it easier to empty the bowels and provides vitamin C, rutin, and several other flavonoids that can help strengthen veins.

LEMONS

Lemons' vitamin C, rutin and certain other flavonoids strenghen veins; their fibre helps prevent constipation; and their antioxidants reduce inflammation.

+ ACTION: Include the zest and juice of a lemon in your daily diet.

GARLIC

This might help because its fibre, flavonoids and vitamin C are anti-inflammatory.

+ ACTION: Include garlic in your diet or take a garlic supplement. You need water- and oil-soluble sulphur compounds (pp.78–9).

OLIVE OIL

Like lemons, this too contains rutin.

+ ACTION: Include 2 tablespoons of olive oil in your daily diet.

SPICES AND TEAS

Coriander contains rutin, which may help. If the veins are inflamed, use anti-inflammatory teas and spices.

+ ACTION: Include coriander and anti-inflammatory teas in your diet. Also apply them in a compress or a poultice (p.96).

Warts, including verrucas

Warts arise from infection of the skin with certain strains of human papilloma virus and are most common on the hands. A verruca is a wart on the sole of the foot. Around one in three untreated warts disappear within 3 months; the rest are likely to disappear within 2 years.

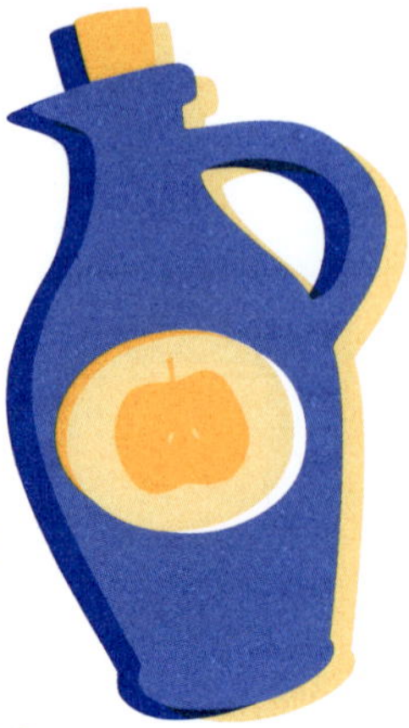

APPLE CIDER VINEGAR

Wart-removing products containing salicylates are a common treatment. Apple cider vinegar contains small amounts of salicylates and there are many reports of its repeated application curing warts. Some podiatrists treat warts with dichloroacetic acid – a more corrosive relative of salicylates.

+ ACTION: Before bedtime, soak some cotton wool in apple cider vinegar and apply to the wart. Cover with a sticking plaster overnight. Repeat each night for 2 weeks.

LEMONS

Both lemon juice and lemon oil are reputed to help cure warts.

+ ACTIONS: Drink the juice of half a lemon twice a day at least. Apply 1 drop of lemon essential oil to your wart and cover with a sticking plaster. Repeat each day for 2 weeks.

OLIVE OIL

Olive oil's flavonoids can help stop wart viruses multiplying.

+ ACTIONS: Take at least 2 tablespoons of extra-virgin olive oil each day to help prevent warts. To treat a wart, apply extra-virgin olive oil then cover with a sticking plaster. Repeat twice daily for 3–6 weeks.

GARLIC

Garlic's antiviral effects are a good enough reason to try it for warts and verrucas. Several studies now provide backing:

- In a study of 28 people, warts vanished within 1–2 weeks in those who applied an oil-soluble garlic extract twice a day.[216]
- In another study, involving five children with warts on their hands, the warts were treated with garlic. Each night, a clove's cut surface was rubbed over each wart and the wart covered overnight with a sticking plaster. All the warts disappeared within 7–12 weeks. The treatment was well tolerated apart from in one child, who had local itching.[217]

+ ACTIONS: First, do a patch test (p.82) to check garlic won't irritate your skin. Smear a little petroleum jelly ("Vaseline") onto the skin around the wart. Apply garlic oil macerate or garlic oil to the wart (p.80). Cover with a large sticking plaster and repeat each day until the wart goes (probably 7–10 days, though it may take several weeks to disappear). Include garlic in your daily diet or take a garlic supplement. Make sure your supplement has both oil- and water-soluble sulphur compounds (pp.78–9).

Wind

Wind in the gastro-intestinal tract is usually perfectly normal and expelled upwards (by burping) and downwards (by flatulence). People with a lot of wind may complain of feeling "bloated" – meaning they have abdominal discomfort and swelling.

SPICES

Digestive and carminative spices should help trouble from excess wind.
+ ACTION: Include these spices in your diet. For example, drink aniseed tea. And chew aniseeds, cardamom pods or fennel seeds after a meal.

TEAS

Digestive teas should help.
+ ACTION: Include these teas in your diet (p.99).

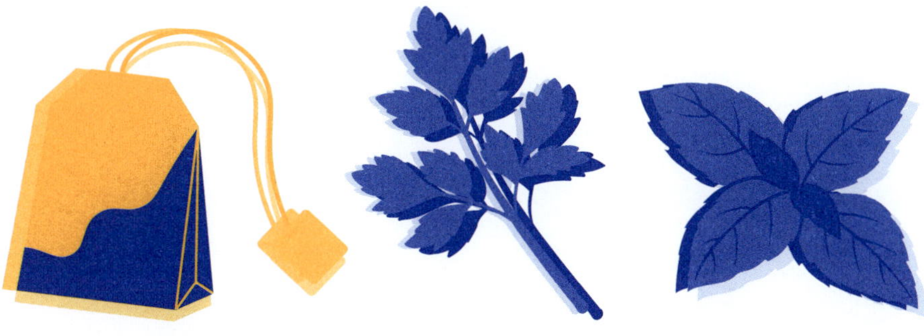

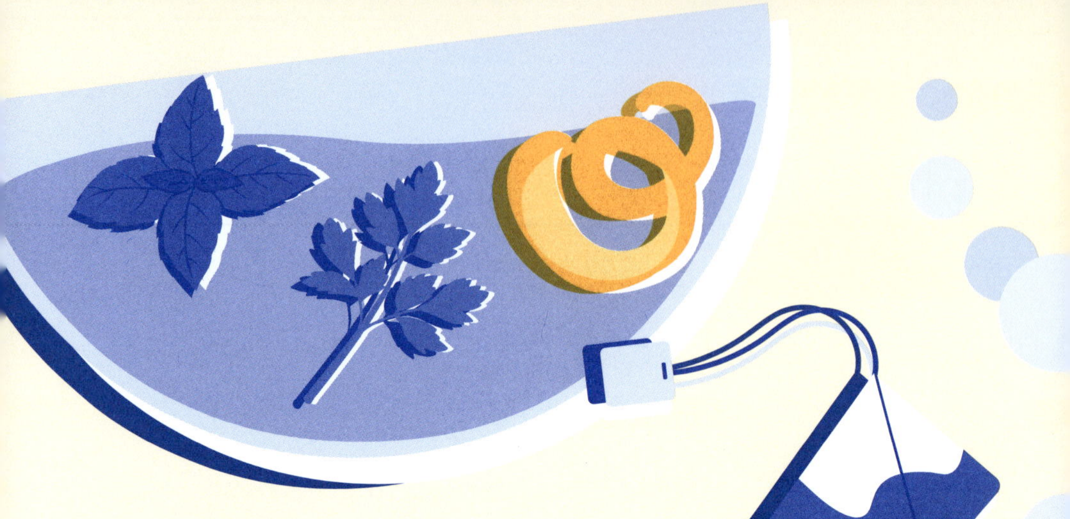

CHAPTER 3
CLEAN BEAUTY

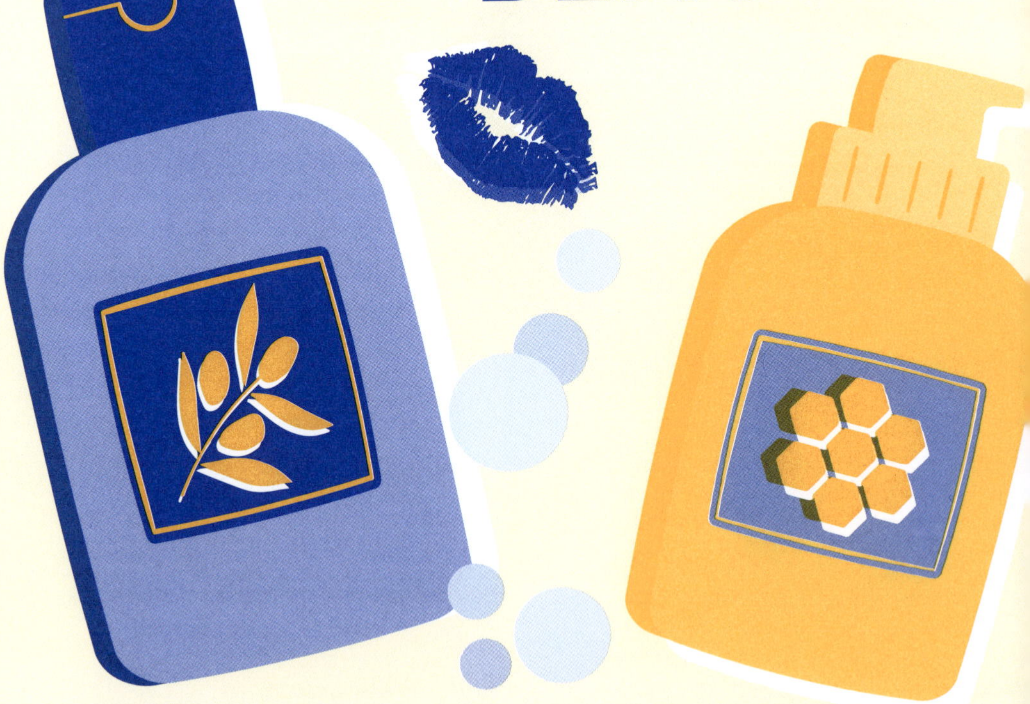

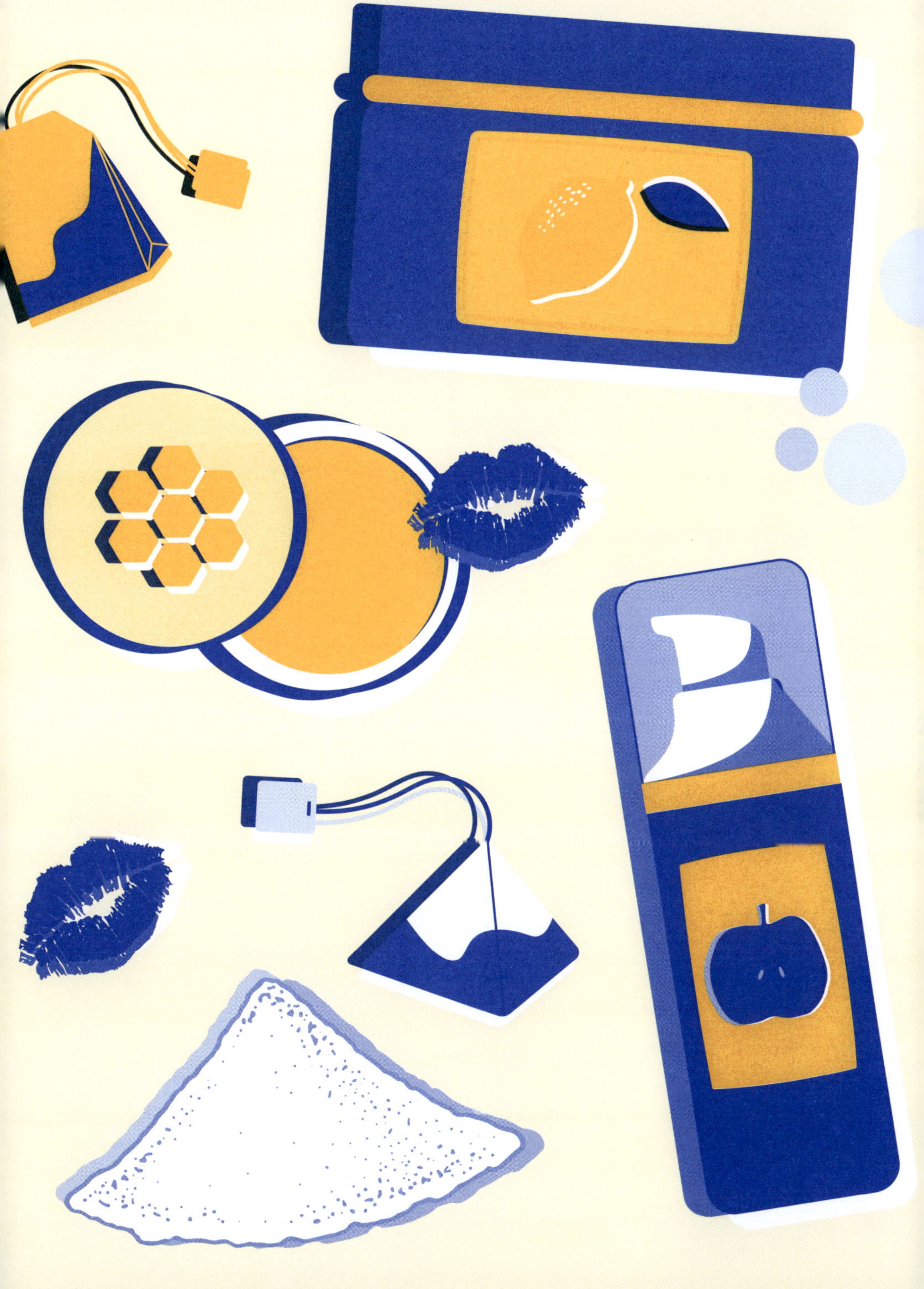

HERO INGREDIENTS FOR CLEAN BEAUTY

We've seen how our "cupboard heroes" have multiple uses for health and wellbeing, but they also have a wealth of benefits for achieving "clean" beauty – a concept that has become increasingly popular in recent times. These humble ingredients can work wonders for the face, body, scalp, hair and nails. In this chapter, you'll find tips for using the eight heroes for personal care and in recipes for toiletries.

The importance of our skin's pH

The skin's slightly acidic and oily surface layer is called the "acid mantle" or hydrolipid film. It is made of water and sebum (an oily liquid made by the skin's sebaceous glands). Its acidity results from:

- Fatty acids in sebum ("skin oil")
- Lactic acid and various amino acids in sweat
- Amino acids and pyrrolidine carboxylic acid from "cornifying" (hardening) skin cells

Acidity is measured in terms of pH – "potential of hydrogen", indicating hydrogen-ion concentration. A score below 7 is acidic, 7 is neutral, above 7 is alkaline. The further below 7, the more acidic; the further above 7, the more alkaline. The optimal pH value of skin is between 4.5 and 5.75. A woman's skin is marginally less acidic than that of a man. The skin in the armpits and around the genitals is less acidic than the skin covering the rest of the body.

NORMAL SKIN ACIDITY

Normal skin acidity helps activate enzymes that enable the production of the lipids (oily fats) found in the skin's hydrolipid film (oily layer). It also encourages skin to repair itself after mechanical or chemical damage. These two factors are important because having intact healthy skin means the skin loses relatively little water (other than in perspiration), and potentially harmful substances and micro-organisms are less able to get in. Normal acidity also encourages a normal skin flora – the populations of "skin-friendly" bacteria and, in smaller amounts, viruses, fungi and even mites – that inhabit healthy skin and help prevent potentially harmful micro-organisms multiplying and causing infections. Any loss of normal skin acidity encourages drying, cracking and itching of the skin.

Knowing your soaps

Most soaps – even those marketed as "mild", "baby" or "beauty" soaps – have an alkaline pH of 7–9, so washing with them destroys the skin's acid mantle. Healthy, unbroken skin can restore its normal acidity but this generally takes between half an hour and two hours or more. What's more, twice-daily washing with alkaline soap slightly reduces the restored acidity level. Certain soaps are even more alkaline, with a pH of 9.5–11, so compromise skin acidity even more. Very few bar soaps have a pH similar to that of normal skin. However, the pH of many liquid soaps, non-soap cleansers and bath and shower gels is closer to that of normal skin.

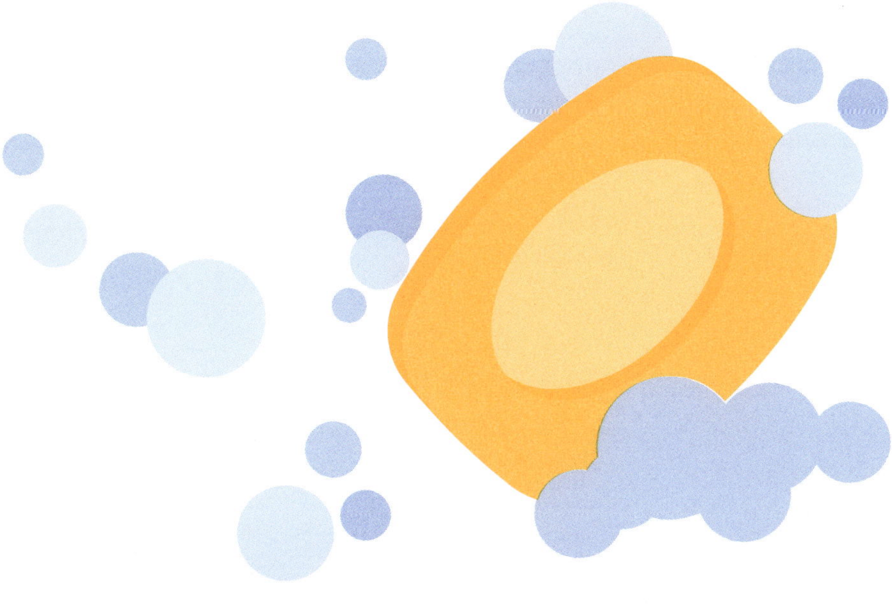

APPLE CIDER VINEGAR

With an acid concentration of about 5 per cent, this can help maintain skin's natural acidity, so it's no wonder that apple cider vinegar is a popular beauty aid. Most other vinegars are more acidic, so are unsuitable for skincare. If you want to continue using alkaline soap, rinse your skin afterwards with a home-made skin splash containing apple cider vinegar to restore normal skin acidity. Or use a home-made skin cleanser containing the vinegar to compensate for the loss of normal acidity that accompanies washing with most types of soap.

Apple cider vinegar can also restore acidity to hair washed with an alkaline shampoo, making it shinier than it would otherwise be and enhancing natural highlights. Most shampoos are alkaline and can leave newly washed hair dull and lacklustre. They also temporarily destroy the scalp's normal acidity, leaving it prone to dryness, irritation and infection.

In addition to these beauty benefits, apple cider vinegar's antibacterial properties give it deodorizing power useful for armpits and feet.

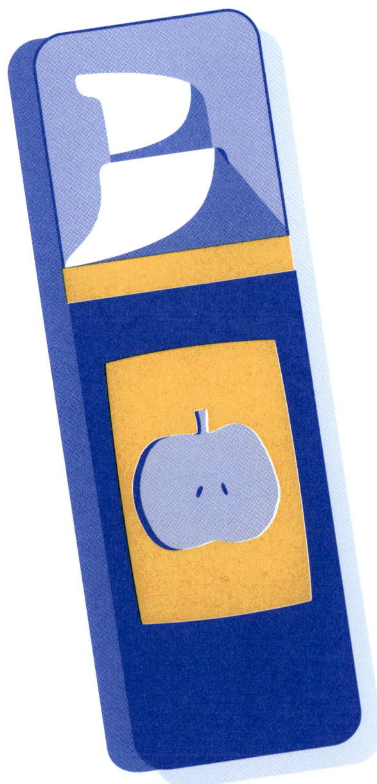

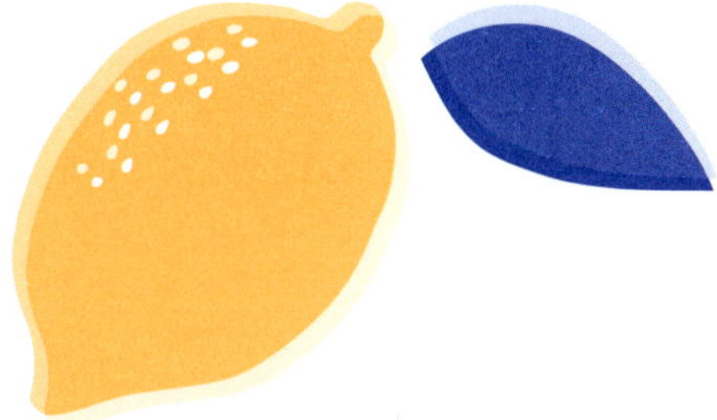

LEMONS

Lemon juice can cleanse, soften and moisturize your skin, condition and lighten your hair and deodorize your body. Its oil is moisturizing and toning; its fresh fragrance can lift the spirits; and it's lovely for a massage when diluted with a carrier oil such as sweet almond, apricot kernel, grapeseed, jojoba, macadamia nut, olive oil, peach kernel, shea butter or wheatgerm. If you like to wash with alkaline soap, rinse your skin afterwards with diluted lemon juice, as its organic acids can help maintain or restore the skin's natural acidity.

Lemon juice is moisturizing as its acidity helps maintain the skin's barrier function, so reducing water loss. Also, its citric acid is an alpha-hydroxy acid (AHA, used in many commercial skincare preparations), so has an intrinsic moisturizing action. It is also an exfoliator, meaning it loosens dead skin cells so they can flake off. All this smooths rough skin, softens hard skin and helps cracked skin heal. The moisturizing, smoothing and softening properties of lemon juice make it an excellent aid for a manicure or pedicure.

Citric acid's softening effect helps explain why applying lemon juice makes blackheads easier to remove with gentle fingertip pressure or a blackhead extractor. What's more, the astringent properties of citric acid can reduce large ("open") pores. And the vitamin C and other antioxidants in lemon juice help prevent lipids in sebum being oxidized and therefore blackened by air to create a blackhead.

Lemons' rutin and certain other flavonoids can strengthen the walls of capillaries, our tiniest blood vessels, making them less likely to become enlarged and therefore visible.

CAUTION: Avoid putting lemon essential oil neat on your skin within 12 hours of exposing it to direct sunlight. If you can't avoid it, use no more than 1 drop per 2 teaspoons of sweet almond or other carrier oil (p.86), so it's unlikely to trigger a photosensitive reaction.

BICARBONATE OF SODA (BAKING SODA)

Also called sodium bicarbonate, this can be a surprisingly good beauty aid and is also useful for other personal care. Adding it to water softens the water, so you need less soap to wash your face and body and less shampoo to wash your hair. This is good because the more soap or shampoo you use, the more you strip valuable natural oils and acidity from your skin and scalp.

Its very mild abrasiveness helps cleanse skin thoroughly. And its tiny particles have gentle exfoliating properties, helping to dislodge dead cells and clear blackheads.

Its presence in certain toothpastes helps remove plaque (the sticky film of food residues and bacteria on teeth) and tartar (or "calculus" – the hard, calcium-impregnated plaque along the gum margins that encourages gum disease). Its alkalinity helps by neutralizing the acidity released as mouth bacteria break down sugars and other refined carbohydrates. This is important, as acidity encourages dental decay.

Its alkalinity has antiseptic and antifungal actions that can help prevent or treat skin and scalp infections. It also has a deodorant action thought to result from neutralization of odoriferous short-chain fatty acids in sweat.

Finally, on a fun note, bicarbonate of soda is a common ingredient in the effervescent balls of bath salts known as "bath bombs" that fizz when thrown into bath water and elevate a bathing experience to a whole new level.

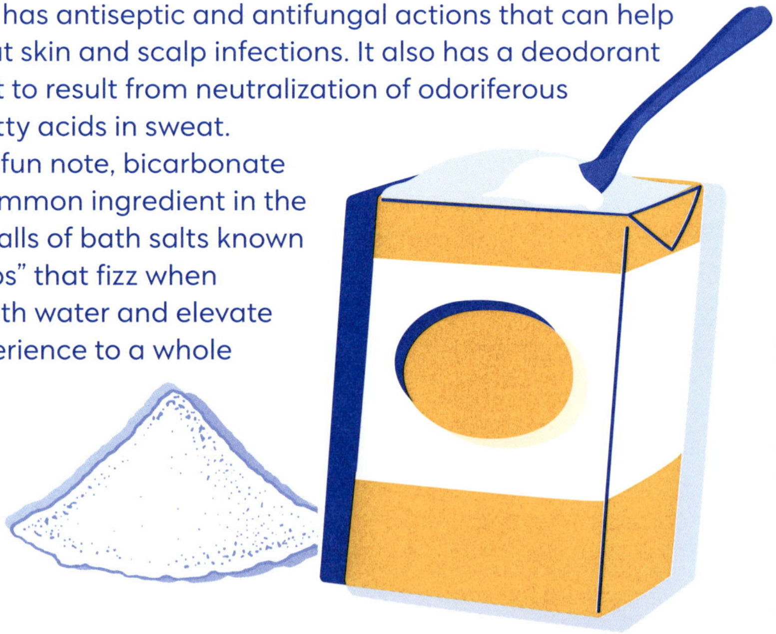

OLIVE OIL

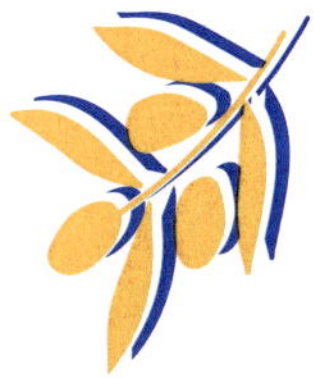

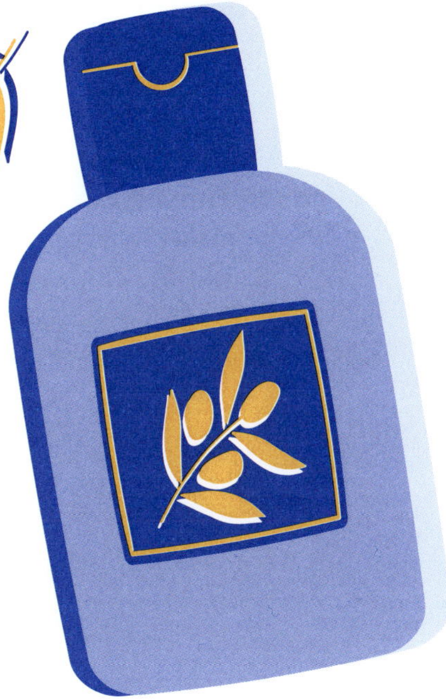

The ancient Greeks and Romans used this to cleanse and moisturize their skin, appreciating the lovely soft sheen it delivered. Over the millennia olive oil has also been used to make a variety of beauty products – including soaps, shower gels, exfoliating scrubs, shampoos, moisturizers, hand creams, moisturizing "dry" oils, nail oils, lip balms, massage oils and after-sun soothing lotions and creams.

Applying it to the skin helps prevent moisture loss and soothes inflammation, while its slight acidity has a mild antimicrobial effect. Most important, applying it to skin does not compromise normal skin acidity, so it is gentle compared with some commercial toiletries, such as most soaps. As oil is insoluble in water, its acidity cannot be measured as pH. Instead, it's calculated in terms of the percentage of free fatty acids it contains. Better-quality oils are less acidic; poorer-quality oils more acidic.

Extra-virgin olive oil is the best choice of olive oil for skin care as it is the richest in skin-friendly substances. These include antioxidants (which help protect sebum from oxidation), anti-inflammatories (for example, monounsaturated fat, and polyphenols) and antimicrobials (such as polyphenols).

Olive oil softens, moisturizes and soothes skin, and helps maintain its elasticity and counter infection. It gives nails sheen and softens and nourishes cuticles. It also conditions hair and makes it shine.

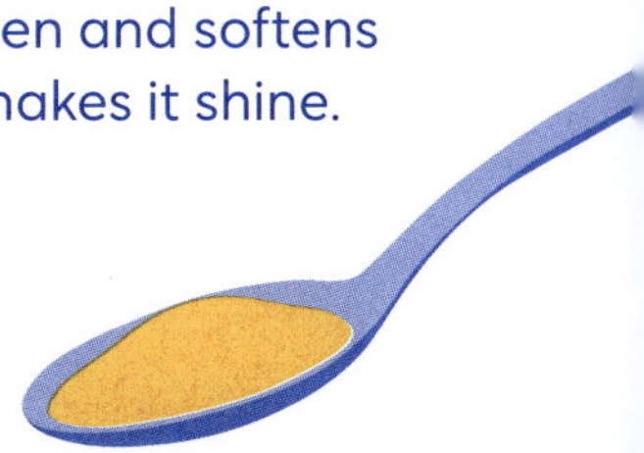

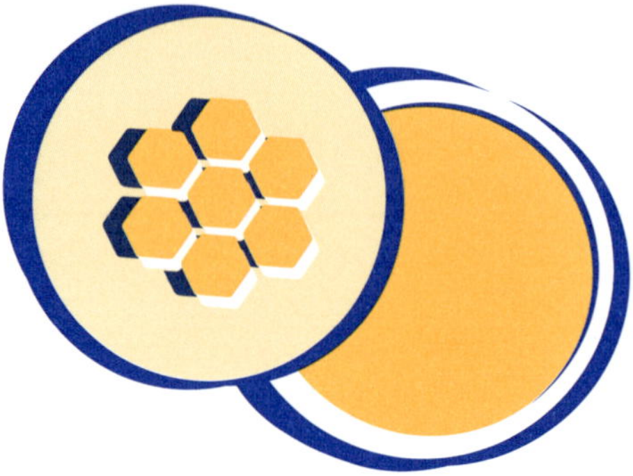

HONEY

This ingredient has many uses beyond the kitchen. It helps cleanse, soften, moisturize, soothe and tone skin and condition hair and nails. Its moisturizing properties make it an excellent aid in a manicure or pedicure and its acidity maintains or restores the skin's natural acidity. Its moisturizing power results partly from it helping to prevent water evaporating from skin; partly from it being a humectant (attracting water from the air); and partly from its acidity. Applying honey to dry skin stimulates skin-oil (sebum) production. Also, honey's humectant effect soothes puffy skin by drawing out water.

Honey's flavonoids improve "broken veins" (over-dilated capillaries). They also help heal cracked or sore skin, have antimicrobial powers and, as antioxidants, reduce damage from polluted air and encourage healthy turnover of skin cells.

Honey is an excellent face-mask ingredient, not only because of its effects on the skin but also because it enables other ingredients, such as oil, ground nuts, egg yolk or clay, to stick to the skin, so keeping the mask in place. Added to this, its fragrance can lift the spirits.

When it comes to hair care, honey has many benefits. A "honey rinse" (a dilute solution of honey in water) can restore acidity to freshly washed hair. This is good because most shampoos are alkaline so temporarily destroy the scalp's normal acidity, leaving it prone to dryness, irritation or even infection. Shampoo residues can also make hair look dull but a honey rinse helps restore the shine. It can also make hair stronger and more elastic as honey attracts and retains moisture within the hair shafts themselves.

When using honey in beauty products, it's often easier to use runny honey. If you use raw honey, you get the added benefit of extra fragrance as it contains the maximum levels of volatile aroma compounds.

SPICES

These aromatic ingredients can add fragrance to beauty and grooming products, wardrobes, drawers and linens, as well as to a hot bath. Toothpaste, for example, may contain cardamom, cinnamon or mastic. And some perfumes, soaps and other toiletries are scented with cinnamon and cloves. "Old Spice", for example, has been a favourite brand of men's shaving creams, deodorants and soaps for many years. In addition, many spice oils have antibacterial and antifungal effects on the skin.

Some particularly small molecules in spice-containing creams and massage oils can enter the skin and very small amounts can pass through the skin into the blood.

Effects of spice oil aromas and of spice oils on skin

SPICE	EFFECTS OF AROMA	EFFECTS WHEN USED ON SKIN
Aniseed	Invigorating, uplifting, calming	Relaxes muscles
Caraway	Calming	Relieves itching, skin regenerating
Cardamom	Calming, uplifting, aids concentration and alertness	Warming
Celery seed	Calming	Relaxes muscles
Cinnamon bark	Invigorating, uplifting, may boost sex drive	Warming, relaxes muscles, anti-inflammatory
Clove bud	Invigorating, uplifting, may boost sex drive	Eases muscle and joint pain, relieves itching
Coriander	Invigorating, uplifting, may boost sex drive	Warming, anti-inflammatory
Cumin	Invigorating, uplifting	Warming
Dill seed	Calming	Promotes wound healing

Fennel seed	Invigorating	Skin-toning
Galangal	Invigorating	Warming
Ginger	Uplifting, may boost sex drive	Warming, anti-inflammatory
Juniper berry	Calming	Astringent, anti-inflammatory
Lemongrass	Invigorating	Deodorant, relaxes muscles
Nutmeg	Calming, uplifting	Warming, anti-inflammatory
Black pepper	Invigorating, uplifting	Warming, skin-toning, relaxes muscles
Vanilla	Calming, uplifting, may boost sex drive	Anti-inflammatory

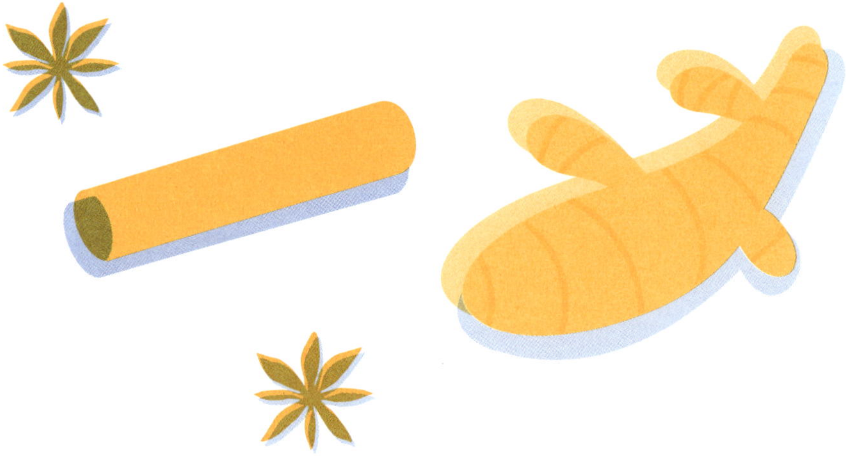

TEAS

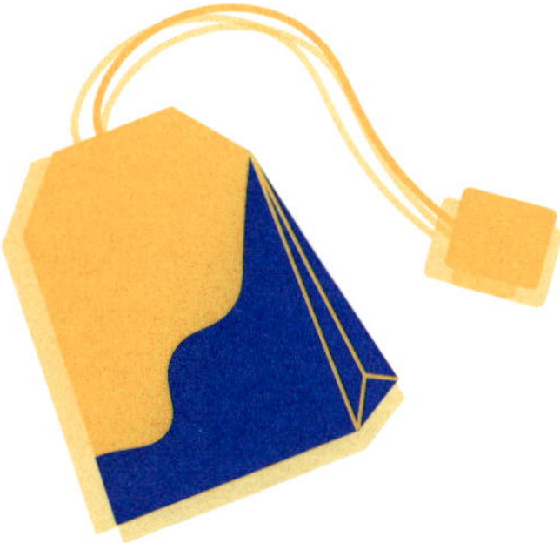

The bioactive constituents of *Camellia-sinensis* tea and certain other herb teas can help nurture and beautify skin and hair. Indeed, many of these bioactives are important ingredients of certain commercially made beauty products.

Skin-friendly constituents of selected teas

Certain teas (see the chart next page) are particularly valued for having these properties:

Anti-inflammatory, collagen-promoting and moisturizing – the antioxidants (such as polyphenols and flavonoids) in all teas soothe skin by helping protect it from free-radical damage; they also promote collagen production and help skin retain moisture. Butterfly pea tea, for example, can improve skin hydration by as much as 70 per cent.
Astringent – their caffeine and tannins reduce oiliness, and help close pores and tighten skin.
Emollient – their allantoin and mucilage hydrate, protect and soothe skin.
Moisturizing and exfoliating – their allantoin and alpha-hydroxy acids (AHAs) can help skin shed dead cells; promote new skin-cell production; hydrate and therefore "plump" skin; moisturize cracked, dry, flaking or hard skin; improve skin texture; tone, smooth and soften skin; reduce fine lines and wrinkles; and reduce visible sun damage.
Improve photo-aged skin – their allantoin promotes new-cell growth; their antioxidants help protect against sun damage and wrinkles; certain alpha-hydroxy acids (AHAs), including citric acid, increase the production of collagen and polysaccharides, making skin thicker and more supple.
Discourage "broken veins' – diosmin, hesperidin, rutin and certain other flavonoids strengthen blood vessel walls, so may shrink the dilated capillaries (tiny blood vessels) sometimes called "broken veins".

	Alpha-hydroxy acids (AHAs)	Antibacterials	Allantoin	Caffeine or tannin	Diosmin, hesperidin or rutin	Mucilage
Calendula		●			●	●
Chamomile		●		●	●	
Chickweed		●			●	●
Cornsilk			●	●		
Dandelion		●		●		●
Elderflower		●		●	●	●
Hibiscus	●	●				
Lavender	●		●			
Linden			●	●	●	
Nettle	●		●	●	●	
Passionflower				●		
Peppermint	●		●	●		
Rooibos		●				
Rosehip	●	●		●	●	
Rosemary	●		●	●		
***Camellia-sinensis* tea**	●	●		●	●	
Thyme	●		●			
Verbena					●	●

CLEAN BEAUTY PREPARATIONS USING CUPBOARD HEROES

It's amazing how many beauty preparations you can create at home at a fraction of the price you'd pay in a pharmacy or other store, or online. Here is a list of ways of making preparations for face, hair, teeth and body care. Our cupboard heroes each have a turn to be the star of a recipe – starting with apple cider vinegar and ending with teas.

Facial skincare and problem-solving

APPLE CIDER VINEGAR SKIN TONER

If you use cleansing cream or lotion, follow with a skin toner made by adding 4 tablespoons of apple cider vinegar to 285ml (½ pint) of cold water. Keep this in a capped glass or plastic bottle, and apply daily with a soft cotton cloth or cotton wool. For a scented toner, put the above toner in a saucepan and add ½ tablespoon of dried rosemary leaves or lavender flowers, or 1 tablespoon of fresh leaves or flowers. Simmer for 5 minutes, then cool and bottle.

LEMON CLEANSER

Steam-clean your face by putting 900ml (30fl oz/3¾ cups) of just-boiled water in a bowl and adding the peel of ½ a lemon, 1 teaspoon of dried (or 2 of chopped fresh) mint, 1 teaspoon of dried (or 2 teaspoons of chopped fresh) parsley and, for dry skin, the contents of a capsule of evening primrose oil. Sit for 5 minutes with your face over the bowl, plus a towel over your head and the bowl to trap the scented steam. Then rinse your face with lukewarm water.

LEMON TONER

Mix the juice of a lemon with twice its volume of water, then refrigerate in a covered container. After cleansing your face, apply some of this with cotton wool and let dry.

LEMON MOISTURIZER

Smooth lemon juice over your skin, wait for half an hour, then rinse off. To soften hard skin on your elbows, sit with each elbow in a squeezed-out half-lemon shell for half an hour.

LEMON JUICE BLACKHEAD CLEARER

Smooth lemon juice over the affected skin and let it dry. Repeat each day as necessary.

LEMON SALT EXFOLIATOR

Rub damp skin with lemon-scented salt. To make this, put 225g (8oz/1 cup) of sea salt crystals into a bowl and stir in ½ a teaspoon of lemon essential oil. Keep the mixture in a screw-top jar.

LEMON MASK FOR SMOOTHING FINE LINES AND WRINKLES

Mix in a bowl 1 well-beaten egg white, 1 teaspoon of egg yolk, 1 tablespoon of lemon juice and a drop of vitamin E oil from a capsule. Apply to your face, then lie down for half an hour. Wash and dry your skin then apply some moisturizer.

BICARBONATE OF SODA BLACKHEAD CLEARER

Once or twice a day, cleanse and dry your face. In a small bowl, mix 1 tablespoon of bicarbonate of soda with about 1 teaspoon of water to make a paste. Rub this over your skin to help loosen and remove blackheads, leave for 10–20 minutes, then rinse. Now help restore your skin's natural acidity by patting on a little apple cider vinegar.

BICARBONATE OF SODA EXFOLIATOR

Mix 3 parts of bicarbonate of soda with 1 part of water. Gently rub this paste into cleansed skin, then rinse off.

To smooth roughened lips, rub them with a paste made by mixing bicarbonate of soda with lemon juice. Rinse, then apply some lip balm.

OLIVE OIL MOISTURIZER

Apply olive oil to your skin to help prevent moisture loss and to soften it and give it a sheen. For a soothing, softening moisturizing cream, put 1 tablespoon of beeswax pellets (available from health food

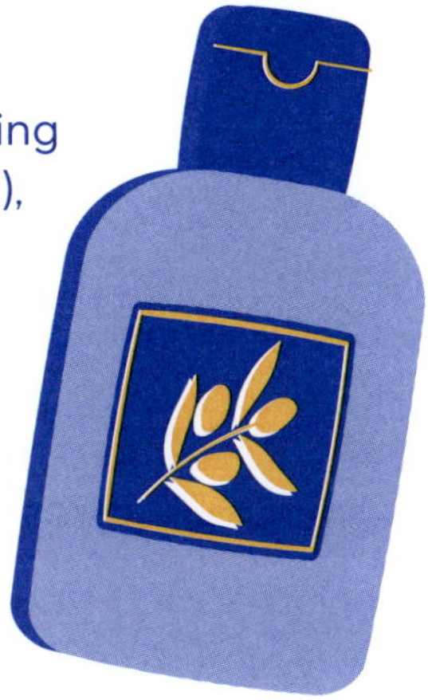

stores, or online) in a basin and melt them by standing the basin in the top of a double boiler ("bain-marie"), or in a pan containing enough boiling water to come no more than halfway up the basin. Beat in 3 tablespoons of olive oil. Remove from the heat and beat in 1 teaspoon of apple cider vinegar and 2 teaspoons of water. Stir the resulting cream until lukewarm, then stir in 3 drops of an essential oil with skin-regenerating properties, choosing from chamomile, frankincense, lavender, neroli, rose, sandalwood or ylang-ylang. Apply to your skin.

For a soothing, moisturizing skin milk, mix in a bowl 2 tablespoons of olive oil, 2 teaspoons of clear honey, 1 teaspoon of apple cider vinegar and 1 tablespoon of full-fat plain bio yoghurt. Apply with a ball or pad of cotton wool.

To soften dry skin on your elbows or feet, gently massage in a small amount of olive oil.

OLIVE OIL EYE MAKEUP REMOVER

To remove eye makeup, pour a little olive oil on a ball or pad of cotton wool and smooth this over your eyelids.

OLIVE OIL FACE MASK

Make a moisturizing, soothing and rejuvenating mask by mixing In a small bowl 1 tablespoon of olive oil, 1 tablespoon of clear honey, 1 tablespoon of plain full-fat bio-yoghurt and 1 egg yolk. Apply this mask to your face, then relax for 30 minutes before rinsing it off with warm water.

HONEY CLEANSER

To make a honey-water cleanser, dissolve 1 teaspoon of runny honey in 4 tablespoons of warm water. To make a honey-milk cleanser, dissolve 1 teaspoon of runny honey in 4 tablespoons of warm milk. Gently smooth either of these over your face to loosen grime and dead skin. Rinse with warm or cool water.

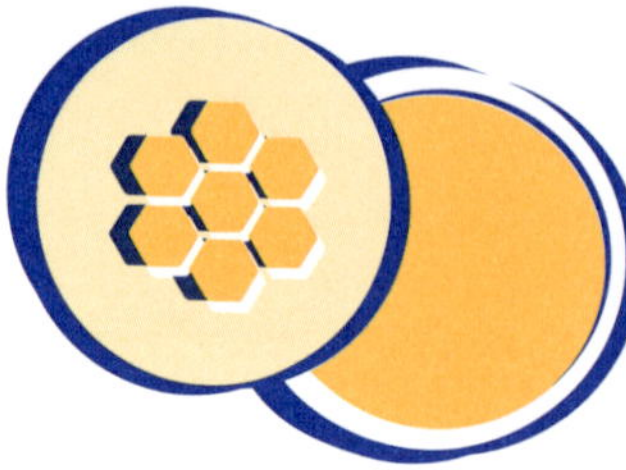

HONEY TONER

Use 2 teaspoons of runny or thick honey. Or peel and purée 5cm (2in) of cucumber, then mix with 1 teaspoon of runny honey. Apply either of these to your face, leave for 5 minutes, then rinse off with cold water.

HONEY MOISTURIZER

According to your skin type, mix 1 teaspoon of runny honey with:

- **For normal skin:** 1 teaspoon of milk
- **For dry skin:** 1 teaspoon of full-fat plain bio yoghurt and 1 teaspoon of sweet almond oil
- **For oily skin:** 1 teaspoon of olive oil and 1 teaspoon of lemon juice
- **For ageing skin:** 1 teaspoon of full-fat plain bio yoghurt, 1 teaspoon of sweet almond oil, the contents of a vitamin E capsule and 1 drop of frankincense essential oil

Add fragrance to any of the first three recipes by stirring in 5–6 drops of neroli, rose or ylang-ylang essential oil. The fourth recipe has fragrance from its frankincense oil. Smooth the chosen mixture into your skin. For convenience, you could make several batches at once: put the mixture into a sterilized jar with a tightly fitting lid and keep it in the fridge for up to 2 weeks.

HONEY EXFOLIATING SCRUB

According to your skin type, mix 1 tablespoon of runny honey with:

- **For normal or oily skin:** 2 tablespoons of ground almonds and 1 teaspoon of lemon juice
- **For dry skin**: 2 tablespoons of coarse sea salt and 1 tablespoon of olive oil

Rub your choice of mixture on to your skin, then rinse with warm water.

THREE HONEY FACE MASKS

According to your skin type, mix 2 tablespoons of honey with:

- **For normal skin:** 1 tablespoon of olive oil, an egg yolk and a handful of fine oatmeal
- **For dry skin:** 1 tablespoon of olive oil, 2 egg yolks and a mashed banana
- **For oily skin:** 2 whisked egg whites, 1 tablespoon of lemon juice and a handful of fine oatmeal

Apply to your face then relax for 30 minutes before rinsing with warm water.

INTENSE HONEY FACE MASK

Mix in a bowl 2 tablespoons of bran, 1 teaspoon of runny honey and 3 tablespoons of a tea appropriate to your skin type (see “Cleansing, toning and moisturizing with teas”, p.302). Apply the mask to your face, leave on for 10 minutes, then rinse with warm water.

MOISTURIZER WITH SPICES

Moisturizing spice oils include allspice, caraway, cardamom, celery seed, coriander, dill seed and nigella oils. Caraway aids skin regeneration; celery seed is anti-inflammatory; nigella reduces wrinkles and eases joint and muscle pain. Buy a small pot of unperfumed skin cream and stir in a few drops of your chosen spice oil, or make it yourself, following these instructions.

Put 1 tablespoon of your chosen spice oil and 6 tablespoons of a “carrier oil” (p.86) into the upper part of a double boiler (“bain-marie”) or into an electric yogurt maker. Mix well. Heat until the mixture darkens. Beat in 1 teaspoon of apple cider vinegar and 2 teaspoons of water. Thicken the cream by adding 1 tablespoon of beeswax pellets and stirring until they melt. Transfer to a small container with a lid. Cool, cover and store in the refrigerator for up to 4 weeks.

LIQUORICE FOR FRECKLES AND BROWN PATCHES

Liquorice can sometimes lighten freckles or other brown patches because its best-known flavonoid, glabridin, helps prevent the enzyme tyrosinase in skin cells called melanocytes from making the pigment

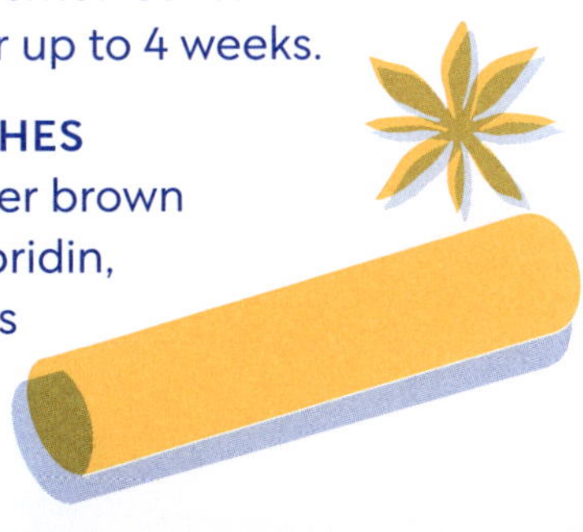

melanin. Put a few drops of liquorice extract on to some cotton wool and smooth it over your face. Do this twice a day.

SOOTHING SPICE FACE MASK
Fenugreek's gum softens and moisturizes skin. And mango's lupeol soothes inflamed skin (by replenishing antioxidants) and aids skin regeneration (by increasing skin cell production). Mix in a bowl 1 tablespoon each of olive oil, runny honey, plain full-fat bio-yoghurt and powdered fenugreek or mango. Apply the mixture to your face then relax for 30 minutes before rinsing with warm water.

JUNIPER FACIAL SAUNA FOR GREASY SKIN
Juniper's tannins help close pores and make skin less greasy. Make 300ml (½ pint/1½ cups) of juniper berry tea in a bowl. Lean over the bowl with a towel loosely draped over both your head and the bowl, and let the fragrant steam bathe your face for 5 minutes.

CLEANSING, TONING AND MOISTURIZING WITH TEAS
Use your chosen tea warm or cool. Apply it as a "splash" while leaning over a washing basin or dab it on with a cotton pad. Then let your skin dry naturally. For example, if you have:

- **Oily skin:** cleanse and tone with a tea containing an astringent – such as chamomile, cornsilk, lavender, mint, rosemary or thyme.
- **Dry skin:** cleanse and moisturize with a mucilage-containing tea free from astringents and AHAs – such as calendula, chickweed, passionflower or rooibos.
- **Mature skin:** cleanse and moisturize with a tea containing mucilage and/or blood vessel strengtheners but free from astringents and AHAs – such as calendula, chickweed or passionflower. If your skin isn't dry, cornsilk is a good choice as it contains allantoin.

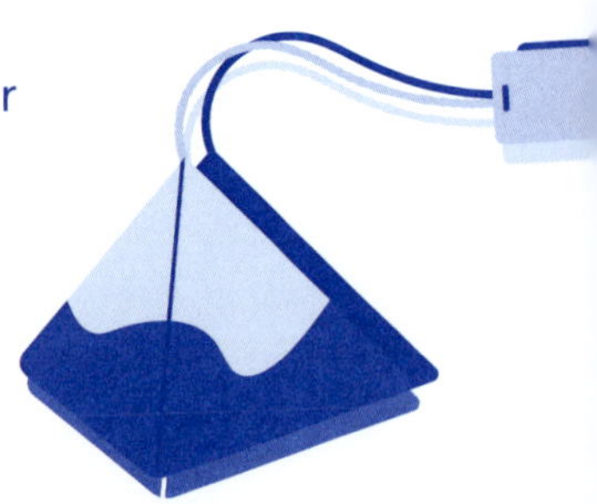

TEA BAGS FOR FINE LINES AROUND THE EYES
Used teabags containing one of the teas for mature skin (see "Cleansing, toning and

moisturizing with teas", above) can help smooth "laughter lines". Lie down, rest the teabag over your closed eyes for 10 to 15 minutes and relax.

Dental care and lips

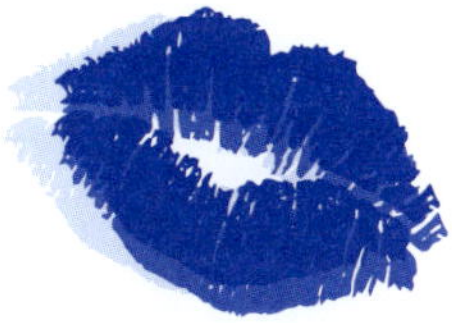

DENTAL CARE WITH BICARBONATE OF SODA

Coat toothbrush bristles with bicarbonate of soda then brush your teeth without water. (This "dry-brushing" is more effective at removing plaque than "wet-brushing".) Bicarbonate of soda cleans and brightens teeth. It also counteracts the acidity that induces tooth decay produced by mouth bacteria from traces of sugars and other refined carbohydrates.

To make a fresher-tasting paste, mix equal amounts of bicarbonate of soda and fine sea salt. Salt boosts the flow of saliva (which has antibacterial properties, so helping prevent tooth decay) and its sodium helps to counteract acidity.

Make a whitening toothpaste by mixing bicarbonate of soda with 3 per cent hydrogen peroxide solution. Rinse your mouth thoroughly with water afterwards. Use it once a week. Hydrogen peroxide is available from certain pharmacies.

Make a cleansing, refreshing mouthwash by mixing ½ a teaspoon of bicarbonate of soda into ¼ a glass of warm water. Take a mouthful and swish it around your mouth.

HONEY LIP BALM

Put 2 tablespoons of beeswax into a basin and stand it in a pan of boiling water until the beeswax melts. Remove from the heat, let it cool, then stir in 4 tablespoons of olive oil, 3 drops of an essential oil (such as lavender or chamomile) and 2 teaspoons of honey. Store in a small, sterilized jar with a tightly fitting lid for up to 2 weeks. Apply as necessary.

You can also smooth olive oil directly on to dry or sore lips to soothe and soften them or help them to heal.

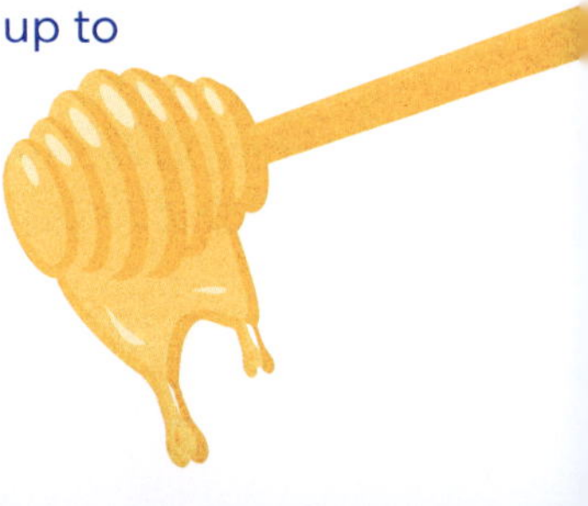

Body cleansing and care

APPLE CIDER VINEGAR AND OATMEAL CLEANSING RUB

Make a cleansing rub by moistening ½ a cup of oatmeal with apple cider vinegar. If you want to cleanse your whole body, use 1 cup of oatmeal. Add 1 cup of apple cider vinegar to the bathwater and use a washcloth to cleanse your skin.

APPLE CIDER VINEGAR RINSE

Wash in a shower or unplugged bathtub, rinsing your whole body with water. Then fill the bathtub with water, add ½ a cup of apple cider vinegar, lie down and relax.

Alternatively, wash in the bathtub or shower, then fill a large plastic jug with warm water and ½ a cup of apple cider vinegar. Use this to rinse yourself.

APPLE CIDER VINEGAR DEODORANT

Wash your armpits, then apply either neat vinegar, or vinegar in which you have steeped some rosemary or mint leaves, or lavender flowers, for 2 weeks.

To combat foot odour, soak your feet for 5 to 10 minutes in a basin of water containing ½ a cup of apple cider vinegar.

LEMON JUICE DEODORANT

Lemon juice has antibacterial properties, so can act as a deodorant. Rub a lemon's cut surface over each armpit or add the juice of a lemon to your bathwater.

LEMON MASSAGE OIL

Make a soothing massage oil by mixing a few drops of lemon oil into a carrier oil (p.86). For extra fragrance add a few drops of geranium, lavender, neroli, rose, sandalwood or ylang-ylang oil.

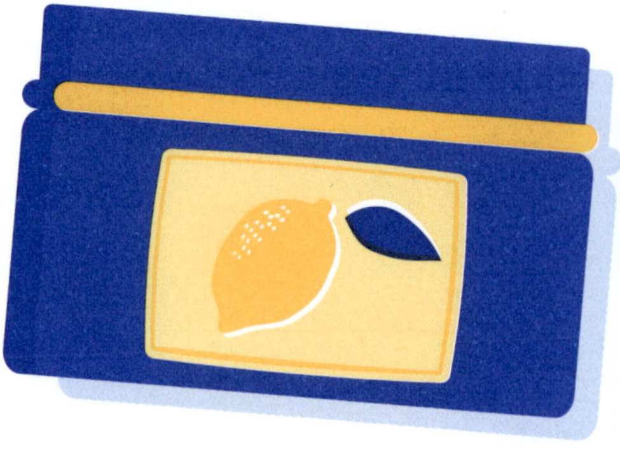

DEODORIZING WITH BICARBONATE OF SODA

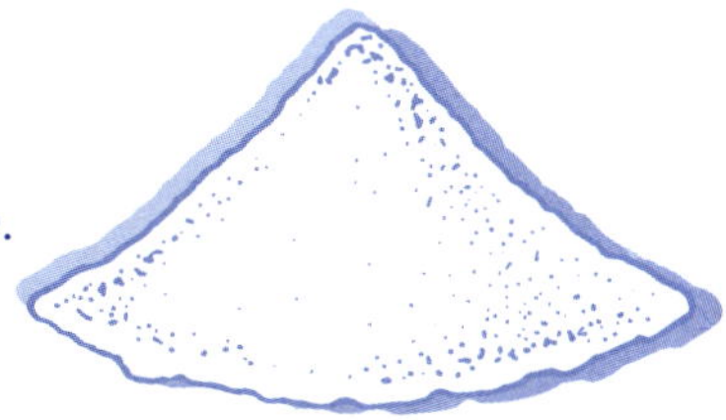

- Adding ½ a cup of bicarbonate of soda to your bathwater will help keep you odour-free.
- You can also make a deodorant paste as follows: in a small bowl, mix ½ a teaspoon of bicarbonate of soda, 1 or 2 drops of water and, if required, 1 drop of a fragrant essential oil such as lavender. Smooth a little of this deodorant paste under your arms.
- Try using bicarbonate of soda as a dry deodorant: sprinkle bicarbonate of soda between the toes, or into tights or socks, as an alternative to talcum powder to help keep feet fresh and dry.
- To reduce odour, shake a little bicarbonate of soda on a new sanitary pad before use.

BATHING WITH BICARBONATE OF SODA

To soften bathwater for a spa-style bath: add ½ a cup of bicarbonate of soda and ½ a cup of sea salt to the water. Adding a few drops of fragrant oil will make bath time particularly sybaritic: cedarwood, frankincense and lavender essential oils are relaxing; geranium, jasmine, neroli and ylang-ylang uplifting; cardamom stimulating and refreshing.

To make "bath bombs" (colourful, fragrant shapes, made of bath salts, that fizz in bathwater), mix in a bowl 2 cups of bicarbonate of soda, and 1 cup of citric acid – from a pharmacy or online. Add 10 drops of your choice of fragrant essential oil, plus, if desired, a few drops of food colouring. Now add about 1 teaspoon of almond oil or baby oil, a few drops at a time, until the mixture is crumbly but clumps together when firmly squeezed. Firmly press into moulds such as plastic egg boxes, silicone or other non-stick fairy-cake moulds, little yogurt pots, or special moulds from craft stores. Leave to dry for a week. Then, when you bathe, put a bath bomb in the water and watch it fizz as its citric acid and bicarbonate of soda react with the water to release bubbles of carbon dioxide.

OLIVE OIL EXFOLIATOR

Mix 1 tablespoon of caster sugar with enough olive oil to make a firm paste. Rub this on to your skin until the sugar dissolves, then rinse off with warm water.

OLIVE OIL BATH OIL

For a fragrant bath oil, add 2 tablespoons of olive oil and 6 drops of essential oil (such as geranium, neroli or lavender) to the tap water as it runs into your bath. Take care in the bath, as the oil will make it slippery.

OLIVE OIL MASSAGE OIL

Mix in a small bowl or bottle 2 tablespoons of olive oil and 10 drops of one or more fragrant essential oils. Cedarwood, frankincense and lavender oils are said to be relaxing; geranium, jasmine, neroli and ylang-ylang uplifting; cardamom stimulating.

HONEY BATH MILK

Use 4 tablespoons of runny honey, or mix 2 tablespoons of runny honey with 285ml (½ a pint) of full-cream milk or buttermilk (or 3 tablespoons of full-cream milk powder). Stir your chosen mixture into a bath of water. For extra fragrance, stir 5–6 drops of neroli, rose or ylang-ylang essential oil into the mixture.

MASSAGE OIL WITH SPICES

Mix 2 teaspoons of a carrier oil (p.86) with 3–5 drops of a spice oil (such as coriander, juniper berry or vanilla).

SPICED PERFUME

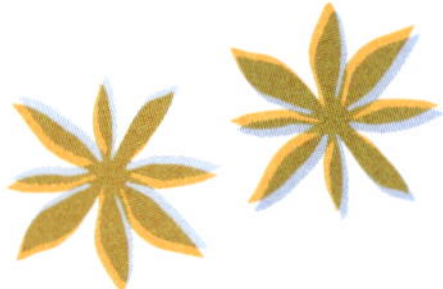

Put 2 drops of a massage oil containing your chosen spice on your wrists, temples and throat.

SPICES FOR THE BATHTUB

Add up to 15 drops of your selected spice oil to warm bathwater for a delightful aroma.

TEA DEODORANT

After washing and drying your armpits, smooth on some chamomile, ginger, lemongrass or linden tea and let your skin dry naturally. These teas contains farnesol, an aromatic antioxidant which has antibacterial activity and is included in some commercially produced deodorants.

TEA FOR A RELAXING OR INVIGORATING BATH

Depending on your mood, add to a bath of comfortably hot water a teabag (or 570ml (1 pint) of made tea) containing either relaxing herbs (such as calendula, chamomile, chickweed, cornsilk, elderflower, lavender, linden, passionflower, rooibos or verbena) or invigorating ones (such as lemongrass, mint, rosemary, rosehip, tea or thyme). Then soak in the water and enjoy its relaxing or invigorating scent. Ideally, choose a tea appropriate for your skin type (p.302).

Hair care

HAIR RINSE WITH APPLE CIDER VINEGAR

Mix in a jug or bowl 570ml (1 pint) of warm water and 2 tablespoons of apple cider vinegar, then use this to rinse your hair after shampooing.

LEMON JUICE FOR DIFFERENT TYPES OF HAIR

After shampooing, rinse your hair with water containing a squeeze of lemon juice for its beneficial citric and other acids; also note these specific benefits:

- **For greasy hair:** it reduces the alkalinity of traces of shampoo. It also dissolves soap residues from the shampoo. All this helps give hair an attractive shine and texture.
- **For dry hair:** it “binds” traces of heavy metals and shampoo that would further dry hair.
- **For bleached or coloured hair:** it precipitates proteins, helping to counteract damage by the bleach or colouring agent.
- **For a sun-kissed effect**: to achieve natural-looking, subtle highlights, rinse clean, wet hair with ¾ cup of water mixed with 4 tablespoons of lemon juice. Sit in the sun until your hair is dry. (And remember to apply sunscreen to your face and other sun-exposed skin.)

HAIRCARE WITH BICARBONATE OF SODA

Remove a build-up of products, such as hairsprays and hair gels, by squeezing into a bowl your usual amount of shampoo plus 1–2 teaspoons of bicarbonate of soda, then mixing well. Use this to wash your hair, then rinse well. Follow this by conditioning your hair.

Dry-clean greasy hair by sprinkling it with bicarbonate of soda, rubbing it through with your hands, then brushing thoroughly.

OLIVE OIL HAIR TREATMENT

Put 3 tablespoons of olive oil into a small bowl, then pour the oil over your hair and gently rub it in. Put a shower cap or plastic carrier bag over your hair and cover with a towel wrapped turban-style. Relax for 30 minutes, then shampoo your hair.

OLIVE OIL, LEMON AND CIDER VINEGAR SHAMPOO

Put 2 tablespoons of olive oil, 1 egg, 1 tablespoon of lemon juice, and ½ a teaspoon of cider vinegar into a bowl, blend with a fork or small whisk and use as normal shampoo.

HAIR CARE WITH HERBAL TEAS

Use herb teas to:

- **Darken greying hair** – 12 hours before you need it, steep either 2 rosemary teabags, or 2 tablespoons of dried rosemary or 6 of fresh rosemary, in 1 cup of boiling water. Let it stand for 12 hours, then strain it. After shampooing, pour it through your hair. Don't rinse it out with water, but simply dry your hair with an old towel. This has only a very slightly darkening effect, but repeating it may produce some further darkening.

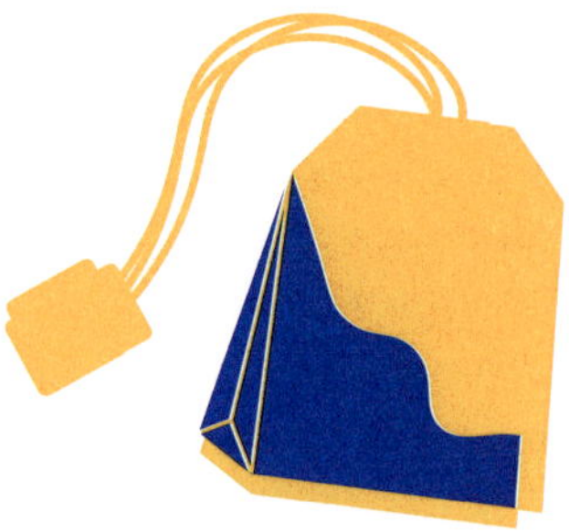

- **Enhance hair growth** – after shampooing, apply linden tea and wait for 5 minutes before rinsing.
- **Give shine to natural highlights in blonde hair** – after shampooing, apply

calendula or chamomile tea and wait for 5 minutes before rinsing.

- **Reduce hair loss** – for general loss, calendula, nettle, rosemary and thyme teas may help. For male-pattern loss (from oversensitivity to the hormone dihydrotestosterone in men and women), chickweed, corn, dandelion, dong quai, elderflower and red clover teas (thanks to their sterols), and tea (thanks to its caffeine and epigallocatechin gallate), may help. After shampooing, apply one of them and wait 5 minutes before rinsing.
- **Help dry hair shine** – after shampooing, rinse with warm tea, then dry your hair with an old towel.
- **Scent hair** – after shampooing, rinse with rosemary tea.

HONEY HAIR CONDITIONER/RINSE/COLOUR-ENHANCER

Stir 2–3 teaspoons of runny honey into 4 cups of warm water until the honey dissolves. Apply to your hair after shampooing. There is no need to rinse it off with water, and the honey won't leave your hair feeling sticky. To enhance your hair colour at the same time, add to the above mixture:

- *If blonde*, add 1 teaspoon of lemon juice.
- *If brunette*, add 1 teaspoon of apple cider vinegar.

INTENSIVE PRE-WASH HONEY HAIR CONDITIONER

Mix 2 tablespoons of honey with 1 tablespoon of olive oil. Consider adding 1 tablespoon of buttermilk for its moisturizing power and because its lactic acid could increase hair strength and elasticity. Wet your hair and massage in the conditioner. Relax for 20 minutes, then wash your hair with a mild shampoo.

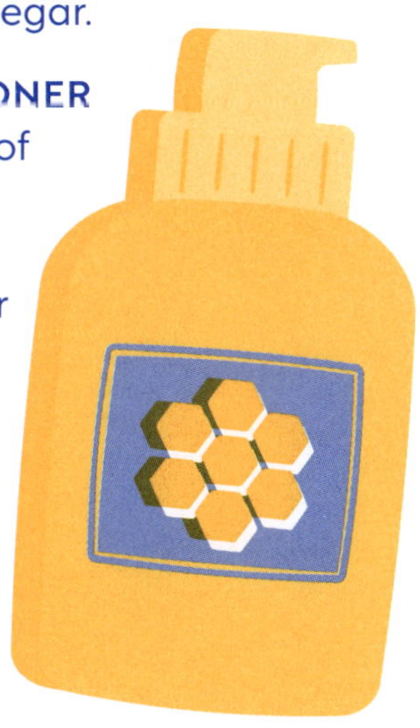

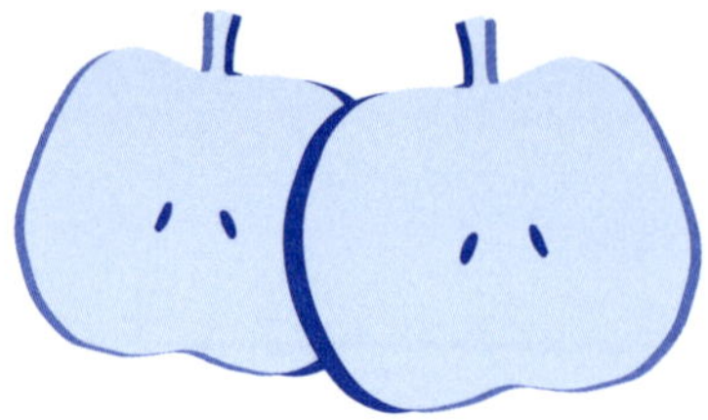

Nail, hand and foot care

SKIN CLEANSING

Make a cleansing rub for soiled hands by moistening half a cup of oatmeal with apple cider vinegar and rubbing the mixture all over your hands. Rinse, and enjoy the smoothing effects as well as the cleanliness!

MANICURE OR PEDICURE

Soften cuticles and whiten stained hands and nails by soaking them for 10 minutes in a bowl of warm water containing the juice of half a lemon. Gently push back your cuticles, then rub a strip of lemon peel on your nails to make them shine.

NAIL AND CUTICLE OIL

Mix 1 teaspoon of olive oil and 1 drop of frankincense, lemon or neroli essential oil in an eggcup. Stir the fragrant oil, then gently rub it on to your fingernails and toenails.

Smooth cuticles by wetting them, rubbing in a little bicarbonate of soda, then rinsing, drying and applying moisturizer.

FOOT CARE

Soothe aching feet by adding 4 tablespoons of bicarbonate of soda to a washing-up bowl of warm water. Put this on the floor, sit on a chair and soak your feet for 10 to 15 minutes. Add several drops of essential oil for fragrance (p.306).

HAND CARE WHEN WASHING UP

If you dislike wearing rubber gloves, help to keep your hands soft by adding 1 tablespoon of bicarbonate of soda to the washing-up water.

SOFTENING DRY, ROUGH OR HARD SKIN

Make a skin-softening paste by stirring olive oil into 1 or 2 tablespoons of bicarbonate of soda. If you like fragrance, add a few drops of lavender, neroli or rose essential oil. Smooth the paste over your hands, elbows, the soles of your feet or other areas of dry, rough or hard skin. Wait for 30 minutes, then rinse off the paste with warm water and smooth in some moisturizing cream.

HAND CREAM MADE WITH SEVERAL "HEROES'

Put 1 tablespoon of beeswax pellets into the upper part of a double boiler and half-fill the bottom pan with water. Bring the water to the boil and simmer until the beeswax melts. Beat in 3 tablespoons of olive oil. Remove the bowl and stir in 1 tablespoon of honey, 1 tablespoon of rose water and 1 teaspoon of cider vinegar. Cool, stirring, until lukewarm, then stir in 3 drops of essential oil, choosing from chamomile, frankincense, lavender, neroli, rose, sandalwood or ylang-ylang, which add fragrance and encourage skin regeneration. Cool and store in a sterilized jar with a tightly fitting lid for up to 2 weeks. Smooth into your hands after washing and drying them.

HONEY NAIL CONDITIONER

Mix 2 teaspoons of thick honey with 2 teaspoons of olive oil and 1 drop of frankincense, lemon or neroli essential oil. Massage this mixture into your cuticles, leave for 20 minutes, then rinse.

Natural shaving products

SHAVING WITH BICARBONATE OF SODA

Mix bicarbonate of soda with water to form a loose paste and apply this to your skin before shaving as an alternative to soap lather or shaving cream or gel. This is less drying to the skin than most soaps as it doesn't reduce the skin's natural oils and acidity.

Soothe or help prevent a shaving rash by smoothing on a paste made from bicarbonate of soda and water, as above.

OLIVE OIL SHAVING CREAM

Mix 1 tablespoon each of olive oil and liquid soap, then apply to your skin. This makes skin slippery and ready for the razor; the oil also has antibacterial and soothing qualities.

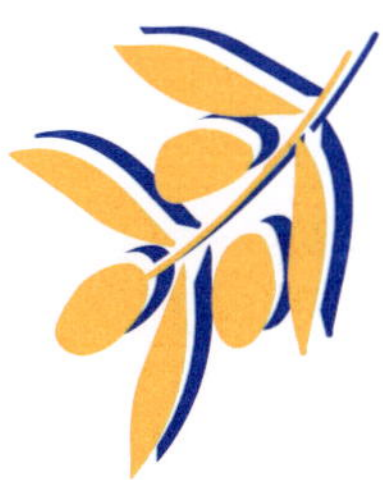

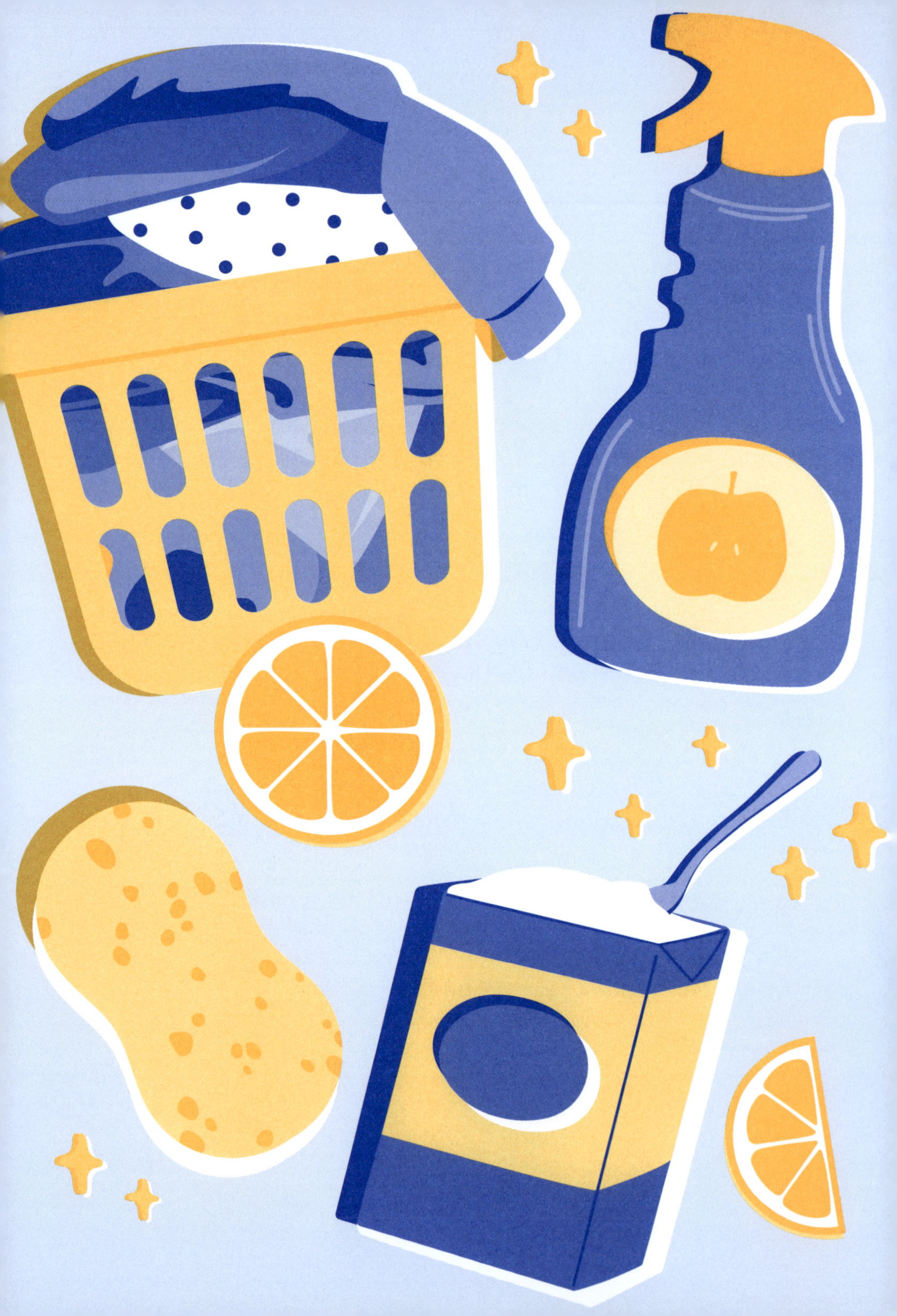

CHAPTER 4
GREEN CLEANING

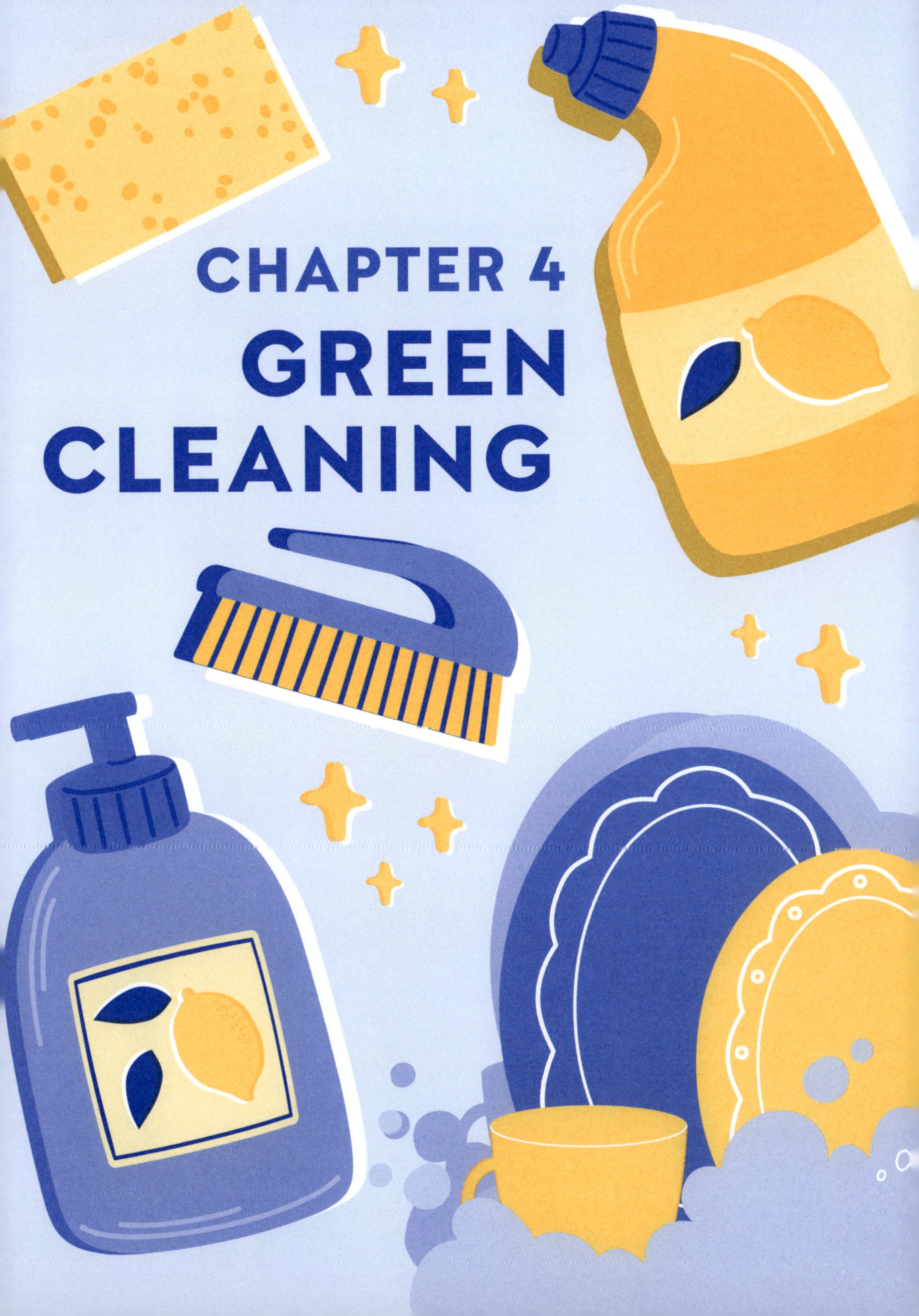

GREEN CLEANING PREPARATIONS USING OUR "CUPBOARD HEROES"

You can use six of our "cupboard heroes" – apple cider vinegar, lemon juice, bicarbonate of soda, olive oil, spices and teas – to make "green" cleaning products. Now, more than ever, people are seeking natural alternatives to chemical products in a bid to reduce the impact on personal and environmental health.

Here we will look at how to use these heroes in "natural" recipes for various sorts of cleaning, including in the kitchen and bathroom, as well as for laundry and polishing.

CAUTION: Bear in mind these provisos so you don't damage furniture, worktops or cookware:

- Don't use vinegar or lemon juice on waxed stone, or wood, as they could cause dulling or other damage over time.
- Don't use bicarbonate of soda to clean surfaces made of sealed stone (for example, granite, marble or quartz countertops or floors), as its mild abrasiveness could gradually strip the protective sealant. Use products specially formulated for sealed stone instead.

If unsure whether a home-made cleaning product will be safe on a particular surface, try it on a small, inconspicuous area first.

General household cleaning

Below you can see how each of our six "heroes" can be used for general household cleaning. There are also some basic recipes for cleaning staples, which will be referenced throughout:

- Basic cleaning fluid
- Extra-strength cleaning fluid
- Basic cleaning paste
- Extra-strength cleaning paste
- Cream cleaner
- Scouring powder

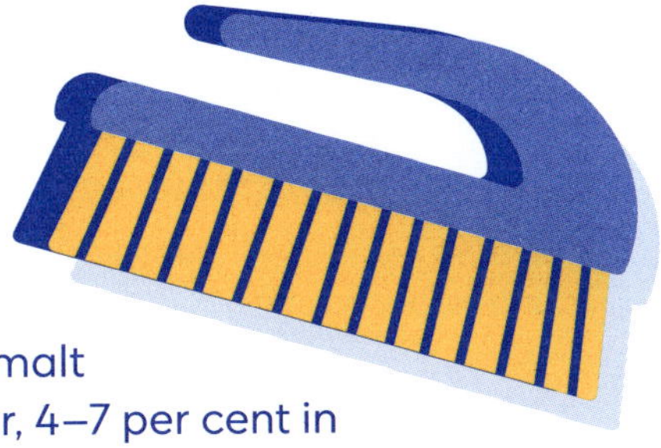

APPLE CIDER VINEGAR

Acetic acid and polyphenols are responsible for vinegar's cleaning power. All vinegars contain roughly the same concentration of acetic acid (5 per cent in malt vinegar, 5–6 per cent in apple cider vinegar, 4–7 per cent in white vinegar). Vinegar's acetic acid helps break down greasy deposits on surfaces in the bathroom and kitchen. It also helps breaks down calcium-containing deposits, so can help dissolve limescale in kettles and on showerheads, on taps and around plugholes. When vinegar is used in laundering, its acetic acid can brighten, whiten and soften fabrics and help remove unwanted odours. This is because it dissolves soap and detergent residues that could otherwise dull colours and make clothes feel stiff. All this is especially useful if you live in an area with hard water.

All vinegars also have antibacterial activity, thanks to the joint action of their acetic acid and polyphenols. The concentration of polyphenols in apple cider vinegar is about three times as high as in malt vinegar and white vinegar. Apple cider vinegar – though more expensive – is the better choice when cleaning surfaces and items in the kitchen and bathroom.

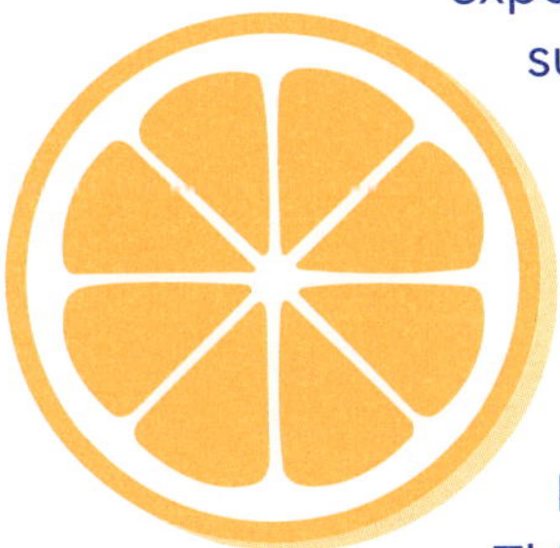

LEMONS

Lemons can help keep your home fresh, clean and sparkling. Bottled lemon juice is fine for household tasks.

BICARBONATE OF SODA

This powder has degreasing, water-softening and deodorizing qualities and is mildly abrasive. It also helps remove stains, particular those from oil and grease, and from tea, coffee and chocolate. Keep it in a flour shaker so it's ready to use.

OLIVE OIL

Its fats and fragrance make it a useful ingredient in a household polish.

SPICES

Spices such as caraway, cardamom, cinnamon, clove, juniper berry, mace and nutmeg give welcome fragrance to furniture polish and pot pourris. Several spices, including caraway, cinnamon, cloves, mace and nutmeg, are said to repel clothes moths.

TEA

Used tea leaves of any sort can help absorb unwanted odours.

BASIC CLEANING FLUID

Put 600ml (21fl oz/2½ cups) of warm water into a large bowl and stir in 1 tablespoon of bicarbonate of soda and two squeezes of washing-up liquid.

- **Use and storage:** Make enough for a particular cleaning job and use it from the bowl. Alternatively, pour it into a spray bottle and shake before use.

EXTRA-STRENGTH CLEANING FLUID

To the basic cleaning fluid recipe above, add the strained juice of 2 lemons. It will fizz with carbon-dioxide bubbles when first mixed.

- **Use:** Mix enough for a particular cleaning job and use while still fizzing.

BASIC CLEANING PASTE

Put some bicarbonate of soda into a bowl and stir in water to make a paste. The amounts depend on the job to be done. The proportions are three parts bicarbonate of soda to one part water. Mix in a few drops of lemon, tea tree, lavender or other essential oil for fragrance, if wanted. This paste is excellent for cleaning adherent grime, such as in a bath.

- **Use and storage:** Make enough for a particular cleaning job and use it from the bowl. If the paste starts to dry, add more water.

EXTRA-STRENGTH CLEANING PASTE

Use vinegar instead of water in the basic cleaning paste recipe above.

The resulting fizzing with carbon-dioxide bubbles can ease the cleaning of hard-to-reach places, such as plugholes and drains. This is because the force of the bubbling helps loosen dirt or staining and the bubbles' changeable shape helps squeeze the mixture into corners and through narrow gaps.

Note, though, that baking soda cuts through grease better when used without vinegar, and vinegar breaks down mineral deposits better when used without baking soda. The best plan is to use baking soda and vinegar separately. Mix them only when you require the mechanical action generated by the resulting bubbles to lift stains or unclog drains.

- **Use and storage:** Make enough for a particular cleaning job and use it from the bowl. If the paste starts to dry, add more water.

CREAM CLEANER

Make the basic cleaning paste recipe, then stir in extra water until it has the consistency of thick cream. Add a few drops of lemon, tea-tree, lavender or other essential oil for fragrance, if wanted.

- **Use and storage:** Make enough for a particular job and use it from the bowl. Or pour it into a labelled squeezy bottle and put the top on after any fizzing has stopped. Shake well before use.

SCOURING POWDER

This recipe includes borax substitute, which has bleaching, stain-removing, deodorizing and disinfecting qualities, and salt, which has degreasing and cleaning qualities. Mix equal amounts of bicarbonate of soda, borax substitute (available online or in hardware stories) and table salt in a bowl. Apply with a scrubbing brush, a cloth or, for small hard-to-reach areas, an old toothbrush.

- **Use and storage:** Make enough for a particular job and use it from the bowl. Or put it into a labelled jar or plastic container.

In the kitchen

FRUITS AND VEGETABLES

To get rid of dirt, pesticide traces and micro-organisms before eating fruits and vegetables:

- Wash them in a solution made by dissolving 1 teaspoon of bicarbonate of soda in 455ml (16fl oz/2 cups) of water. Leave to soak for 10–15 minutes, then rinse.
- Shake a little bicarbonate of soda on to a wet vegetable brush and gently scrub them.

SOILED OR SMELLY HANDS

- Wash very soiled hands with soap, rinse, then sprinkle them with bicarbonate of soda. Rub your hands together, then rinse again and dry.
- If your hands are stained (for example, after peeling red onions), rub them with lemon juice to remove the stains.
- Rid your hands of the smell of onions, garlic or fish by pouring vinegar into your cupped hand. Rub your hands together then rinse well with plenty of soapy water.
- Remove the odour of fish, onion or garlic from your hands by rubbing them with fresh lemon juice.

BLOCKED OR SMELLY DRAINS

- Help keep sink and basin drains clear by pouring ½ a cup of bicarbonate of soda down the plughole, then ½ a cup of hot vinegar (heated for one minute in the microwave). Leave for half an hour and then flush with a kettle of just-boiled water.
- Deodorize a sink's drain by mixing the juice of a lemon into a glass of water and pouring the mixture down the plughole.

SMELLY FACE FLANNEL, SPONGE, OR DISHCLOTH

Immerse a smelly face flannel, sponge or dishcloth in a solution of half-and-half vinegar and water. Leave it to deodorize for 2 hours then rinse well with water.

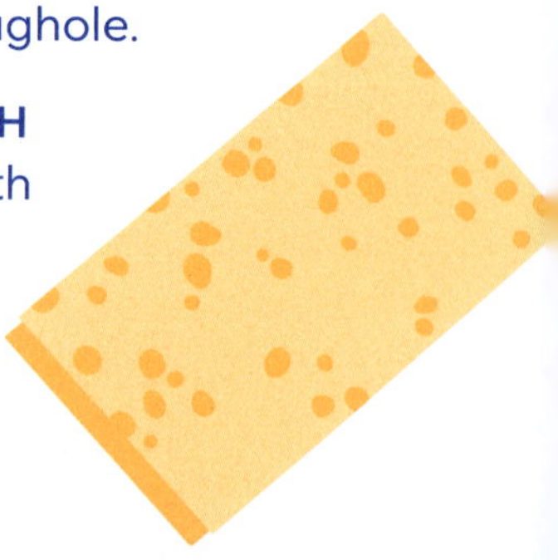

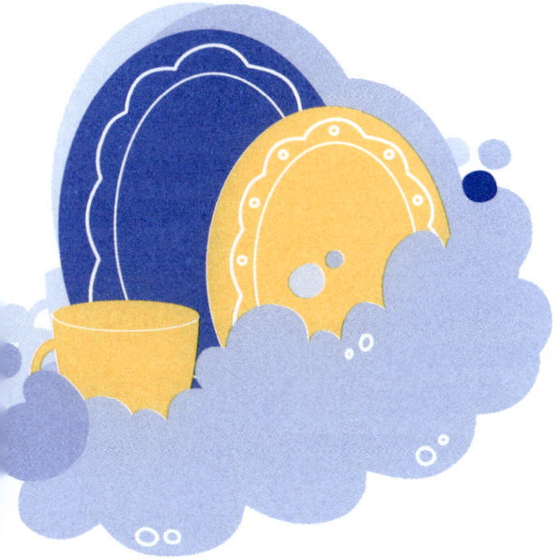

WASHING DISHES

Add one of these helpful degreasing aids to washing-up water, as they reduce the amount of washing-up liquid needed.

- ½ a cup of vinegar
- The juice of ½ a lemon
- 50g (1¾oz/¼ cup) of bicarbonate of soda plus the juice of ½ a lemon

STAINED SAUCEPANS

Clean stained stainless-steel or copper-coated pans and bowls with a paste of salt and vinegar.

STAINED TEA OR COFFEE POTS

Help clean away brown stains in a tea or coffee pot by filling it with half-and-half vinegar and water. Leave for half an hour, then rinse.

WOODEN CHOPPING BOARDS AND BUTCHER'S BLOCKS

- Disinfect these with lemon juice, as this contains citric and other acids – and bacteria dislike an acidic environment.
- Spring-clean a wooden chopping board or butcher's block by sprinkling it with bicarbonate of soda, then spraying with vinegar. Leave for 30 minutes before rinsing with hot water.
- Rub a little olive oil into the surface of a newly cleaned chopping board or butcher's block to help keep the wood in good condition.
- Deodorize a cutting board that smells of garlic or onions by sprinkling bicarbonate of soda on to a damp sponge, rubbing this over the board, then rinsing clean.

STAINED PLASTIC FOOD CONTAINERS

Make a paste of 1 tablespoon of bicarbonate of soda plus a few drops of fresh lemon juice, then rub this over the stains.

STAINED LAMINATE WORKTOPS

Put fresh lemon juice on to stains on a laminate worktop. Leave for 45 minutes. Then sprinkle with bicarbonate of soda, scrub gently and rinse.

KITCHEN SURFACES

Use lemon essential oil to clean kitchen surfaces, as its limonene is a solvent that effectively removes greasy marks.

- Put a few drops of lemon essential oil into a bowl of hot water and use this to clean kitchen surfaces or other surfaces especially likely to be contaminated with bacteria. Several of the oil's constituents, including limonene, have antibacterial properties.
- Add a splash of vinegar to soapy water then use this to wipe kitchen worktops or other hard surfaces to rid them of food smells or other unwanted odours.

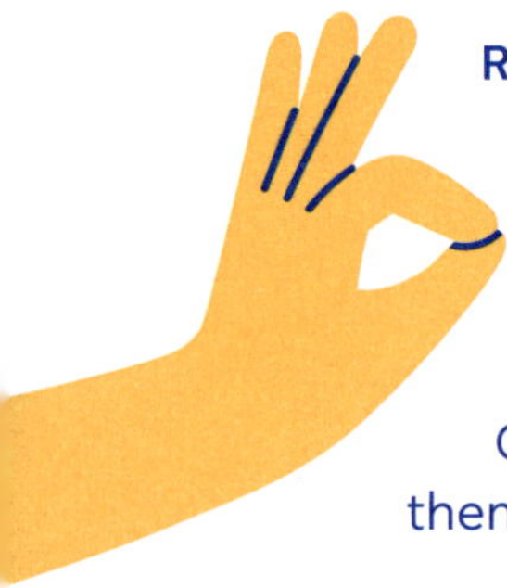

RUBBER GLOVES

Sprinkle a little bicarbonate of soda into rubber gloves to keep them fresh and make them easy to put on and take off.

SPONGES AND CLOTHS

Clean and deodorize sponges and cloths by soaking them in basic cleaning fluid (p.316), then rinse and dry.

KITCHEN SINK

Clean the kitchen sink with extra-strength cleaning fluid (p.316) or rub with bicarbonate of soda sprinkled on a damp sponge or cloth.

BLOCKED SINK AND WASTE PIPES

- Help clear a blockage by pouring down the plughole 200g (7oz/ 1 cup) of bicarbonate of soda, followed by 240ml (8fl oz/1 cup) of hot vinegar. Wait 30 minutes, then flush with a kettle of just-boiled water. If necessary, use a sink plunger.
- Freshen waste pipes and prevent them becoming blocked by pouring down the plughole 100g (3½oz/½ cup) of bicarbonate of soda followed by a full kettle of just-boiled water. Do this each month.

BURNT-ON SAUCEPAN STAINS

Get rid of burnt-on food residues by:

- Brushing or scrubbing a saucepan with bicarbonate of soda or scouring powder (p.317).
- Wetting the saucepan with hot water then sprinkling on a thick layer of bicarbonate of soda. Leave overnight, then brush or scrape off the residues.
- Putting 240ml (8fl oz/1 cup) of water into the saucepan, adding 1 tablespoon of white vinegar and bringing to the boil. Add 2 tablespoons of bicarbonate of soda and wait for the fizzing to subside, then brush or scrape off the residues.

CAUTION: Don't use bicarbonate of soda on a non-stick pan, as it could damage its surface. Don't scour saucepans with an enamelled interior.

TEA AND COFFEE STAINS

- Use a damp sponge to rub bicarbonate of soda onto stains in cups and mugs. Leave for 30 minutes, then rinse.
- Fill a cup or mug with warm water and add ½ a teaspoon of bicarbonate of soda. Leave for 30 minutes, then rinse.
- Fill a coffee pot or teapot with hot water and add 2 teaspoons of bicarbonate of soda and 2 teaspoons of vinegar. Leave for 30 minutes, then rinse.
- Fill a glass and metal (but not aluminium) cafetière with hot water, stir in 1 teaspoon of bicarbonate of soda and 1 teaspoon of vinegar. Leave it to soak for 30 minutes before rinsing.

FRUIT DRINK OR FRUIT JUICE STAINS

Clean washable surfaces with water, then sprinkle with bicarbonate of soda. Leave for 30 minutes, then wipe clean.

Appliances

WASHING MACHINE

- Clean the drum and the inside of the door with basic cleaning fluid or, for stubborn marks, basic cleaning paste (p.316).
- Or put 50g (1¾oz/¼ cup) of bicarbonate of soda into the washing-powder dispenser and 240ml (8fl oz/¼ cup) of white vinegar into the fabric-softener dispenser before running the machine on a short cycle.

- Deodorize the washing-machine drum and the inside of the door by wiping with basic cleaning fluid (p.316).
- Or clean the washing machine and its dispenser with a brush and soapy water, then add a cup of vinegar to the empty machine and run a cycle to remove the odour.
- If the washing-machine dispenser is furred up with limescale, clean with a brush and soapy water, then add a cup of vinegar to the dispenser and run a cycle to help remove the deposits.

DISHWASHER

Mix 2 tablespoons of bicarbonate of soda with 2 tablespoons of borax substitute (p.317) to make dishwashing powder.
To help prevent unwanted odours:

- Put 2 tablespoons of bicarbonate of soda into the dishwasher-powder (or tablet or pod) dispenser and run a rinse cycle.
- Clean inside and out with basic cleaning fluid or extra-strength cleaning fluid and wipe clean.
- Sprinkle 100g (3½oz/½ cup) of bicarbonate of soda into the bottom of the dishwasher after emptying it.
- Clean with a brush and soapy water, then add a cup of cider vinegar to the empty machine and run a cycle.

REFRIGERATOR AND FREEZER

- Clean it by wiping inside and out with basic cleaning fluid (p.316), then rinsing.
- Rub stained areas with some basic cleaning paste (p.316), then wipe off.
- Make a refrigerator or freezer smell sweet by keeping a small bowl of bicarbonate of soda inside. Stir it every few days and replace every 2–3 months.
- Keep your fridge smelling sweet by keeping ½ a lemon on a saucer inside.

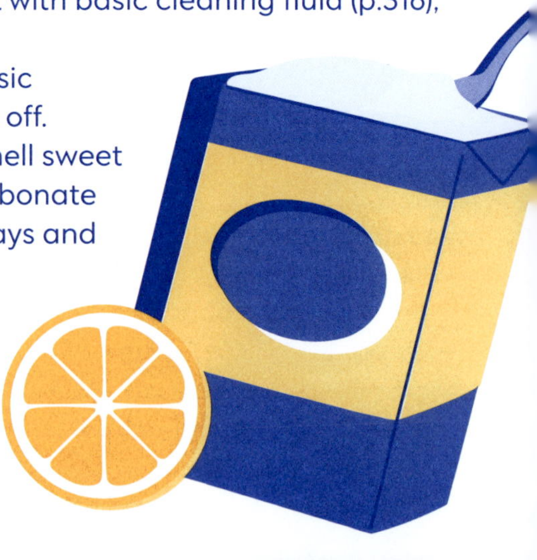

OVEN

Baking soda and vinegar are good for oven cleaning as they are non-toxic. (In contrast, most oven-cleaning products contain chemicals such as caustic soda, sodium hydroxide or ethylene glycol, which can be hazardous if used incorrectly.)

To clean an oven:

- Remove the oven racks and clean them separately (see below).
- Use a sponge or brush to spread basic cleaning paste (p.316) over the oven walls, avoiding the heating elements and the light.
- Leave for at least 12 hours.
- Wipe off most of the paste with a damp cloth.
- Use a spray bottle to spray vinegar on to the oven walls.
- Wipe the oven clean with a damp cloth, a hob scraper or wet paper towels.

To clean stainless steel oven racks:

- Sprinkle them with bicarbonate of soda.
- Wait for at least 12 hours.
- Spray with vinegar.
- When the foaming stops, soak the racks in hot water to make the grease and other burnt food deposits easier to scrub away.

HOB, SPLASHBACK AND GRILL

To clean these:

- Rub on bicarbonate of soda with a damp sponge or cloth, then wipe clean.
- Or use a damp cloth plus lemon juice.
- If very soiled, use extra-strength cleaning paste (p.316).
- Degrease and clean an encrusted barbecue grill by applying extra-strength cleaning paste (p.316), leaving for several hours, brushing with a wire brush, then wiping clean.

MICROWAVE OVEN

- Clean inside a microwave oven by wiping with basic cleaning fluid (p.316).

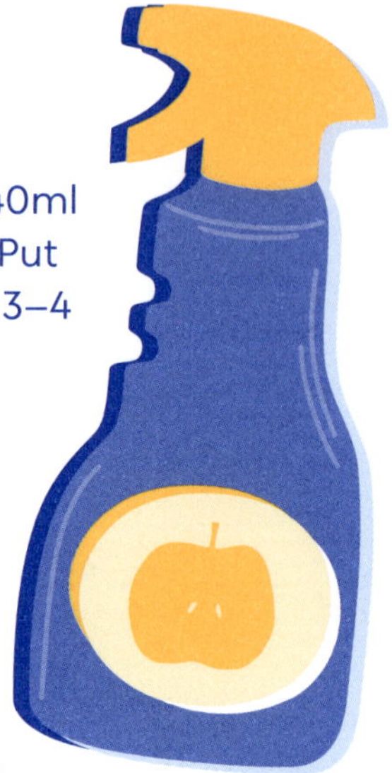

- Or put 1 tablespoon of bicarbonate of soda and 240ml (8fl oz/1 cup) of water into a microwaveable bowl. Put this in the oven. Set the oven so the liquid boils for 3–4 minutes. Wipe the inside of the oven with a damp cloth or kitchen paper.
- To clean and deodorize a microwave oven, mix 30g (1oz) of bicarbonate of soda, 1 teaspoon of vinegar and 6 drops of lemon essential oil. Use a sponge to apply this paste to the inside of the microwave oven. Rinse with water and leave the door open for 15 minutes to allow for drying.

In the bathroom

SURFACES

Clean with hot water to which you have added a few drops of lemon essential oil, as its limonene is a solvent that efficiently removes greasy marks. Also, several constituents of lemon oil, including limonene, have antibacterial properties.

CLEANING THE BATH

- When you have a bath, add 2 tablespoons of bicarbonate of soda to the water. This will help prevent a scummy ring forming inside the bath as the water drains away.
- Clean the bath, basin, taps, tiles and mirrors by applying basic cleaning paste (p.316) with a damp cloth or sponge. Then rinse.
- Or rub with a damp cloth or sponge sprinkled with bicarbonate of soda, then rinse.

SHOWER SCREEN

For heavier soiling, or to clean glass shower screens, rub on extra-strength cleaning paste (p.317), leave for 30 minutes, then rinse. Dry a glass shower screen with a barely damp towel.

SHOWER CURTAIN

- Clean a mildewed shower curtain by putting it in the washing machine along with a large bath towel. Add 1 cup of bicarbonate of soda to the washing powder or liquid detergent in the washing-machine dispenser. Then wash the load on a low-temperature setting, adding ½ a cup of cider vinegar to the fabric-softener dispenser during the rinse cycle. Don't spin fast, or the curtain could become permanently creased. Hang up to dry.

- Clean a non-machine-washable shower curtain by soaking it for 30 minutes in a bath of warm water containing 1 cup of bicarbonate of soda. Rinse and drip-dry.

SHOWER HEAD

Help prevent hard water's mineral salts blocking a shower head by pouring 50g (1¾oz/¼ cup) of bicarbonate of soda and 240ml (8fl oz/1 cup) white vinegar into a strong, intact plastic bag. Tie this around the shower head and leave for 30 minutes. Remove the bag. Then run the water for a few seconds.

TILE GROUTING

- Use an old firm-bristled toothbrush to apply extra-strength cleaning paste (p.317) to soiled tile grout. Leave for 30 minutes, then rinse.
- For particularly grimy grout, mix 3 parts bicarbonate of soda with 1 part bleach and scrub this over the grout with a toothbrush. Wait for 30 minutes, then rinse.

CAUTION: Use extra-strength cleaning paste only on grout that has been sealed. If you don't know if it has been sealed, put a few drops of water on the grout and wait for 5 minutes The grout is unsealed if the water soaks in or leaves a dark mark.

TOILET

- Clean a lavatory cistern and bowl by putting 200g (7oz/1 cup) of bicarbonate of soda into the cistern overnight, then flushing next morning. Repeat once a month.
- Clean a lavatory bowl by sprinkling bicarbonate of soda on to a damp scrubbing brush and scrubbing under the rim.
- Treat a stained lavatory bowl by rubbing with extra-strength cleaning paste (p.317).

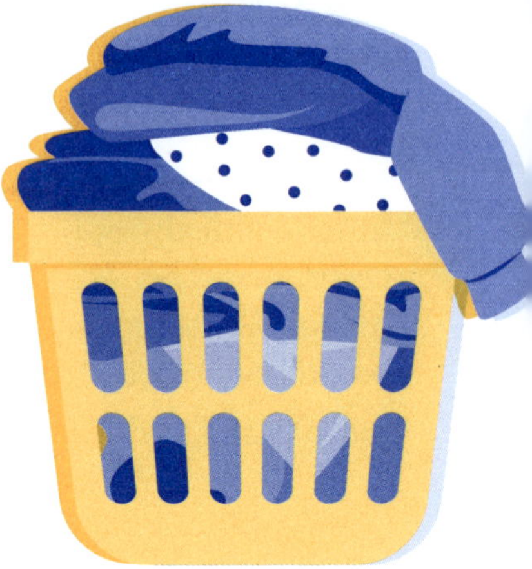

Laundry and stain removal

LAUNDRY BASKET FRESHENING

Keep a laundry basket fresh by sprinkling a little bicarbonate of soda into it each day.

FABRIC SOFTENING

- Mix 2 tablespoons of vinegar, 2 tablespoons of bicarbonate of soda and 4 tablespoons of water. Add to the final rinse water if washing by hand, or to the fabric-softener dispenser of a washing machine.
- Make fabric softener (conditioner) by putting 1 cup of bicarbonate of soda, 1 cup of vinegar and 2 cups of water into a bottle. The bottle should be large enough to accommodate the effervescence produced when bicarbonate of soda mixes with vinegar. Gently shake the bottle. Add 60ml (2fl oz/¼ cup) of this mixture to your washing machine's fabric softener dispenser when you do a wash, or put it into the final rinse water if handwashing. Bicarbonate of soda helps make towels soft and fluffy.
- For a fragranced fabric softener, use the above recipe but add 3–4 drops of lemon, lavender or rose essential oil.

WHITENING

- Help whiten white clothes by adding ½ a cup of bicarbonate of soda to the washing powder dispenser, or, if washing by hand, to the final rinse water.
- Alternatively, add ¼ cup of bicarbonate of soda to a basin of cold water, immerse the clothing and soak overnight. Next morning, wash as usual.
- For greater whitening action, add the juice of a lemon and ¼ cup of bicarbonate of soda to a basin of cold water. Soak the clothing overnight and wash it next morning.
- Alternatively, boost the performance of bleach by adding ½ a cup of bicarbonate of soda and ½ a cup of bleach to a bowl of water.

- Whiten cloth nappies by adding ½ a cup of bicarbonate of soda to the washing powder dispenser, or to the washing powder if handwashing.
- Use bicarbonate of soda to make chlorine bleach more effective: add ½ a cup along with the usual amount of bleach.

COLOUR SETTING

When washing coloured fabric, add a cup of cider vinegar to help set the dye so it won't leach out and stain other fabrics.

GENERAL STAIN REMOVAL

- Rub soiled collars and cuffs with a paste of equal parts of vinegar and bicarbonate of soda. Wait 30 minutes then wash as normal.
- Try removing ink, grass, coffee, tea, fruit and berry stains from fabric by soaking the stain in vinegar for an hour, then washing.
- To remove stains from white laundry, mix 1 tablespoon each of lemon juice and cream of tartar (also known as potassium bitartrate, potassium hydrogen tartrate or tartaric acid) and apply the mixture to the stain. Leave for a few minutes, then rinse with water. For persistent or extensive staining on a fabric that is washable in very hot water, boil the item in a pan containing 5 tablespoons of cream of tartar to every 1.1 litre (2 pints/4.8 cups) of water, then rinse.
- You can also dampen the stain and sprinkle it with cream of tartar. Carefully hold the stained area in the steam from a boiling kettle, then rinse well with water.
- For stains on fabrics that can be washed in hot water, pour 240ml (8fl oz/1 cup) of lemon juice into the washing machine during the wash cycle.
- Sprinkle lemon juice over berry stains on clothing or other fabric to fade the stains.
- If clothing is stained with something acidic (such as fruit juice or tomato ketchup), pre-treating it with bicarbonate of soda before washing will help prevent the acid eating into the fabric; it

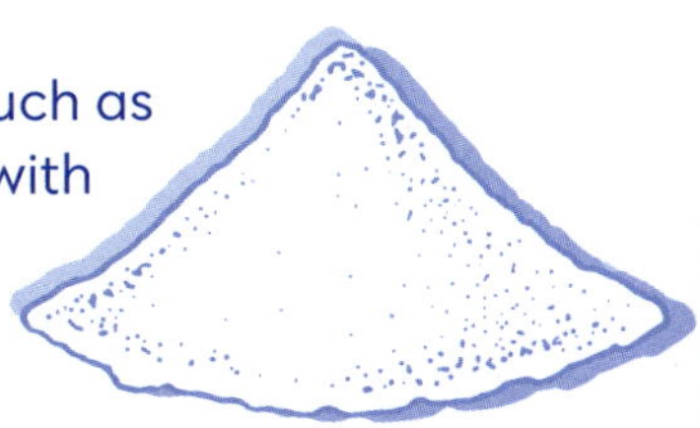

should also loosen the stain. Sprinkle with bicarbonate of soda, spray with water then leave for 30 minutes before washing. This is also effective for acidic sweat, vomit and urine stains.

- Rub a tar stain with basic cleaning paste (p.316) then wash it with bicarbonate of soda and water.

PERSPIRATION STAINS ON CLOTHES

- Reduce these by soaking garments for several hours in a basin of water containing ½ a cup of vinegar.
- You can also try scrubbing the stains gently with half-and-half lemon juice and water.

RUST AND MILDEW STAINS ON CLOTHES

- For washable clothing, sprinkle the stained area generously with salt, then squeeze fresh lemon juice over it. Leave the item for several hours, ideally in direct sunlight. Keep the stain moist by applying more lemon juice as necessary. Brush off the salt then launder as usual.
- Add ½ a cup of bicarbonate of soda along with your usual amount of liquid washing detergent to the washing machine or hand-wash bowl for more effective washing power. This also helps shift many other stains.
- Remove a rust stain by soaking the clothing in lemon juice then sprinkling with a thick layer of bicarbonate of soda. Leave overnight, then rinse and wash.

BLOOD STAINS ON CLOTHES

Remove a blood stain by putting ½ a cup of bicarbonate of soda and ½ a cup of white vinegar into a bowl of cold water and soaking the item in this mixture overnight. Wash as normal the next day.

GREASE STAINS ON CLOTHES

- Apply a paste of bicarbonate of soda and water, leave for 30 minutes then add ½ a cup of bicarbonate of soda to the washing machine (or

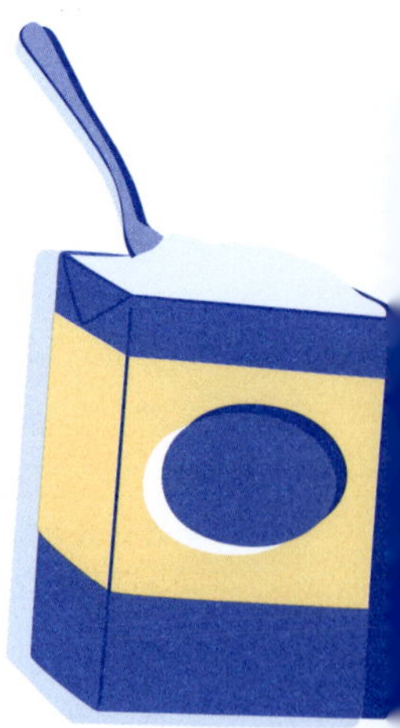

a bowl if hand-washing) along with the liquid detergent. Run your usual cycle.

- Make a paste from 2 parts of bicarbonate of soda, 1 part of cream of tartar and a little water and rub this on a grease mark before washing.

MILDEW SMELL ON CLOTHES

Try soaking the item in basic cleaning fluid (p.316) overnight, then washing.

CHEWING GUM ON CLOTHES

Loosen chewing gum or its stains by rubbing with vinegar before laundering.

Air freshening and scent

DEODORIZING WITH BICARBONATE OF SODA

Bicarbonate of soda is a brilliant natural ingredient for neutralizing all kinds of unpleasant smells. It acts against odours from acidic substances (such as in sweat, urine or vomit) and alkaline ones (such as ammonia from wet nappies).

EASY AIR FRESHENERS

- Half-fill a spray bottle with water and add a teaspoon of bicarbonate of soda and a tablespoon of vinegar. Shake the open bottle to mix the contents. When the foaming stops, fill the bottle with water and put on the cap. Use as an air freshener to help eliminate the smell of smoke, pets, cooking and other unpleasant odours.
- Make a fragrant freshener by adding to a saucepan 1.1 litres (2 pints) of water, 2 tablespoons of vinegar and 50g (2oz) fresh, or 25g (1oz) dried, lavender, thyme, rosemary or cloves. Bring to the boil and simmer for 10 minutes. Cool, strain, put into a spray bottle and use as desired.
- Leave a small open pot of bicarbonate of soda in each room to act as an air freshener by neutralizing any unwanted odours. This is more effective than using commercial air fresheners, which mostly act by producing a masking scent.

- Make a fragranced air freshener by adding a few drops of lemon, geranium, lavender, neroli, rose or other essential oil to a small pot of bicarbonate of soda.

KITCHEN SMELLS

- Prevent unpleasant smells in a larder or store cupboard by keeping a small, open bowl of bicarbonate of soda there. Stir every few days and replace every 2–3 months.
- Eliminate stale smells from plastic bowls or food containers by filling them with hot water and stirring in 1 tablespoon of bicarbonate of soda. Soak for 30 minutes, then rinse. If the smell persists, repeat, adding 1 tablespoon of vinegar and a few drops of washing-up liquid along with the bicarbonate of soda.
- Half-fill a ceramic diffuser's bowl with water, add a few drops of lemon essential oil and light the tea light. The oil's vapour is said to help lift the spirits, clear the mind and improve concentration.
- Add a few drops of lemon essential oil to a spray bottle half-filled with water, shake well and spray to make the air in a room smell fragrant.
- Add strips of dried lemon peel to a bowl of fragrant dried flowers or leaves to scent a room. Sprinkle a few drops of lemon essential oil over the bowl's contents every couple of weeks to refresh the aroma. See also "Pot pourri" below.
- Stud a lemon with cloves, then tie a ribbon around it so you can hang it up to release its lovely fresh scent.

ABSORB UNWANTED SMELLS

Keep unused teabags in an airtight container so you can put them in a shallow dish to absorb formaldehyde from fresh paint or glue; newly-cut particle board, plywood or pressed-wood products; and urea-formaldehyde-foam insulation, which is now banned in certain countries.

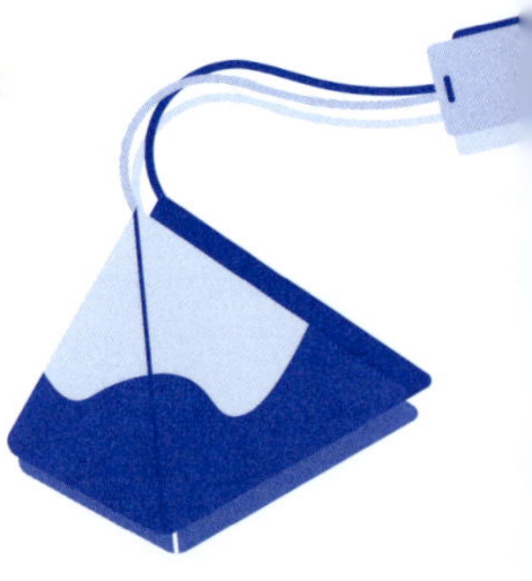

WARDROBES AND DRAWERS

- Keep a wardrobe smelling sweet by putting an open bowl of bicarbonate of soda inside. Add a few drops of lemon, geranium, lavender, neroli, rose or other essential oil for a nice fragrance.

- Alternatively, use scraps of fabric to make little bags which you can fill with bicarbonate of soda and, perhaps, a few drops of fragrant essential oil. Tie up with ribbon and keep inside a wardrobe or drawer.
- Sprinkle bicarbonate of soda into garment storage bags to help prevent musty smells.
- Leave thinly pared strips of lemon peel to dry over several days, then put them in your wardrobe or chest of drawers to scent your clothes.

PET SMELLS

- Sprinkle bicarbonate of soda over a tray of cat litter to help neutralize unpleasant smells.
- Remove a "wet-dog" smell by sprinkling bicarbonate of soda over the dog's coat, waiting 30 minutes, then brushing it out.
- Make a dog's or cat's bedding smell better by sprinkling it with bicarbonate of soda, leaving it for 1 hour, then vacuuming it.

HUMIDIFIER

Add a few drops of lemon juice to the water container.

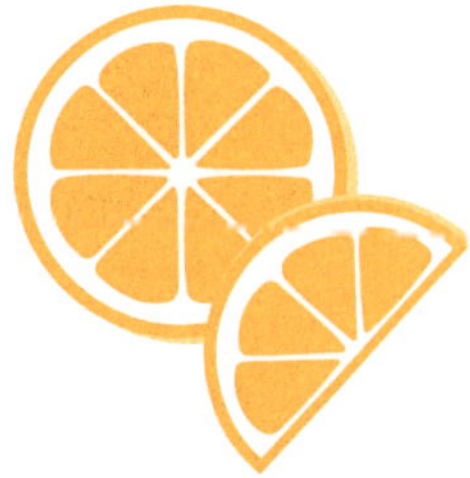

VACUUM CLEANER

Freshen the bag by sprinkling a few drops of lemon essential oil on to a paper tissue and putting this into it.

WASTE DISPOSAL UNIT IN SINK

- Make this smell fresh by putting the peel of a lemon through it and then rinsing with water.
- Add a small handful of bicarbonate of soda to help prevent an unpleasant smell.
- Every week, pour in 2 tablespoons of bicarbonate of soda and 1 tablespoon of white vinegar and run hot water from the tap as you operate the disposal unit.

BLANKETS

Make a stored blanket smell sweeter by shaking bicarbonate of soda over it, then rolling it up. Leave overnight, then shake it next morning and tumble it in the tumble drier, set to cold.

CAR CARPET

Deodorize by sprinkling with bicarbonate of soda, leaving for at least 30 minutes, then vacuuming.

VOMIT ODOUR

Neutralize a sour odour from cleaned-up vomit stains by sprinkling generously with bicarbonate of soda. Leave for several hours, then vacuum clean.

SHOES

Sprinkle in bicarbonate of soda, leave overnight, then next morning tap out the surplus.

NOTE: Doing this with leather shoes could stiffen the leather.

SMOKE

Put bicarbonate of soda into ashtrays to combat the tobacco smell.

CAMPING GEAR

Sprinkle tents, waterproofs and other gear with bicarbonate of soda before storing.

VAPORIZER

Add up to 5 drops of your chosen essential oil to an oil vaporizer to impart a pleasant scent to a room.

POT POURRI

Mix 2 cups of dried and fragrant plant material (such as rose petals, lavender flowers, marigold flowers, bay leaves, lemon or rose geranium leaves, lemon balm leaves, pine needles and fir cones) with 50g (2oz) of coarse sea salt. Leave in a dry place for 3 days.

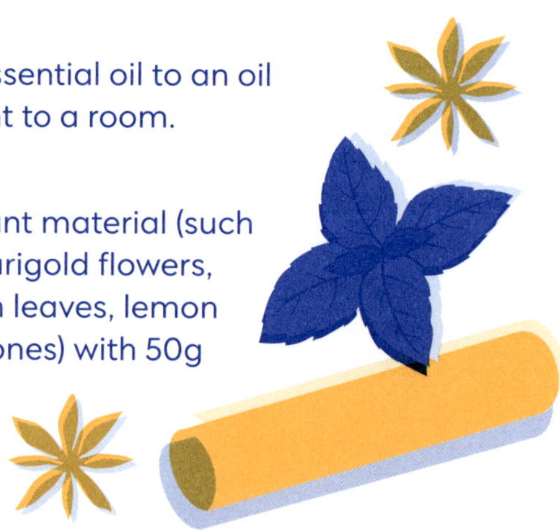

In another bowl, mix 2 tablespoons each of coarsely crushed allspice berries and whole cloves, with 3 cinnamon sticks each broken into several pieces. Add all this to the plant material. Sprinkle the mixture with 2 tablespoons of brandy and transfer to a decorative container. Refresh the scent every few weeks by stirring 1 tablespoon of brandy into the pot pourri.

POMANDER

A pomander will scent your wardrobe and deter moths.

- Stud an orange with cloves, starting each hole with a thick needle. Mix 2 teaspoons each of orris root (from a pharmacy or the internet) and ground cinnamon. Sprinkle the fragrant mixture over the orange.
- Put the orange on a plate and leave in a cool, dry place for 4 weeks to harden, turning it every few days.
- Wrap narrow coloured ribbon around the orange, finished with a loop for hanging.

SPICE BAGS FOR DRAWERS AND CUPBOARDS

To scent clothes and linens and keep moths away, mix 1 teaspoon each of ground caraway, cloves, nutmeg (or mace) and cinnamon. Stir in 1 tablespoon of orris root (from a pharmacy or the internet). Put the fragrant mixture into a small cloth bag and secure with a drawstring.

SCENTED SACHETS

Remove and dry the contents of used teabags, then use them to fill small cotton bags to create scented sachets for wardrobe or bedroom drawers.

Polishing

WOODEN FURNITURE

- Give extra shine to wooden furniture by adding a few drops of vinegar to a commercial polish.
- Polish wooden furniture with half-and-half mixture of vinegar and paraffin.

- To make a furniture polish, combine in a glass jar 2 parts of olive oil with 1 part of strained fresh lemon juice. This polish accentuates the beauty of the wood; it also nourishes it and prevents it from drying out.
- Make a polish for furniture, wooden floors and other hard surfaces by mixing 1 part of olive oil with 1 part of vinegar or lemon juice. Apply this, wait for 5–10 minutes, then burnish the wood with a soft cloth.
- For aromatic sheeny wood, put 2 tablespoons of unscented beeswax or other furniture polish into a small bowl and use a fork to mix in 1 teaspoon of finely ground allspice, caraway, cardamom, cinnamon, clove, ginger, juniper berry or nutmeg.
- Put 2 *Camellia-sinensis* teabags into a bowl, add 5 cups of just-boiled water and let the tea cool. Clean wooden furniture with a cloth soaked in the tea and squeezed out. Then dry it with an old towel.

CAUTION: Before trying these natural polishing methods, first do a trial patch test somewhere out of sight.

SURFACES

Use lemon essential oil to polish surfaces, as its limonene acts as a solvent, dissolving old wax, fingerprints and grime.

MIRRORS

Make a strong brew of *Camellia-sinensis* tea, let it cool, soak a cloth in it, squeeze out the cloth and use it to clean mirrors. Polish the mirror with a soft, lint-free cloth.

LEATHER SHOES, JACKETS, SOFAS AND CHAIRS

If the leather is faded or cracked, use a soft cloth to rub in a light coat of olive oil. Leave it for 30 minutes, then carefully wipe off any excess with a soft absorbent cloth or a paper towel. This will moisturize and soften the leather and restore some of its natural colour.

CAUTION: Test it on a small, inconspicuous area first. Some leather types may darken with oil, and delicate leathers could be damaged.

Metal and rust removal

USING BICARBONATE OF SODA TO CLEAN AND SHINE METALS

This helps clean and shine silver, chrome and copper by removing oxidation and tarnish. It has even been used to clean the copper Statue of Liberty in New York!

CAUTION: Don't use bicarbonate of soda on anything made of aluminium, as it removes the metal's thin protective coating of aluminium oxide. (This coating prevents aluminium reacting to acid from sweaty hands or city air – which would soon make it look patchy.)

ALUMINIUM OR CHROME

Polish the dulled surfaces of aluminium or chrome objects by rubbing with the cut surface of half a lemon, then buffing with a cloth.

COPPER AND BRASS

- To brighten copper and brass items, first make a paste from equal parts of salt, flour and vinegar. Let it dry for 10 minutes, then apply it, then buff with a polishing cloth.
- Brighten copper cookware or ornaments by dipping the cut surface of half a lemon into salt or bicarbonate of soda, then rubbing this over the surface. The lemon acids dissolve the tarnish, and the salt and bicarbonate of soda act as a mild abrasive to clear it away. Rinse with water and dry with a cloth or a paper towel.

RUST REMOVAL

- Help remove rust from small metal objects by immersing them in vinegar for several hours.
- Help remove rust from metal by applying basic cleaning paste (p.316) with a damp cloth. Scrub lightly with a piece of aluminium foil, then rinse and dry with kitchen paper.

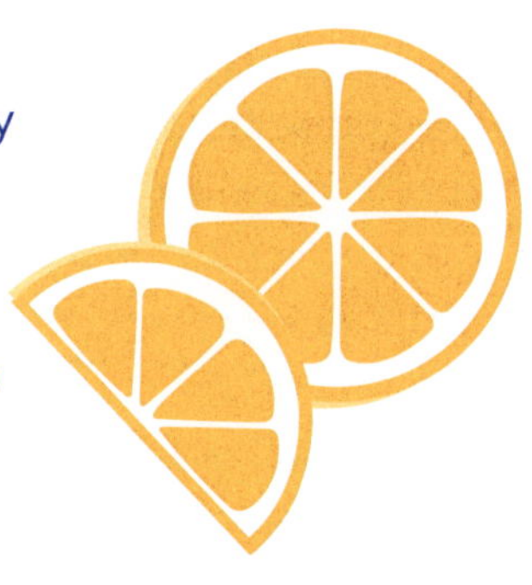

STORING SCOURERS

Store steel wool pan scourers in a sprinkling of bicarbonate of soda to prevent rust.

SILVER (THOUGH NOT SILVER JEWELLERY WITH PEARLS OR OPALS)

- Scrub a silver item with an old toothbrush and basic cleaning paste (p.316). Rinse with warm water, dry with kitchen paper, then polish with a soft cloth.
- Put tarnished silver on aluminium foil in a bowl of warm water containing 1 teaspoon of bicarbonate of soda per cup of water, or put the silver item into warm water in an aluminium container. Wait 5–15 minutes, then remove, rinse, dry with kitchen paper and polish with a soft cloth. Silver reacts with oxygen and sulphur gases in the air to form a tarnish containing silver sulphide. In turn, aluminium reacts with silver sulphide to form aluminium sulphide, leaving sparkly bright pure silver.

CAR BUMPERS AND HUBCAPS:

Clean chrome on these, or on a bicycle, by rubbing bicarbonate of soda over them with a damp sponge. Rinse, then polish with a soft dry cloth.

STAINLESS STEEL

Make stainless steel shine by rubbing on bicarbonate of soda with a damp sponge, then rinsing and drying.

GOLD JEWELLERY

De-grime gold jewellery by putting it into a bowl, sprinkling it with bicarbonate of soda, then pouring white vinegar over it. Rinse and dry.

CAUTION: Don't do this if the jewellery contains pearls or opals, or if gemstones have been glued in place rather than captured in metal "claws".

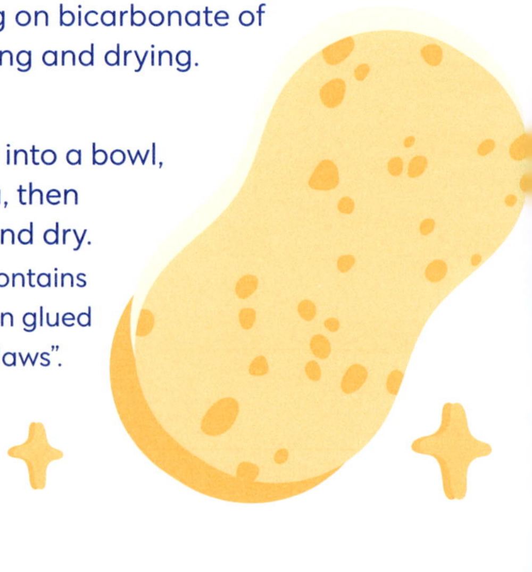

Walls, floors, windows and mirrors

USING BICARBONATE OF SODA FOR CLEANING WALLS

Bicarbonate of soda helps to clean paint, laminate, other plastic, glass, granite, other stone, composite, rubber, brick, steel, fibreglass and washable wallpaper.

CAUTION: If using bicarbonate of soda on bare wood, be sparing with the water and dry well to avoid water marks.

WALLS

- Remove crayon marks on a painted or papered wall by sprinkling bicarbonate of soda on to a damp sponge, rubbing the wall very gently with this, then wiping clean.
- Banish grease or scuff marks on washable walls by wiping with bicarbonate of soda on a damp sponge. Then rinse and wipe dry.
- Wipe with basic cleaning fluid (p.316), then rinse.
- Use a damp sponge or cloth to rub heavily-soiled or stained areas with bicarbonate of soda, then rinse.

FLOORS

- Freshen and clean floors by adding a cup of vinegar to the cleaning water.
- To clean wooden, laminate or ceramic-tiled floors, pour into a spray bottle 1 cup of white vinegar, 1 cup of water, 5 drops of lemon essential oil, 2 drops of tea tree essential oil and 5 drops of lavender essential oil. Spray the mixture on to the floor and wipe clean with a microfibre cloth or a mop.
- For a fresh-smelling floor cleaner, add 4 tablespoons of white vinegar and 10 drops of lemon essential oil to a bucket of water and mop the floor with the solution.
- Sprinkle bicarbonate of soda on to floors or worktops or in cupboards to repel unwanted insects.
- Eradicate water spots on wooden floors by dabbing with a sponge or cloth dampened with basic cleaning fluid (p.316). Wipe clean and repeat several times to remove all traces of bicarbonate of soda. Dry well.

CAUTION: Don't wet the wood too much, as this could make more water spots!

- Apply extra-strength cleaning paste (p.317) to ink stains on hard floors, then rinse and dry.
- Mop or wipe floors with 100g (3½oz/½ cup) of bicarbonate of soda dissolved in a bucket of hot water.

CARPETS AND RUGS

- To freshen these, mix 10 drops each of lemon and lavender essential oils into 125g (4½oz/1 cup) of bicarbonate of soda. Put this mixture in a covered container and leave overnight so the bicarbonate of soda absorbs the oil. Next day, sprinkle it over the carpet or rug, leave for an hour, then vacuum up the powder.
- Remove wine, grease and certain other stains from carpets by lightly wetting the stains, then sprinkling them with bicarbonate of soda. Leave to dry, then vacuum up the residue.
- Deodorize carpets and rugs by shaking bicarbonate of soda over them, waiting at least 30 minutes, then vacuuming.
- After cleaning spilt drink or food from a carpet, sprinkle liberally with bicarbonate of soda, wait 30 minutes, then vacuum. This makes an unpleasant smell less likely to linger.

GLASS

- Clean streaks and dirt from window glass, spectacle lenses or mirrors with a mixture of 1 part of vinegar to 3 parts of water applied with a microfibre cloth. Then dry with newspaper or a slightly damp towel.
- To clean windows, rub the cut surfaces of a lemon quarter over the glass, wipe off with a damp cloth, then dry with a dry cloth.

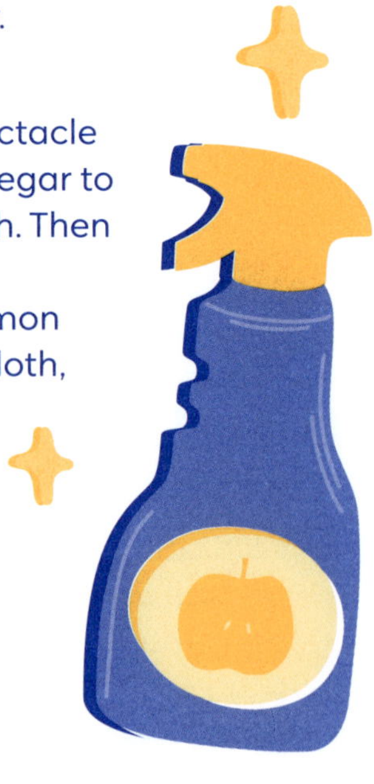

Repelling insects

DOG FLEAS

Repel fleas by adding ½ a cup of cider vinegar to the final rinsing water when shampooing your dog.

KITCHEN INSECTS

- If kitchen or other cupboards are infested with insects, wipe inside the cupboards with lemon essential oil on a cloth. Its limonene is toxic to insects but not to humans.
- Sprinkle lemon juice around door thresholds and on windowsills, as its scent will deter the entry of insects.

ANTS

Leave a rotten lemon out to repel ants.

CLOTHES MOTHS

Make your own mothballs. These smell sweet to humans but abhorrent to clothes moths, so will help protect your precious knits from moth holes. Put knots in sealed plastic bags to be absolutely safe.

- Buy some cedarwood balls from a hardware store or the internet. Put them into a bowl, sprinkle with 1 teaspoon of black pepper, cedar, clove, cinnamon or lemon oil, and stir.
- Leave these balls for a week, stirring each day, to let the oil soak in. Then scatter in drawers, shelves or cupboards. Refresh with oil twice a year.
- You can also put strips of dried lemon peel into small muslin bags and place them in cupboards and drawers to repel clothes moths.

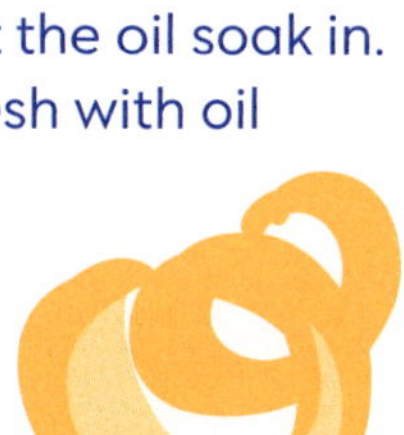

INSECTS ON A CAR WINDSCREEN

Remove smears left by cleaning off dead insects by applying bicarbonate of soda on a damp sponge, then rinsing and wiping clean.

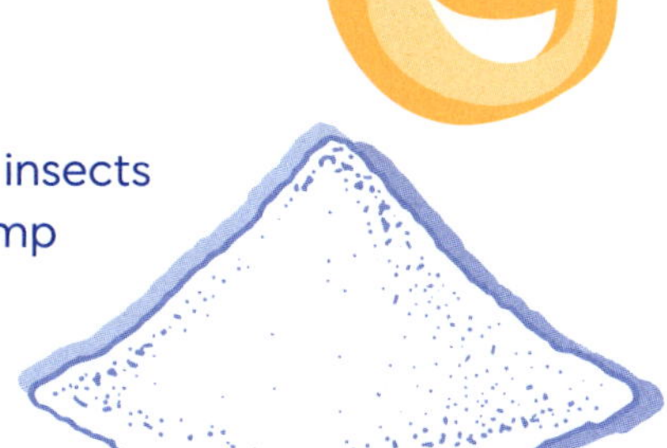

Home hacks

LIMESCALE REMOVAL

- To remove limescale from around a plughole or tap, rub with the cut end of half a lemon, then rinse.
- Soften limescale around taps by covering overnight with a paper towel soaked in vinegar. The limescale should then be much easier to remove.
- Help clear limescale from a steam-iron's reservoir by filling it with vinegar. Turn on the iron, let it steam until dry, then rinse the reservoir with clean water.

SALT-STAINED SHOES

Wipe these with a solution made by stirring 1 tablespoon of vinegar into 1 cup of water.

TIGHTS

Make tights longer lasting and less ladder-prone by adding a tablespoon of vinegar to the final rinsing water after washing.

PAINT SMELLS

Reduce the odour of fresh paint by standing a bowl of vinegar somewhere safe.

WINDSCREEN ANTI-ICER

Mix 3 parts of vinegar with 1 part of water and use this to wipe over your windscreen.

BABY EQUIPMENT AND TOYS

- Use a cloth to wipe sticky toys and baby equipment with basic cleaning fluid (p.316). Rinse and dry.
- Wash a plastic paddling pool and remove any mildew with basic cleaning fluid (p.316).
- Rub clean high chairs, car seats, buggies and plastic mattress protectors with a damp sponge sprinkled with bicarbonate of soda, then wipe several times with a clean sponge.

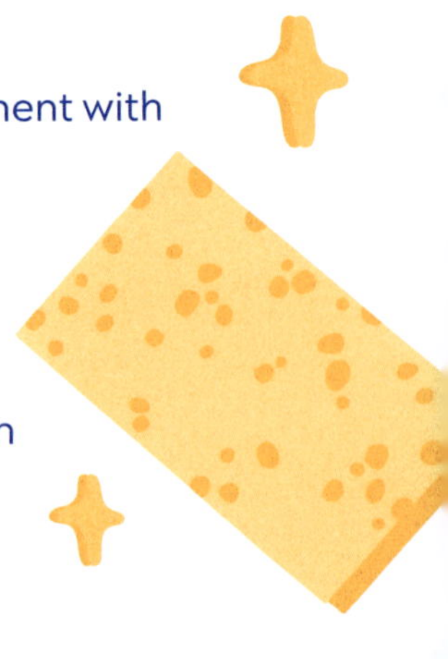

- Freshen stuffed toys by sprinkling with bicarbonate of soda. Wait for 30 minutes, then brush off.

STICKY LABELS AND GLUE REMNANTS

- Loosen these by rubbing gently with vinegar.
- Use vinegar to remove the resin and hardener components of two-part epoxy glue, or even glue that has not yet set.

CAUTION: If glue remnants touch your eye or skin, irrigate the area immediately with plenty of water.

SMALL FIRES

If you don't have a fire extinguisher or a fire blanket at the ready, but do have a large amount of bicarbonate of soda to hand, put out a small grease or oil fire, or an electrical fire, by throwing bicarbonate of soda over it. Water is unsafe for either sort of fire.

CAUTION: Don't use bicarbonate of soda on a fire in a deep-fat fryer, as it could make the flaming grease splatter. Take no risks. If necessary, get yourself and others out of the house and make sure someone calls the fire service without delay.

HAIRBRUSHES, COMBS, TOOTHBRUSHES, MAKE-UP APPLICATORS

Clean these by soaking them in basic cleaning fluid (p.316) for 30 minutes, then rinsing well.

PLANT CARE

- Spray mildewed plant foliage with basic cleaning fluid (p.316) in the evening.
- To treat plant foliage affected by black-spot fungi, add 1 teaspoon of cooking oil to a bottle of basic cleaning fluid (p.316) and spray in the evening.
- Clean vases inside by filling with hot water and adding 2 tablespoons of bicarbonate of soda. Leave for 1 hour, then rinse.

VACUUM FLASK OR WATER BOTTLE

Clean a stained flask or bottle, or one you haven't used for some time, by putting 1–2 teaspoons of bicarbonate of soda into the flask and filling it with hot water. Leave for 30 minutes, then rinse well.

ABOUT THE AUTHOR

Dr Penny Stanway practised for several years as a GP and as a child-health doctor before becoming increasingly fascinated by researching and writing about nutrition and natural approaches to health and wellbeing. She is an accomplished cook who enjoys being creative in the kitchen and sharing food. Penny has written more than 20 books on health, food, and the connections between the two. She lives by the Thames in London and often visits south-west Ireland. Her leisure pursuits include painting, swimming and being with her family and friends.

Author's acknowledgements

Penny would like to thank those involved in creating this book, including Sophie Blackman (the commissioning editor whose vision it was), Daniel Culver and Caitlin Nolan (who edited it), Karen Smith, Francesca Corsini and Steven Williamson (for their design and illustration work) and Caroline Montgomery (her literary agent).

CUPBOARD HEROES REFERENCES

Chapter 1

1 Maximum-free-acidity: International Olive Council, "Guide for the Determination of the Characteristics of Oil-Olives", 2011
Phenol-content: Gorzynik-Debicka, "Potential Health Benefits of Olive Oil and Plant Polyphenols", *International Journal of Molecular Science*, 2018

Chapter 2

MILD ACIDOSIS
1 DiNicolantonio, "Low-Grade Metabolic Acidosis as a Driver of Chronic Disease: A 21st Century Public Health Crisis", *Open Heart*, 2021

AVOID HEATING OLIVE OIL
2 Lozano-Castellón, "Domestic Sautéing with EVOO: Change in the Phenolic Profile", *Antioxidants Basel*, 2020

BENEFITS OF HONEY
3 Al-Kafaween, "Physicochemical Characteristics and Bioactive Compounds of Different Types of Honey and their Biological and Therapeutic Properties: A Comprehensive Review", *Antibiotics*, 2023

Ageing-related health concerns:

APPLE CIDER VINEGAR
4 Ames, "Mineral and Vitamin Deficiencies Can Accelerate the Mitochondrial Decay of Aging", *Molecular Aspects of Medicine*, 2005

LEMONS
5 Enstrom, "Vitamin C Intake and Mortality Among a Sample of the United States Population", *Epidemiology*, 1992
6 Shimizu, "Effects of Lifelong Intake of Lemon Polyphenols on Aging and Intestinal Microbiome in the Senescence-Accelerated Mouse Prone 1", *Scientific Reports*, 2019

OLIVE OIL
7 Donat-Vargas, "Only Virgin Type of Olive Oil Consumption Reduces the Risk of Mortality: Results From a Mediterranean Population-Based Cohort", *European Journal of Clinical Nutrition*, 2022
8 Guasch-Ferré ,"Consumption of Olive Oil and Risk of Total and Cause-Specific Mortality Among US Adults", *Journal of the American College of Cardiology*, 2022

TEAS
9 Xiang, "Tea Consumption and Attenuation of Biological Aging: A Longitudinal Analysis from Two Cohort Studies", *The Lancet Regional Health – Western Pacific*, 2023

Age-related cognitive decline

OLIVE OIL
10 Fazlollahi, "The Effects of Olive Oil Consumption on Cognitive Performance: A Systematic Review", *Nutrients*, 2023
11 Solfrizzi, "Dietary Fatty Acids, Age-Related Cognitive Decline, and Mild Cognitive Impairment", *Journal of Nutrition*, 2008

GARLIC
12 Nishiyama, "Beneficial Effects of Aged Garlic Extract on Learning and Memory Impairment in the Senescence-Accelerated Mouse", *Experimental Gerontology*, 1997

Alzheimer's disease

13 Joshi, "Transcriptional Patterns in Stages of Alzheimer's Disease Are

Cell-Type-Specific and Partially Converge with the Effects of Alcohol Use Disorder in Humans", *eNeuro*, 2024

APPLE CIDER VINEGAR

14 Tripathi, "Neuroprotective Efficacy of Apple Cider Vinegar on Zinc-High Fat Diet-Induced Mono Amine Oxidase Alteration in Murine Model of Alzheimer's Disease", *Journal of the American Nutrition Association*, 2022

LEMONS

15 Zhang, "Citrus Consumption and Incident Dementia in Elderly Japanese: the Ohsaki Cohort 2006 Study", *British Journal of Nutrition*, 2017

16 Youdim, "Interaction Between Flavonoids and the Blood-Brain Barrier: In Vitro Studies", *Journal of Neurochemistry*, 2003

17 Heo, "Apple Phenolics Protect In Vitro Oxidative Stress-Induced Neuronal Cell Death", *Journal of Agricultural and Food Chemistry*, 2004

OLIVE OIL

18 Breslin, "Alzheimer's-Associated Aβ Oligomers Show Altered Structure, Immunoreactivity and Synaptotoxicity with Low Doses of Oleocanthal", *Toxicology and Applied Pharmacology*, 2009

19 Lourida, "Mediterranean Diet, Cognitive Function, and Dementia", *Epidemiology*, 2013

HONEY

20 Al-Himyari, "The Use of Honey As a Natural Preventive Therapy of Cognitive Decline and Dementia in the Middle East", *Alzheimer's and Dementia*, 2009

GARLIC

21 Chauhan, "Amelioration of Early Cognitive Deficits by Aged Garlic Extract in Alzheimer's Transgenic Mice", *Phytotherapy Research*, 2007

TEAS

22 Baranowska-Wójcik, "Regardless of the Brewing Conditions, Various Types of Tea are a Source of Acetylcholinesterase Inhibitors", *Nutrients*, 2020

23 Feng, "Tea Drinking and Cognitive Function in Oldest-Old Chinese", *Journal of Nutrition, Health and Aging*, 2013

24 Razazan, "Activation of Microbiota Sensing–Free Fatty Acid Receptor 2 Signaling Ameliorates Amyloid-B Induced Neurotoxicity by Modulating Proteolysis-Senescence Axis", *Aging Neuroscience*, 2021

25 Rini, "Literature Study: The Effect of Butterfly Pea Flowers (Clitoria ternatea L.) on Human Health", *Oshada*, 2025

26 Moss, "Acute Consumption of Peppermint and Chamomile Teas Produce Contrasting Effects on Cognition and Mood in Healthy Young Adults", *Plant Science Today*, 2016

27 Akhondzadeh, "Melissa Officinalis Extract in the Treatment of Patients With Mild To Moderate Alzheimer's Disease", *Journal of Neurology, Neurosurgery and Psychiatry*, 2003

Anaemia

HONEY

28 Al-Waili, "Effects of Daily Consumption of Honey Solution on Hematological Indices and Blood Levels of Minerals and Enzymes in Normal Individuals", *Journal of Medicinal Food*, 2003

ANXIETY

29 Ye, "Role of Inflammation in Depression and Anxiety: Tests for Disorder Specificity, Linearity and Potential Causality of Association in the UK Biobank", *eClinicalMedicine*, 2021

HONEY

30 Zamri, "Honey on Brain Health: A Promising Brain Booster", *Frontiers in Ageing Neuroscience*, 2023

31 Chepulis, "The Long-Term Effects of Feeding Honey Compared with Sucrose and a Sugar-Free Diet on Weight Gain, Lipid Profiles, and DEXA Measurements in Rats", *Journal of Food Science*, 2008

Artery disease

32 Zhou, "Association between Dietary Choline Intake and Cardiovascular Diseases: National Health and Nutrition Examination Survey 2011–2016" *Nutrients*, 2023

APPLE CIDER VINEGAR

33 Hadi, "The Effect of Apple Cider Vinegar on Lipid Profiles and Glycemic Parameters: A Systematic Review and Meta-Analysis of Randomized Clinical Trials", *BMC Complementary Medicine and Therapies*, 2021

HONEY

34 Ahmed, "Effect of Natural Honey on Human Platelets and Blood Coagulation Proteins", *Pakistan Journal of Pharmaceutical Sciences*, 2011

35 Yaghoobi, "Natural Honey and Cardiovascular Risk Factors: Effects on Blood Glucose, Cholesterol, Triacylglycerole, CRP, and Body Weight Compared With Sucrose", *Scientific World Journal*, 2008

36 El-Saleh, "Protection by Natural Honey Against Hyperhomocysteinemia in Rats", *Vascular Disease Prevention*, 2006

37 Al-Waili, "Natural Honey Lowers Plasma Glucose, C-Reactive Protein, Homocysteine, and Blood Lipids in Healthy, Diabetic, and Hyperlipidemic Subjects: Comparison With Dextrose and Sucrose", *Journal of Medicinal Food*, 2004

GARLIC

38 Rahman, "Garlic and Cardiovascular Disease: A Critical Review", *Journal of Nutrition*, 2006

39 Sun, "Anti-Hyperlipidemia of Garlic By Reducing the Level of Total Cholesterol and Low-Density Lipoprotein: A Meta-analysis", *Medicine*, 2018

40 Vidyashanka, "Dietary Garlic and Onion Reduce the Incidence of Atherogenic Diet-Induced Cholesterol Gallstones in Experimental Mice", *British Journal of Nutrition*, 2009

41 Hosseini, "Garlic Extract Reduces Serum Angiotensin Converting Enzyme (ACE) Activity in Nondiabetic and Streptozotocin-Diabetic Rats", *Pathophysiology*, 2007

42 Durak, "Effects of Garlic Extract Consumption on Plasma and Erythrocyte Antioxidant Parameters in Atherosclerotic Patients", *Life Sciences*, 2006

Arthritis

43 Pattison, "Dietary Risk Factors for the Development of Inflammatory Polyarthritis: Evidence for a Role of High Level of Red Meat Consumption", *Arthritis and Rheumatism*, 2004

LEMONS

44 Pattison, "Vitamin C and the Risk of Developing Inflammatory Polyarthritis: Prospective Nested Case-Control Study", *Annals of Rheumatic Diseases*, 2004

45 Cerhan, "Antioxidant Micronutrients and Risk of Rheumatoid Arthritis in a Cohort of Older Women", *American Journal of Epidemiology*, 2003

46 Fu, "Hesperidin Protects Against Il-1β-Induced Inflammation in Human Osteoarthritis Chondrocytes",

Experimental and Therapeutic Medicine, 2018

OLIVE OIL

47 De Veto, "Olive Oil and Nuts in Rheumatoid Arthritis Disease Activity", *Nutrients*, 2023

GARLIC

48 Williams, "Dietary Garlic and Hip Osteoarthritis: Evidence of a Protective Effect and Putative Mechanism of Action", *BMC Musculoskeletal Disorders*, 2010

49 Dehghani, "The Effect of a Garlic Supplement on the Pro-Inflammatory Adipocytokines, Resistin and Tumor Necrosis Factor-Alpha, and on Pain Severity, in Overweight or Obese Women With Knee Osteoarthritis", *Phytomedicine*, 2018

Asthma

OLIVE OIL

50 Cazzoletti, "Dietary Fats, Olive Oil and Respiratory Diseases in Italian Adults: A Population-Based Study", *Clinical and Experimental Allergy*, 2019

51 Chatzi, "Protective Effect of Fruits, Vegetables and the Mediterranean Diet on Asthma and Allergies Among Children in Crete", *Thorax*, 2006

GARLIC

52 Fehri, "The Relaxant Effect Induced By Allium Sativum L. Bulb Aqueous Extract on Rat Isolated Trachea", *Pharmacognosy Magazine*, 2011

53 Ahad, "Purified Aged Garlic Extract Modulates Allergic Airway Inflammation in Balb/c Mice", *Iranian Journal of Allergy, Asthma and Immunology*, 2008

Athlete's foot

GARLIC

54 Ledezma, "Efficacy of Ajoene in the Treatment of Tinea Pedis: A Double-Blind and Comparative Study With Terbinafine", *Journal of the American Academy of Dermatology*, 2000

Autoimmune diseases

OLIVE OIL

55 De Vito, "Olive Oil and Nuts in Rheumatoid Arthritis Disease Activity", *Nutrition*, 2023

Bad breath

SODIUM BICARBONATE

56 Westman, "Effect of 6-Month Adherence to a Very Low Carbohydrate Diet Program", *American Journal of Clinical Nutrition*, 2002

Bronchitis and pneumonia

LEMONS

57 Butler, "Dietary Fiber and Reduced Cough with Phlegm: A Cohort Study in Singapore", *American Journal of Respiratory and Critical Care Medicine*, 2004

Burns

HONEY

58 Gupta, "Honey Dressing Versus Silver Sulfadiazene Dressing for Wound Healing in Burn Patients: A Retrospective Study", *Journal of Cutaneous and Aesthetic Surgery*, 2011

Cancer

59 Thomas, "Endogenous Estrogen and Postmenopausal Breast Cancer: A Quantitative Review", *Cancer Causes & Control*, 1997

60 Seo, "Evaluating Flavonoids As Potential Aromatase Inhibitors for Breast Cancer Treatment: In Vitro Studies and in Silico Predictions", *Chemical and Biological Interactions*, 2024

LEMONS

61 Bae, "Dietary Intakes of Citrus Fruit and Risk of Gastric Cancer Incidence: an Adaptive Meta-Analysis of Cohort Studies", *Epidemiology and Health*, 2016

SODIUM BICARBONATE

62 Robey, "Bicarbonate Increases Tumor pH and Inhibits Spontaneous Metastases", *Cancer Research*, 2009

OLIVE OIL

63 Markellos, "Olive Oil Intake and Cancer Risk: A Systematic Review and Meta-Analysis", *PLoS One*, 2022

64 Maroto-Rodriguez, "Association of a Mediterranean Lifestyle With All-Cause and Cause-Specific Mortality: A Prospective Study from the UK Biobank", *Mayo Clinic Proceedings*, 2024

65 Markellos, "Olive Oil Intake and Cancer Risk: A Systematic Review and Meta-Analysis", *PLoS One*, 2022

66 Markellos, "Olive Oil Intake and Cancer Risk: A Systematic Review and Meta-Analysis", *PLoS One*, 2022

67 Stoneham, "Olive Oil, Diet and Colorectal Cancer: An Ecological Study and a Hypothesis", *Journal of Epidemiology and Community Health*, 2000

HONEY

68 Ghashm, "Antiproliferative Effect of Tualang Honey on Oral Squamous Cell Carcinoma and Osteosarcoma Cell Lines", *BMC Complementary and Alternative Medicine*, 2010

69 Tsiapara,"Bioactivity of Greek Honey Extracts on Breast Cancer (MC7), Prostate Cancer (PC-3) and Endometrial Cancer (Ishikawa) Cells: Profile Analysis of Extracts", *Food Chemistry*, 2009

GARLIC

70 Kim, "Garlic Intake and Cancer Risk: an Analysis Using the Food and Drug Administration's Evidence-Based Review System for the Scientific Evaluation of Health Claims", *American Journal of Clinical Nutrition*, 2009

TEAS

71 Al-Ataby, "Daily Consumption of Lemon and Ginger Herbal Infusion Caused Tumor Regression and Activation of the Immune System in a Mouse Model of Breast Cancer", *Frontiers in Nutrition*, 2022

72 Hakim, "Joint Effects of Citrus Peel Use and Black Tea Intake on the Risk of Squamous Cell Carcinoma of the Skin", *BMC Dermatology*, 2001

Chronic metabolic stress and metabolic syndrome

APPLE CIDER VINEGAR

73 Khalil, "Apple Cider Vinegar for Weight Management in Lebanese Adolescents and Young Adults With Overweight and Obesity: A Randomised, Double-Blind, Placebo-Controlled Study", *BMJ Prevention, Nutrition, and Health*, 2023

OLIVE OIL

74 Seidita, "The Clinical Impact of an Extra Virgin Olive Oil Enriched Mediterranean Diet on Metabolic Syndrome: Lights and Shadows of a Nutraceutical Approach", *Frontiers in Nutrition*, 2022

75 Camargo, "Gene Expression Changes in Mononuclear Cells in Patients With Metabolic Syndrome After Acute Intake of Phenol-Rich Virgin Olive Oil", *BMC Genomics*, 2010

76 Babio, "Adherence to the Mediterranean Diet and Risk of Metabolic Syndrome and Its Components", *Nutrition, Metabolism and Cardiovascular Disease*, 2009

HONEY
77 Hashim, "The Mechanism of Honey in Reversing Metabolic Syndrome", *Molecules*, 2021

GARLIC
78 Yoo, "High Dietary Fructose Intake on Cardiovascular Disease Related Parameters in Growing Rats", *Nutrition, Metabolism and Cardiovascular Diseases*, 2016

Cold sores

HONEY
79 Al-Waili, "Topical Honey Application Vs. Acyclovir for the Treatment of Recurrent Herpes Simplex Lesions", *Medical Science Monitor*, 2004

Colds, flu, laryngitis, sore throat, sinusitis

LEMONS
80 De Vrese, "Effect of Lactobacillus gasseri PA 16/8, Bifidobacterium Longum SP 07/3, B. Bifidum MF 20/5 on Common Cold Episodes: A Double Blind, Randomized, Controlled Trial", *Clinical Nutrition*, 2005

GARLIC
81 Josling, "Preventing the Common Cold With a Garlic Supplement: A Double-Blind, Placebo-Controlled Survey", *Advances in Therapy*, 2001

Convulsions

82 Yuen, "Low-Grade Chronic Metabolic Acidosis Is a Contributory Mechanism in the Development of Chronic Epilepsy", *Epilepsy and Behavior*, 2006

Coughs

LEMONS
83 Butler, "Dietary Fiber and Reduced Cough With Phlegm: A Cohort Study in Singapore", *American Journal of Respiratory and Critical Care Medicine*, 2004

HONEY
84 Paul, "Effect of Honey, Dextromethorphan, and No Treatment on Nocturnal Cough and Sleep Quality for Coughing Children and Their Parents", *Archives of Pediatric Adolescent Medicine*, 2007

Cuts & grazes

HONEY
85 Al-Waili, "Effects of Topical Honey on Post-Operative Wound Infections Due to Gram Positive and Gram Negative Bacteria Following Caesarean Sections and Hysterectomies", *European Journal of Medical Research*, 1999

Depression

LEMONS
86 Kiecolt-Glaser, "Olfactory Influences on Mood and Autonomic, Endocrine, and Immune Function", *Psychoneuroendocrinology*, 2008

OLIVE OIL
87 Sánchez-Villegas, "Association of the Mediterranean Dietary Pattern With the Incidence of Depression: The Seguimiento Universidad De Navarra/University of Navarra Follow-Up (Sun) Cohort", *Archives of General Psychiatry*, 2009

GARLIC
88 Dhingra, "Evidences for the Involvement of Monoaminergic and Gabaergic Systems in Antidepressant-Like Activity of Garlic Extract in Mice", *Indian Journal of Pharmacology*, 2008

Diabetes type 2

APPLE CIDER VINEGAR

89 Cheng, "A Systematic Review and Meta-Analysis: Vinegar Consumption on Glycaemic Control in Adults With Type 2 Diabetes Mellitus", *Journal of Advanced Nursing*, 2020

90 Johnston, "Vinegar Improves Insulin Sensitivity to a High-Carbohydrate Meal in Subjects With Insulin Resistance or Type 2 Diabetes", *Diabetes Care*, 2004

91 Ogawa, "Acetic Acid Suppresses the Increase in Disaccharidase Activity That Occurs During Culture of Caco-2 Cells", *Journal of Nutrients*, 2000

OLIVE OIL

92 Liu, "Compound from Olives Shows Promise for Treating Obesity and Diabetes", presented at the annual meeting of the American Society for Nutrition, 2024

93 Esposito, "Effects of a Mediterranean-style Diet on the Need for Antihyperglycemic Drug Therapy in Patients With Newly Diagnosed Type 2 Diabetes: A Randomized Trial", *Annals of Internal Medicine*, 2009

94 Martinez-González, "Adherence to Mediterranean Diet and Risk of Developing Diabetes: Prospective Cohort Study", *British Medical Journal*, 2008

HONEY

95 Ahmad, "Natural Honey Modulates Physiological Glycemic Response Compared to Simulated Honey and D-Glucose", *Journal of Food Science*, 2009

96 Yaghoobi, "Natural Honey and Cardiovascular Risk Factors: Effects on Blood Glucose, Cholesterol, Triacylglycerole, CRP, and Body Weight Compared With Sucrose", *Scientific World Journal*, 2008

97 Agrawal, "Subjects With Impaired Glucose Tolerance Exhibit a High Degree of Tolerance to Honey", *Journal of Medicinal Food*, 2007

GARLIC

98 Padiya, "Garlic Improves Insulin Sensitivity and Associated Metabolic Syndromes in Fructose Fed Rats", *Nutrition, Metabolism and Cardiovascular Diseases*, 2011

Fatigue

99 Myhill, "Chronic Fatigue Syndrome and Mitochondrial Dysfunction", *International Journal of Clinical Experimental Medicine*, 2009

100 Ames, "Mineral and Vitamin Deficiencies Can Accelerate the Mitochondrial Decay of Aging", *Molecular Aspects of Medicine*, 2005

APPLE CIDER VINEGAR

101 Fushimi, "Acetic Acid Feeding Enhances Glycogen Repletion in Liver and Skeletal Muscle of Rats", *Journal of Nutrition*, 2001

LEMONS

102 Fushimi, "Acetic Acid Feeding Enhances Glycogen Repletion in Liver and Skeletal Muscle of Rats", *Journal of Nutrition*, 2001

HONEY

103 Dr Richard Kreider, University of Memphis Exercise and Sport Nutrition Laboratory, 39 athletes ate protein, sugar, maltodextrin or honey after weight lifting; only honey maintained optimal blood sugar for two hours; study presented at the National Strength and Conditioning Association's annual meeting, Orlando, 2000. https://www.eurekalert.org/news-releases/635281

GARLIC
104 Morihara, "Aged Garlic Extract Ameliorates Physical Fatigue", *Biological & Pharmaceutical Bulletin*, 2006

Fibromyalgia

105 Çakit, "Coexistence of Fibromyalgia and Metabolic Syndrome in Females: The Effects on Fatigue, Clinical Features, Pain Sensitivity, Urinary Cortisol and Norepinephrine Levels: a Cross-Sectional Study", *Archives of Rheumatology*, 2020
106 Nadal-Nicolás, "Vegetarian and Vegan Diet in Fibromyalgia: A Systematic Review", *International Journal for Environmental Research and Public Health*, 2021
107 Goesling," Associations Between Pain, Current Tobacco Smoking, Depression, and Fibromyalgia Status Among Treatment-Seeking Chronic Pain Patients", *Pain Medicine*, 2015

SPICES
108 Shen, "Bioactive Compounds for Fibromyalgia-like Symptoms: A Narrative Review and Future Perspectives", *International Journal of Environmental Research and Public Health*, 2022

Fluid retention

GARLIC
109 Hosseini, "Garlic Extract Reduces Serum Angiotensin Converting Enzyme (ACE) Activity in Nondiabetic and Streptozotocin-Diabetic Rats", *Pathophysiology*, 2007
110 Pantoja, "Diuretic, Natriuretic and Hypotensive Effects Produced By Allium Sativum (Garlic) in Anaesthetized Dogs", *Journal of Ethnopharmacology*, 1991

Fungal infections

HONEY
111 Koc, "Antifungal Activity of Turkish Honey against Candida spp. and Trichosporon spp: An in Vitro Evaluation", *Medical Mycology*, 2009

Gallstones

GARLIC
112 Vidyashankar, "Regression of Preestablished Cholesterol Gallstones By Dietary Garlic and Onion in Experimental Mice", *Metabolism*, 2010

Gastroenteritis

HONEY
113 Haffejee, "Honey in the Treatment of Infantile Gastroenteritis", *British Medical Journal*, 1985

Hair loss

114 Bassino, "Protective Role of Nutritional Plants Containing Flavonoids in Hair Follicle Disruption: A Review", *International Journal of Molecular Sciences*, 2020
115 Chaksupa, "Effects of Alcoholic Extract from Clitoria Ternatea Flowers on the Proliferation of Human Dermal Papilla Cells and Hair Growth in C57BL/6Mlac Mice", *Pharmaceutical Sciences Asia*, 2022

HONEY
116 Al-Waili, "Therapeutic and Prophylactic Effects of Crude Honey on Chronic Seborrheic Dermatitis and Dandruff", *European Journal of Medical Research*, 2001

Hay fever

OLIVE OIL
117 Chatzi, "Protective Effect of Fruits, Vegetables and the Mediterranean Diet

on Asthma and Allergies Among Children in Crete", *Thorax*, 2006

HONEY

118 Saarinen, "Birch Pollen Honey for Birch Pollen Allergy: A Randomized Controlled Pilot Study", *International Archives of Allergy and Immunology*, 2011

119 Rajan, "Effect of Ingestion of Honey on Symptoms of Rhinoconjunctivitis", *Annals of Allergy, Asthma and Immunology*, 2002

Heart disease

120 Poole-Wilson, "Acidosis and Contractility of Heart Muscle", *Ciba Foundation Symposium*, 1982

APPLE CIDER VINEGAR

121 Hu, "Dietary Intake of Alpha-Linolenic Acid and Risk of Fatal Ischemic Heart Disease Among Women", *American Journal of Clinical Nutrition*, 1999

LEMONS

122 Vita, "Polyphenols and Cardiovascular Disease: Effects on Endothelial and Platelet Function", *American Journal of Clinical Nutrition*, 2005

123 Knekt, "Flavonoid Intake and Coronary Mortality in Finland: A Cohort Study", *British Medical Journal*, 1996

124 Baekey, "Grapefruit Pectin Inhibits Hypercholesterolemia and Atherosclerosis in Miniature Swine", *Clinical Cardiology*, 1988

OLIVE OIL

125 Ke, "Olive Oil Intake and Cardiovascular Disease, Cancer, and All-Cause Mortality: A Systematic Review and Dose-Response Meta-Analysis of Prospective Cohort Studies", *Food and Function*, 2024

126 Sarapis, "Extra Virgin Olive Oil High in Polyphenols Improves Antioxidant Status in Adults: A Double-Blind, Randomized, Controlled, Cross-Over Study (OLIVAUS)", *European Journal of Nutrition*, 2022

127 Guasch-Ferré, "Olive Oil Intake and Risk of Cardiovascular Disease and Mortality in the PREDIMED Study", *BMC Medicine*, 2014

128 Martínez-González, "Mediterranean Diet and the Incidence of Cardiovascular Disease: A Spanish Cohort", *Nutrition, Metabolism and Cardiovascular Diseases*, 2010

High blood pressure

129 Jhang, "Diet-Dependent Net Acid Load and Risk of Incident Hypertension in United States Women", *Hypertension*, 2010.

130 Schorr, "Effect of Sodium Chloride- and Sodium Bicarbonate-Rich Mineral Water on Blood Pressure and Metabolic Parameters in Elderly Normotensive Individuals: a Randomized Double-Blind Crossover Trial", *Journal of Hypertension*, January 1996

APPLE CIDER VINEGAR

131 Shahinfar, "Dose-Dependent Effect of Vinegar on Blood Pressure: A GRADE-Assessed Systematic Review and Meta-Analysis of Randomized Controlled Trials", *Complementary Therapies in Medicine*, 2022

132 Kondo, "Antihypertensive Effects of Acetic Acid and Vinegar on Spontaneously Hypertensive Rats", *Bioscience, Biotechnology, and Biochemistry*, 2001

LEMONS

133 Yamamoto, "Short-Term Effects of Glucosyl Hesperidin and Hesperetin on Blood Pressure and Vascular Endothelial Function in Spontaneously Hypertensive

Rats", *Journal of Nutritional Science and Vitaminology*, 2008
134 Nakamura, "Antihypertensive and Vasorelaxant Effects of Citric Acid and Lemon Juice in Spontaneously Hypertensive Rats: In Vivo and Ex Vivo Studies", *Nutrients*, 2023

OLIVE OIL

135 Flynn, "Olive Oil As Medicine: The Effect on Blood Pressure", *UC Davis Olive Center Report*, 2015
136 Psaltopoulou, "Olive Oil, the Mediterranean Diet, and Arterial Blood Pressure: the Greek European Prospective Investigation into Cancer and Nutrition (EPIC) Study", *American Journal of Clinical Nutrition*, 2004
137 Ruíz-Gutiérrez, "Plasma Lipids, Erythrocyte Membrane Lipids and Blood Pressure of Hypertensive Women After Ingestion of Dietary Oleic Acid from Two Different Sources", *Journal of Hypertension*, 1996.

GARLIC

138 Ried, "Garlic Lowers Blood Pressure in Hypertensive Subjects, Improves Arterial Stiffness and Gut Microbiota: a Review and Meta-Analysis", *Experimental and Therapeutic Medicine*, 2019
139 Wang, "Effect of Garlic on Blood Pressure: a Meta-Analysis", *Journal of Clinical Hypertension*, 2015
140 Ried, "Aged Garlic Extract Lowers Blood Pressure in Patients With Treated but Uncontrolled Hypertension: A Randomised Controlled Trial", *Maturitas*, 2010

High cholesterol

APPLE CIDER VINEGAR

141 Hadi, "The Effect of Apple Cider Vinegar on Lipid Profiles and Glycemic Parameters: A Systematic Review and Meta-Analysis of Randomized Clinical Trials", *BMC Complementary Medicine and Therapies*, 2021
142 Cheng, "A Systematic Review and Meta-Analysis: Vinegar Consumption on Glycaemic Control in Adults With Type 2 Diabetes Mellitus", *Journal of Advanced Nursing*, 2020

LEMONS

143 Kurowska, "Hypolipidemic Effects and Absorption of Citrus Polymethoxylated Flavones in Hamsters With Diet-Induced Hypercholesterolemia", *Journal of Agricultural and Food Chemistry*, 2004
144 Aslani, "Effect of Garlic and Lemon Juice Mixture on Lipid Profile and Some Cardiovascular Risk Factors in People 30–60 Years Old with Moderate Hyperlipidaemia: A Randomized Clinical Trial", *International Journal of Preventive Medicine*, 2016
145 Kurowska, "Regulation of Apo B Production in HepG2 Cells by Citrus Limonoids", *ACS Symposium Series*, 2000
146 Walaszek, "D-Glucaric Acid Content of Various Fruits and Vegetables and Cholesterol-Lowering Effects of Dietary D-Glucarate in the Rat", *Nutrition Research*, 1996

OLIVE OIL

147 Swain, "Characteristics of the Diet Patterns Tested in the Optimal Macronutrient Intake Trial to Prevent Heart Disease (OmniHeart): Options for a Heart-Healthy Diet", Johns Hopkins University, 2008
148 Cicero, "Changes in LDL Fatty Acid Composition as a Response to Olive Oil Treatment Are Inversely Related to Lipid Oxidative Damage: The EUROLIVE

Study", *Journal of the American College of Nutrition*, 2008
149 Pérez-Jiménez, "The Influence of Olive Oil on Human Health: Not a Question of Fat Alone", *American Journal of Clinical Nutrition*, 2007
150 Covas, "The Effect of Polyphenols in Olive Oil on Heart Disease Risk Factors: A Randomized Trial", *Annals of Internal Medicine*, 2006
151 Ruano, "Phenolic Content of Virgin Olive Oil Improves Ischemic Reactive Hyperemia in Hypercholesterolemic Patients", *Journal of the American College of Cardiology*, 2005

HONEY
152 Mushtaq, "80 Obese and 80 Normal-Weight Volunteers 80g Honey 4 Weeks Lower Total Cholesterol Higher HDL Cholesterol", *Pakistan Journal of Zoology*, 2011
153 Hegazi , "Influence of Honey on the Suppression of Human Low Density Lipoprotein (LDL) Peroxidation (In Vitro)", *Evidence Based Complementary and Alternative Medicine*, 2009

Infection

APPLE CIDER VINEGAR
154 Yagnik, "Antibacterial Apple Cider Vinegar Eradicates Methicillin Resistant Staphylococcus Aureus and Resistant Escherichia Coli", *Nature*, 2021

OLIVE OIL
155 Medina, "Antimicrobial Activity of Olive Oil, Vinegar, and Various Beverages Against Foodborne Pathogens", *Journal of Food Protection*, 2007

HONEY
156 Almasaudi, "The Antibacterial Activities of Honey", *Medical Sciences*, 2000

GARLIC
157 Rouf, "Antiviral Potential of Garlic (Allium Sativum) and Its Organosulfur Compounds: a Systematic Update of Pre-Clinical and Clinical Data", *Trends in Food Science & Technology*, 2020

Inflammation

OLIVE OIL
158 Beauchamp, "Phytochemistry: Ibuprofen-Like Activity in Extra-Virgin Olive Oil", *Nature*, 2005

HONEY
159 Yagoobi, "Natural Honey and Cardiovascular Risk Factors; Effects on Blood Glucose, Cholesterol, Triacylglycerole, CRP, and Body Weight Compared With Sucrose", *Scientific World Journal*, 2008
160 Waili, "Natural Honey Lowers Plasma Prostaglandin Concentrations in Normal Individuals", *Journal of Medicinal Food*, 2003

GARLIC
161 Vaidya, "Garlic: Source of the Ultimate Antioxidants—Sulfenic Acids", *Angewandte Chemie*, 2009
162 Aggarwal, "Suppresion of the Nuclear Factor-kB Activation Pathway By Spice-Derived Phytochemicals", *Annals of the New York Academy of Sciences*, 2004
163 van Doorn, "Effect of Garlic Powder on C-Reactive Protein and Plasma Lipids in Overweight and Smoking Subjects", *American Journal of Clinical Nutrition*, 2006

Inflammatory bowel disease

OLIVE OIL
164 Hart, "Olive Oil Could Guard Against Developing Ulcerative Colitis", Presented at the Digestive Disease Week

conference, New Orleans, 2010

Kidney stones

165 Della Guardia, "Diet-Induced Acidosis and Alkali Supplementation", *Urology Research*, 2006

Low sex drive

GARLIC

166 Oi, "Garlic Supplementation Increases Testicular Testosterone and Decreases Plasma Corticosterone in Rats Fed a High Protein Diet", *Journal of Nutrition*, 2001

Memory loss

HONEY

167 "The Effects of Long-Term Honey, Sucrose or Sugar-Free Diets on Memory and Anxiety in Rats", *Physiology & Behaviour*, 2009

Macular degeneration – age-related

LEMONS

168 van Leeuwen, "Dietary Intake of Antioxidants and Risk of Age-Related Macular Degeneration", *Journal of the American Medical Association*, 2005

Muscle fatigue & aching

SODIUM BICARBONATE

169 Verbitsky, "Effect of Ingested Sodium Bicarbonate on Muscle Force, Fatigue, and Recovery", *Journal of Applied Physiology*, 1985

OVERWEIGHT AND OBESITY

170 Spencer, "Diet and Body Mass Index in 38000 Epic-Oxford Meat-Eaters, Fish-Eaters, Vegetarians and Vegans", *International Journal of Obesity*, 2003

171 Ellulu. "Obesity and Inflammation: the Linking Mechanism and the Complications", *Archives of Medical Science*, 2016

APPLE CIDER VINEGAR

172 Abou-Khalil , "Apple Cider Vinegar for Weight Management in Lebanese Adolescents and Young Adults With Overweight and Obesity: A Randomised, Double-Blind, Placebo-Controlled Study", *BMJ Nutrition, Prevention & Health*, 2024

173 Kondo, "Acetic Acid Upregulates the Expression of Genes for Fatty Acid Oxidation Enzymes in Liver to Suppress Body Fat Accumulation", *Journal of Agricultural and Food Chemistry*, 2009

174 Wright, "Effect of Food Acids on Postprandial Glucose Levels", *Journal of the Federation of American Societies for Experimental Biology*, 2006

175 Ostman, "Vinegar Supplementation Lowers Glucose and Insulin Responses and Increases Satiety After a Bread Meal in Healthy Subjects", *European Journal of Clinical Nutrition*, 2005

LEMONS

176 Tiwary, "Effect of Pectin on Satiety in Healthy US Army Adults", *Journal of the American College of Nutrition*, 1997

177 Gonzalez, "Calcium Intake and 10-Year Weight Change in Middle-Aged Adults", *Journal of the American Dietetic Association*, 2006

178 Johnston, "Strategies for Healthy Weight Loss: From Vitamin C to the Glycemic Response", American College of Nutrition, 2005

OLIVE OIL

179 Study presented at the annual meeting of the American Society for Nutrition, Chicago, 2024: https://nutrition.org/compound-from-olives-shows-promise-for-treating-obesity-and-diabetes/

180 Almaraz, "Incidence of Obesity Is

Lower in Persons Who Consume Olive Oil", *European Journal of Clinical Nutrition*, 2009
181 Oi-Kano, "Oleuropein, a Phenolic Compound in Extra Virgin Olive Oil, Increases Uncoupling Protein 1 Content in Brown Adipose Tissue and Enhances Noradrenaline and Adrenaline Secretions in Rats", *Journal of Nutritional Science and Vitaminology*, 2008
182 Schwartz, "The Lipid Messenger OEA Links Dietary Fat Intake to Satiety', *Cell Metabolism*, 2008
183 Piers, "Substitution of Saturated With Monounsaturated Fat in a 4-Week Diet Affects Body Weight and Composition of Overweight and Obese Men", *British Journal of Nutrition*, 2003

HONEY

184 Chepulis, "The Effect of Honey Compared to Sucrose, Mixed Sugars, and a Sugar-Free Diet on Weight Gain in Young Rats", *Journal of Food Science*, 2007
185 Yaghoobi, "Natural Honey and Cardiovascular Risk Factors: Effects on Blood Glucose, Cholesterol, Triacylglycerole, CRP, and Body Weight Compared with Sucrose", *Scientific World Journal*, 2008

GARLIC

186 Padiya, "Garlic Improves Insulin Sensitivity and Associated Metabolic Syndromes in Fructose Fed Rats", *Nutrition and Metabolism*, 2011
187 Keophiphath, "1,2-Vinyldithiin from Garlic Inhibits Differentiation and Inflammation of Human Preadipocytes", *Journal of Nutrition*, 2009
188 Oi, "Allyl-Containing Sulfides in Garlic Increase Uncoupling Protein Content in Brown Adipose Tissue, and Noradrenaline and Adrenaline Secretion in Rats", *Journal of Nutrition*, 1999
189 Gargouri, "Ajoene Prevents Fat Digestion By Human Gastric Lipase in Vitro", *Biochimica et Biophysica Acta*, 1989

Osteoporosis

LEMONS

190 Chiba, "Hesperidin, a Citrus Flavonoid, Inhibits Bone Loss and Decreases Serum and Hepatic Lipids in Ovariectomized Mice", *Journal of Nutrition*, 2003

SODIUM BICARBONATE

191 Pizzorno, "Diet-Induced Acidosis: Is It Real and Clinically Relevant?", *British Journal of Nutrition*, 2010

OLIVE OIL

192 Puel, "Major Phenolic Compounds in Olive Oil Modulate Bone Loss in an Ovariectomy/Inflammation Experimental Model", *Journal of Agricultural and Food Chemistry*, 2008
193 Puel, "Mediterranean Diet and Osteoporosis Prevention", *Médecine Science*, 2007

Parkinson's disease

194 Knekt, "Serum Vitamin D and the Risk of Parkinson's Disease", *Archives of Neurology*, 2010

OLIVE OIL

195 Sofi, "Adherence to Mediterranean Diet and Health Status: Meta-Analysis", *British Medical Journal*, 2008

Peptic ulcer

LEMONS

196 Maandalari, "Effectiveness of Citrus Fruits on Helicobacter pylori", *Evidence-based Complementary and Alternative Medicine*, 2017

OLIVE OIL

197 Romero, "In Vitro Activity of Olive Oil

Polyphenols Against Helicobacter Pylori", *Journal of Agriculture and Food Chemistry*, 2007
198 a study in Vrachebnoe delo (English: "Medical Matters"), published in 1986 in Kiev but untraceable by me – found that when people with a peptic ulcer consumed animal fat instead of olive oil, their ulcer size greatly decreased and healing improved.

HONEY
199 Somal, "Susceptibility of Helicobacter pylori to the Antibacterial Activity of Manuka Honey", *Journal of the Royal Society of Medicine*, 1994

Polycystic ovary syndrome

OLIVE OIL
200 Dehghani, "Effect of Extra Virgin Olive Oil Consumption on Glycemic Control: A Systematic Review and Meta-Analysis", *Diabetologia*, 2001

Poor immunity

HONEY
201 Al-Waili, "Effects of Daily Consumption of Honey Solution on Hematological Indices and Blood Levels of Minerals and Enzymes in Normal Individuals", *Journal of Medicinal Food*, 2003

Premature ageing

202 Goraya. "How Metabolic Acidosis and Kidney Disease May Accelerate the Aging Process", *European Journal of Premature Ageing*, 2020

OLIVE OIL
203 Ames, "Mineral and Vitamin Deficiencies Can Accelerate the Mitochondrial Decay of Aging", *Molecular Aspects of Medicine*, 2005
204 Purba, "Skin Wrinkling: Can Food Make a Difference?", *Journal of the American College of Nutrition*, 2001

Garlic

205 Moriguchi, "Aged Garlic Extract Prolongs Longevity and Improves Spatial Memory Deficit in Senescence-Accelerated Mouse", *Biological and Pharmaceutical Bulletin*, 1996

Premature death

OLIVE OIL
206 Sofi, "Adherence to Mediterranean Diet and Health Status: Meta-Analysis", *British Medical Journal*, 2008

Pre-menstrual syndrome

GARLIC
207 Jafari, "Effect of Garlic (Allium sativum) Supplementation on Premenstrual Disorders: A Randomized, Double-Blind, Placebo-Controlled Trial", *Evidence-Based Complementary and Alternative Medicine*, 2021

Psoriasis

SODIUM BICARBONATE
208 Verdolini, "Old Fashioned Sodium Bicarbonate Baths for the Treatment of Psoriasis in the Era of Futuristic Biologics: An Old Ally to Be Rescued!", *Journal of Dermatological Treatment*, 2005

Ringworm

GARLIC
209 Ledezma, "Ajoene in the Topical Short-Term Treatment of Tinea Cruris and Tinea Corporis in Humans: Randomized Comparative Study With Terbinafine", *Arzneimittelforschung*,1999

Strokes

210 He, "Fruit and Vegetable Consumption and Stroke: Meta-Analysis of Cohort Studies", *Lancet*, 2006

OLIVE OIL

211 Samieri, "Olive Oil Consumption, Plasma Oleic Acid, and Stroke Incidence: The Three-City Study", *Neurology*, 2011

212 Sofi, "Adherence to Mediterranean Diet and Health Status: Meta-Analysis", *British Medical Journal*, 2008

213 Correa, "Virgin Olive Oil Polyphenol Hydroxytyrosol Acetate Inhibits in Vitro Platelet Aggregation in Human Whole Blood: Comparison With Hydroxytyrosol and Acetylsalicylic Acid", *British Journal of Nutrition*, 2008

214 Vito, "Polyphenols and Cardiovascular Disease: Effects on Endothelial and Platelet Function", *American Journal of Clinical Nutrition*, 2005

Tooth decay & gum disease

HONEY

215 English, "The Effects of Manuka Honey on Plaque and Gingivitis: A Pilot Study", *Journal of the International Academy of Periodontology*, 2004

Warts & verrucas

GARLIC

216 Dehghani, "Healing Effect of Garlic Extract on Warts and Corns", *International Journal of Dermatology*, 2005

217 Silverberg, "Garlic Cloves for Verruca Vulgaris", letter in *Pediatric Dermatology*, 2002

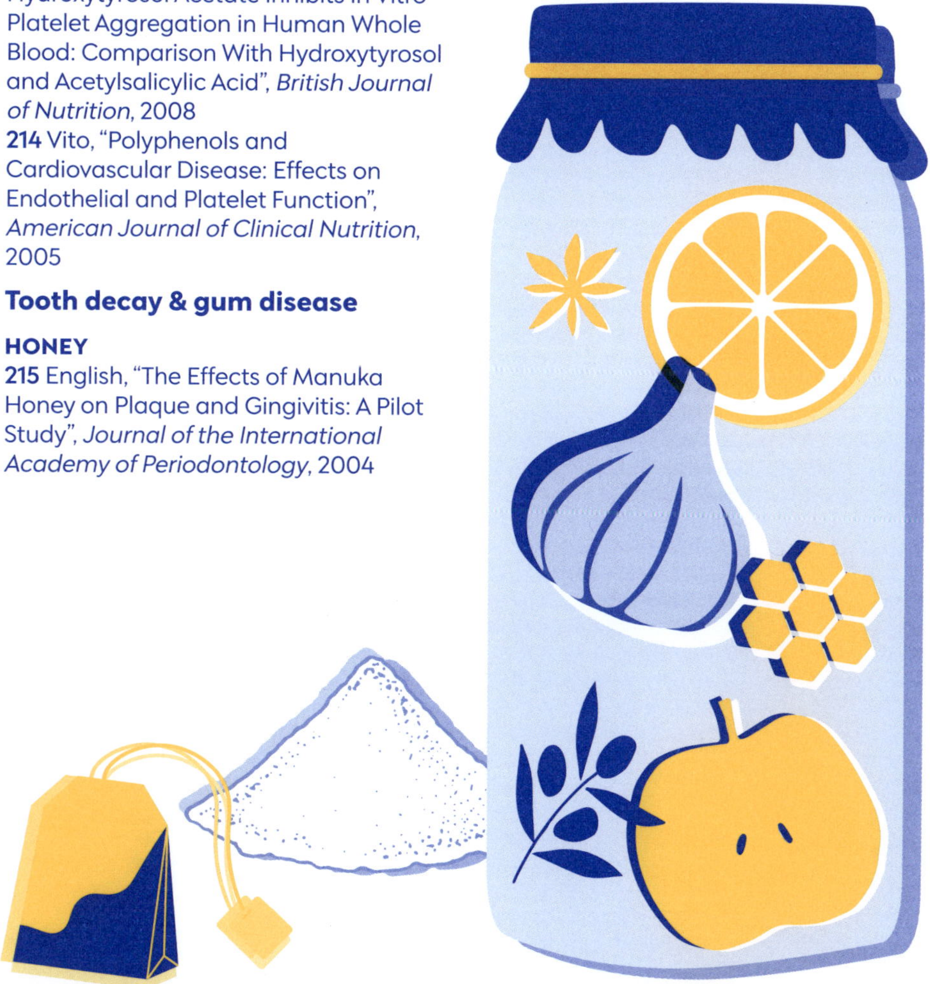

INDEX